the Unofficial Guide™ to Alternative Medicine

Debra Fulghum Bruce
with
Harris H. McIlwain, M.D.

Macmillan • USA

Macmillan General Reference
A Simon & Schuster Macmillan Company
1633 Broadway
New York, New York 10019-6785

ISBN: 0-02862526-9

Manufactured in the United States of America

10 9 8 7 6 5 4 3 2 1

First edition

In memory of my father, Roy Fulghum,
who taught me to always set lofty goals,
work diligently each day,
see stumbling blocks as stepping stones,
and never give up when life got tough.
His life was a true example of faithful persistence
and never ending devotion
that is an inspiration to many.

Acknowledgments

I would especially like to thank my special family—Bob, Rob, Brittnye, and Ashley—for the untiring devotion, inspiration, late night research and copy editing, typing, faxing, creative ideas, and boosts of encouragement that they gave to make this book happen.

To Dr. Harris and Linda McIlwain: Your expertise, research, and devotion to optimal health gave this book a solid backing and for that I am grateful.

To Raymond and Candy: Your e-mails at dawn and late night phone calls kept me working hard and for that I am thankful.

To Stephen G. Prom, Esq., chair of the Health Law Team of the law firm of Brant, Moore, Macdonald & Wells, and Elizabeth Shaw, a third year law student and registered nurse at Baptist/ St. Vincent's Health System, both of Jacksonville, Florida: your expert legal and insurance advice helped to give credibility to this book. I am extremely grateful for your knowledge.

To Dr. Paul Braden: Your answers to questions regarding pharmaceuticals and alternative treatments were most helpful, and I acknowledge your assistance.

My sincere appreciation to my agent, Denise Marcil, and Jeff Rutherford, who believed in this project and in the topic of alternative medicine.

Contents

The *Unofficial Guide* Reader's Bill of Rights

We Give You More Than the Official Line

Welcome to the *Unofficial Guide* series of Lifestyles titles—books that deliver critical, unbiased information that other books can't or won't reveal—*the inside scoop.* Our goal is to provide you with the *most accessible, useful* information and advice possible. The recommendations we offer in these pages are not influenced by the corporate line of any organization or industry; we give you the hard facts, whether those institutions like them or not. If something is ill-advised or will cause a loss of time and/or money, we'll give you ample warning. And if it is a worthwhile option, we'll let you know that, too.

Armed and Ready

Our hand-picked authors confidently and critically report on a wide range of topics that matter to smart readers like you. Our authors are passionate about their subjects, but have distanced themselves enough from them to help you be armed and protected, and help you make educated decisions as you go through your process. It is our intent that, from having read this book, you will avoid the pitfalls everyone else falls into and get it right the first time.

Don't be fooled by cheap imitations; this is the *genuine article Unofficial Guide* series from Macmillan Publishing. You may be familiar with our proven track record of the travel *Unofficial Guides*, which have more than three million copies in print. Each year, thousands of travelers—new and old—are armed with a brand-new, fully updated edition of the flagship *Unofficial Guide to Walt Disney World*, by Bob Sehlinger. It is our intention here to provide you with the same level of objective authority that Mr. Sehlinger does in his brainchild.

The Unofficial Panel of Experts

Every work in the Lifestyle *Unofficial Guides* is intensively inspected by a team of top professionals in their fields. These experts review the manuscript for factual accuracy, comprehensiveness, and an insider's determination as to whether the manuscript fulfills the credo in this Reader's Bill of Rights. In other words, our Panel ensures that you are, in fact, getting "the inside scoop."

Our Pledge

The authors, the editorial staff, and the Unofficial Panel of Experts assembled for *Unofficial Guides* are determined to lay out the most valuable alternatives available for our readers. This dictum means that our writers must be explicit, prescriptive, and above all, direct. We strive to be thorough and complete, but our goal is not necessarily to have the "most" or "all" of the information on a topic; this is not, after all, an encyclopedia. Our objective is to help you narrow down your options to the best of what is available, unbiased by affiliation with any industry or organization.

In each *Unofficial Guide* we give you:

- Comprehensive coverage of necessary and vital information

- Authoritative, rigidly fact-checked data

- The most up-to-date insights into trends

- Savvy, sophisticated writing that's also readable

- Sensible, applicable facts and secrets that only an insider knows

Special Features

Every book in our series offers the following six special sidebars in the margins that were devised to help you get things done cheaply, efficiently, and smartly.

1. "Timesaver"—tips and shortcuts that save you time.

2. "Moneysaver"—tips and shortcuts that save you money.

3. "Watch Out!"—more serious cautions and warnings.

4. "Bright Idea"—general tips and shortcuts to help you find an easier or smarter way to do something.

5. "Quote"—statements from real people that are intended to be prescriptive and valuable to you.

6. "Unofficially..."—an insider's fact or anecdote.

We also recognize your need to have quick information at your fingertips, and have thus provided the following comprehensive sections at the back of the book:

1. **Glossary:** Definitions of complicated terminology and jargon.

2. **Resource Guide:** Lists of relevant agencies, associations, institutions, web sites, etc.

3. **Recommended Reading List:** Suggested titles that can help you get more in-depth information on related topics.

4. **Important Documents:** "Official" pieces of information you need to refer to, such as government forms.

5. **Important Statistics:** Facts and numbers presented at-a-glance for easy reference.

6. **Index.**

Letters, Comments, and Questions from Readers

We strive to continually improve the *Unofficial* series, and input from our readers is a valuable way for us to do that.

Many of those who have used the *Unofficial Guide* travel books write to the authors to ask questions, make comments, or share their own discoveries and lessons. For Lifestyle *Unofficial Guides*, we would also appreciate all such correspondence, both positive and critical, and we will make best efforts to incorporate appropriate readers' feedback and comments in revised editions of this work.

How to write to us:
Unofficial Guides
Macmillan Lifestyle Guides
Macmillan Publishing
1633 Broadway
New York, NY 10019
Attention: Reader's Comments

The *Unofficial Guide* Panel of Experts

The *Unofficial* editorial team recognizes that you've purchased this book with the expectation of getting the most authoritative, carefully inspected information currently available. Toward that end, on each and every title in this series, we have selected a minimum of two "official" experts comprising the "Unofficial Panel" who painstakingly review the manuscripts to ensure: factual accuracy of all data; inclusion of the most up-to-date and relevant information; and that, from an insider's perspective, the authors have armed you with all the necessary facts you need—but the institutions don't want you to know.

For *The Unofficial Guide to Alternative Medicine,* we are proud to introduce the following panel of experts:

David L. Diehl, M.D. David L. Diehl is currently Associate Clinical Professor of Medicine at the UCLA School of Medicine, Director of Gastrointestinal Endoscopy at Olive View–UCLA Medical Center, and Vice-President of the Medical Acupuncture Research Foundation (MARF), a non-profit organization active in promoting acupuncture research. His specialty is gastroenterology. He has practiced acupuncture since 1991, and utilizes acupuncture and herbal medicine in his clinical practice of gastroenterology, besides practicing conventional Western medicine.

Christopher Trahan, O.M.D., L.Ac. Christopher Trahan is a Doctor of Oriental Medicine and a Licensed Acupuncturist (NY, NM) who integrates Chinese Medicine, Western Herbal Medicine, and Homeopathy. He has been in clinical practice since 1979, trained in China and India, and is nationally board-certified in Acupuncture and Chinese Herbal Medicine. He has lectured internationally and has been a faculty member at several institutes of Chinese Medicine.

Introduction

From Ayurveda to reflexology, from black cohosh root to saw palmetto berries, from visualization to aromatherapy to meditation, alternative medicine is a billion-dollar business in today's world. This school of drug-free doctoring, also called "complementary" or "unconventional" medicine, views the mind and the body as an integrated system—meaning they influence each other—and depends on your commitment to staying well, or self-care.

In the past three decades, alternative medicine has soared in popularity and now touts a wide range of nonstandard approaches to personal health and healing. Some, like yoga and herbal treatments, are deeply steeped in ancient Asian traditions; others, like art therapy or mindfully listening to a Windham Hill CD while practicing deep abdominal breathing, are strictly New Age; all, however, have proponents from every walk of life who vouch for their healing powers.

The skyrocketing use of complementary medicine represents a growing dissatisfaction with conventional or allopathic health care. Allopaths, or conventional medical doctors, focus on defining disease based on measurable symptoms and then eliminating those signs; alternative therapists treat the whole person—body, mind, and spirit—with the focus on staying balanced and well.

Although many alternative healers do not have medical degrees, more and more people are turning to alternative medicine because the solutions are appealing and offer hope. Especially with the soaring costs of health care, alternative treatments, which range from herbal supplements to meditation, are relatively affordable, are easily accessible, and allow you to actively participate in key decisions about your health.

Official recognition of alternative therapies is growing. A survey conducted at the American Academy of Family Physicians' annual meeting in 1996 demonstrated that family physicians have great regard for spirituality as a complement to conventional medicine. Ninety-nine percent of physicians surveyed agreed that spiritual beliefs are helpful in complementing medical treatment, in reducing hospital stays, and in enhancing quality of life.

All Stressed Up and No Place to Go

But what is this mind/body interplay that alternative practitioners claim to balance? To begin with, alternative therapies are based on the premise that the mind and the body are interconnected to an extent far surpassing previous assumptions and that physical health and emotional well-being are closely linked. Based on scientific tests, we know that stress can literally wreck your health. In today's pressured society, chronic stress can persist for days, weeks, or even months, tearing at your mind, body, and spirit.

In terms of lost hours due to absenteeism, reduced productivity, and workers' compensation benefits, stress costs American industry more than $300 billion annually. But more than that, stress can make us ill. At least 4 in 10 of all adults suffer adverse health effects from stress, and as many as 9 in 10 of all visits to doctors' offices are for stress-related complaints, according to the American Psychological Association. This is because cortisol, the body's main stress-related hormone, and the autonomic nervous system both are activated during stress. As a result of being bathed in these chemicals, the immune system no longer is able to keep infections or diseases at bay, making us more susceptible to viruses and bacteria.

Symptoms of too much stress include:

- Anger
- Anxiety
- Apathy
- Back pain
- Chest pain or tightness
- Depression
- Headaches
- Heart palpitations
- Hives
- Impotence
- Inability to relax (tension)
- Inability to concentrate
- Insomnia
- Irregular menstrual periods
- Irritable bowel syndrome (IBS)

- Loss of sexual desire
- Loss of sexual function
- Mood swings
- Neck pain
- No energy
- Rapid pulse
- Rashes
- Short temper
- Short-term memory loss
- Weight gain or loss

Many experiments have shown that exposure to viruses and bacteria results in no health problems, provided your immune system is strong. Yet, when faced with chronic stress, your immune system cannot work at full capacity. When your immune system malfunctions, it yields to the development of autoimmune diseases such as some types of arthritis, allergy, or asthma. If your immune system is depleted, your body is at risk of being overwhelmed by invading bacteria and viruses, resulting in cancer or other life-threatening diseases.

Although each person's response to life's stressors is different, many people believe that alternative therapies can put you back in control and that self-efficacy is essential for wellness.

Instead of prescribing an expensive pharmaceutical as the treatment for an illness, alternative practitioners focus on ideas of natural medicine, holism, and wellness—ideas that must be gently explained and taught by the practitioner. In fact, most alternative practitioners take into account all parts of the person, not just the part with the symptom. Think back to the last time you had an excruciating headache. What treatment finally worked to relieve your pain? If you go to a conventional medical doctor with a headache as your symptom, he may run some laboratory tests and then give you a prescription pain reliever or antibiotic for infection. If you see a holistic practitioner with a headache as your symptom, she may review your history, ask questions about your lifestyle, and then prescribe various treatments that would work together to reconnect the mind and the body. These treatments would help you do the following:

- Reduce your tension with biofeedback
- Decrease pain with feverfew, an herb that has been found to help with migraine pain
- Eliminate toxins from your body by increasing fluids
- Visualize being pain free using guided imagery
- Increase healing sleep with hydrotherapy (a warm bath)
- Strengthen the immune system using nutritional supplements

Proponents of alternative treatments claim that these nondrug (or complementary) interventions may allow you to take less medication, have fewer laboratory tests and surgeries, and actively participate in self-care. Although studies have focused on the negative effect of stress hormones that trigger physiological changes in the body, even more recent groundbreaking research reveals that some alternative therapies can literally reconfigure the brain's biology, triggering biochemical and neurological changes that heal the body. This reconfiguring can make a big difference in your overall health or recovery from illness. The outlook for alternative treatments is remarkably optimistic, and we are gaining a better understanding of these nonstandard treatments and how they can increase health and prevent disease. The following are just a few breakthrough studies:

- A new British study revealed that men who ate garlic more than twice a week had only half the risk of prostate cancer of men who never ate garlic. Harvard researchers found that eating tomatoes and tomato products also reduced the risk of prostate cancer.

- Researchers at Cambridge University in England studied 1,100 heart attack victims and found that those who took 400 to 800 International Units (IU) of vitamin E daily had 77 percent fewer nonfatal heart attacks than those on a placebo.

- A researcher at Harvard found that omega-3 fish oil may help regulate the heart's electrical activity. Two to three servings of fatty fish per week offer protection. For vegetarians, canola oil, walnuts, and flaxseed oil also are high in omega-3s.

- A recent Dutch study found that people who ate half an onion a day cut their risk of stomach cancer in half. Quercetin is an antioxidant and is concentrated in onions. Studies show that quercetin has anticancer, antifungal, anti-inflammatory, antiviral, and antibacterial properties.

- A groundbreaking study reported in The Journal of the American Medical Association (1997) revealed that even frequent book reading and singing in a choir can reduce a person's risk of death and can help increase resiliency.

- Researchers believe that ginkgo may help increase mental functioning in people with dementia caused by Alzheimer's disease.

Take Two Bananas and Call Me in the Morning

Forty-seven-year-old Jacob became a believer in alternative medicine after using nutrition therapy—specifically, a low-fat diet high in complex carbohydrates such as whole grains, fruits, and vegetables—and meditation to lower his blood pressure. Jacob's high-stress sales job, in which he flies from city to city throughout the week, kept him in a constant state of anxiety. To control his blood pressure, he ended up taking three different prescriptions that made him feel tired and dull, yet his medical doctor never suggested that job stress could be a contributing factor to his medical condition. A coworker mentioned that he could keep his blood pressure in normal ranges with a low-salt diet, daily exercise, and meditation, so Jacob decided to check out alternative therapies. He met with a Certified Nutritionist, dramatically changed his diet to include more vegetables and fruits, and began a daily walking program. He also learned how to meditate and, instead of taking coffee breaks throughout the day, he went into an empty conference room and quietly imagined peaceful images for 15 minutes. Within three months of changing his lifestyle, Jacob's blood pressure lowered dramatically, and he was able to drop two of his medications. He continues to check in with his internist while sticking to the healthful lifestyle changes that ultimately made the dramatic difference in his health.

As Jacob and millions of others have experienced, alternative therapies can play a successful role in solving many chronic problems such as hypertension, insomnia, or ulcers. In the midst of the appeal and mystery of alternative medicine, however, do not close the door to Western medicine, for this is where we turn for the "big stuff." After all, who are you going to call when you have an acute infection, suspect a mysterious disease, or need an organ transplant? Probably not a shaman! This member of certain tribal societies mediates between the visible and invisible spirit worlds for healing purposes and to control natural events—and he does not have the training to repair an ailing gall bladder or to remove a malignant tumor.

Nonetheless, the reality is that most of us have not needed a vital organ replaced lately. Rather, most of us are just plain burned out and are battling the resulting lifestyle ailments, such as headaches, backaches, cardiovascular disease, arthritis, allergy and asthma, insomnia, and depression, along with diseases that can become chronic or even terminal, such as AIDS and cancer.

Still, let's not forget what happens when a person goes to a medical doctor and laboratory tests cannot verify the disease to be in the body, such as with chronic fatigue or fibromyalgia. This arthritis-like syndrome affects more than 10 million Americans, mostly women, with symptoms of deep muscle pain, unending fatigue, poor sleep quality, and depression, and there is no laboratory test to diagnosis it. While treatment is available to manage symptoms, no cure is in sight at this time. Not surprisingly, many traditional doctors feel that, if the illness has vague symptoms—especially with psychological overtones—and cannot be defined scientifically, perhaps it is not a real illness. Thus, any form of health care intervention that attempts to address these symptoms without a specific diagnosis is branded as alternative. Perhaps, in focusing on isolated systems and the corresponding parts of the body (heart, lungs, liver, and so on), current medicine has lost sight of the fact that we are much more than just the total of our component biological parts.

From Stone Age to New Age

Belief in alternative treatments is not a new revelation. Aristotle gave credence to mind/body therapies with this advice to other physicians: "Just as you ought not to attempt to cure eyes without head or head without body, so you should not treat body without soul." The 2000-year-old Hippocratic writings contain observations that "there is a measure of conscious thought throughout the body." Hippocrates also taught his students to carefully assess their clients' living environment for an understanding of their diseases. The Chinese have used herbs for centuries to treat and cure a host of medical problems; the healing traditions of Ayurvedic medicine, which focuses on balancing the body using methods such as meditation, herbs and minerals, massage, and dietary advice, go back 4,000 years in India's rich history; reflexology, which relieves stress and tension through systematically probing the feet, dates back to at least 2330 B.C. and is even depicted in a wall painting in an Egyptian tomb. From Aristotle's time to the present, medical literature has revealed anecdotal material documenting the use of unconventional treatments as well as the intimate connection between mind, body, and spirit.

Yet it was not until the mid-1960s that Americans became intrigued with alternative medicine. At that time, the Vietnam War was invoking major changes in American society, particularly the exposure to Eastern Asian culture, including medical practices used there. This exposure, along with the increasing costs and mistrust of our nation's health care, began to fuel the rapid adoption of alternative treatment in the United States.

Alternative Medicine Hits the Mainstream

There is a growing body of evidence that our dissatisfaction with conventional medical care has continued to swell in epidemic proportions since the mid-1960s. A poll conducted by the National Coalition on Health Care in Washington, D.C. (1996) resulted in the following provocative statistics:

- A startling 75 percent of Americans are frightened by accounts of medical mistakes that have damaged or killed patients.

- 57 percent fear getting sicker after they are hospitalized.

- 44 percent claim to have had a bad experience with medical treatment.

Combine these spiraling fears with a comprehensive report by the Centers for Disease Control (CDC) stating that annual medical costs for treating the six major chronic diseases (heart disease, cancer, stroke, diabetes, obstructive pulmonary disease, and liver disease), which account for 73 percent of all deaths in our nation, amount to $425 billion.

The CDC adds that these six diseases are, in a large part, preventable. Here's the astounding CDC statistic: Only $287 million were spent on disease prevention in 1994—about 0.07 percent of the amount spent on treatment. This figure breaks down to about $1.21 per person spent annually for disease prevention in our nation. That amount does not even buy a week's supply of immune-boosting antioxidants for one person. Today's consumers are not waiting for their primary care physician or even the latest government studies to outline a plan for prevention of disease. People want to take charge of their health and to be involved in decision making regarding treatment methods, especially the 70 million baby boomers who have always had a problem with authority (remember Kent State and Berkeley?).

Take a Number, Please

Tired of assembly-line medical care in which doctors spend an average of 10 minutes with each patient per visit? Millions are seeking natural and effective ways to prevent, manage, or even cure diseases, using methods that are not always scientifically-based, such as massages with essential oils or copper bracelets to relieve arthritic pain.

According to a recent nationwide poll, more than 4 in 10 adults in the United States (42 percent) now embrace alternative-care therapies. The Landmark Report on Public Perceptions of Alternative Care (1997) reported that nearly half of adults in the United States (45 percent) say they would be willing to pay more in medical insurance each month to have access to alternative care. Of those Americans who use alternative care, almost three-quarters (74 percent) say they use it along with conventional medical care.

Within the realm of conventional medicine, there are some accepted alternative therapies (such as acupuncture, biofeedback, chiropractic, herbal therapy, and nutrition) that many medical doctors will agree to use in conjunction with traditional therapy. In fact, a growing trend at some of the nation's most prestigious teaching hospitals is to blend the two schools of medicine. Beth Israel Hospital in Boston, associated with Harvard Medical School, recently set up a center for alternative medicine. Columbia University has done the same. Even the National Institutes of Health (NIH) has turned its head cautiously toward alternative treatments to sort out the truth from the hype. The NIH's Office of Alternative Medicine, headed by Dr. Wayne B. Jonas, is funding studies aimed at establishing or disproving the clinical basis of different types of alternative therapy. Although this marks a positive step in the right direction, according to naysayers, the amount of money being spent to research unconventional treatments is only about $20 million of the NIH's staggering $13.6 billion annual budget—not nearly enough to make a difference.

Separating Fact from Fiction

When you hear about spinal manipulation to end headaches or foot massages to calm gastrointestinal upsets, you may wonder if alternative medicine really is a radical new prescription. Here is where we must take a clue from those in the know—scientists and conventional medical doctors who express caution because most alternative treatments have not passed clinical trials.

No matter what the advertising flyer at the natural food store claims, even the most popular medicinal herbs with pharmaceutical compounds contain ingredients that have not been tested and are now being scrutinized by the Food and Drug Administration (FDA).

A growing body of scientists and medical doctors are now saying, "Why not?" These professionals believe that, if a therapy is safe with no substantiated harmful side effects, it can be considered along with your scientifically proven conventional treatments. Now, get this straight here: Do not replace your conventional medications. Rather, complement these prescribed treatments with safe alternative therapies. This can be a positive move toward unifying the conventional with the unconventional.

As such, continuing regular medical therapy is important, as is your physician's approval before adding any unproven alternative therapy to your proven medical plan. Just because something is natural does not mean it is always safe. Yes, calcium supplements will ward off osteoporosis, folic acid can help prevent birth defects, garlic may lower cholesterol, ginger calms nausea, and valerian can help you sleep. Nonetheless, some natural supplements and herbs are highly toxic and can raise blood pressure, cause liver damage, and even lead to death. Because of the lack of regulation by the government, most consumers do not know this until they ingest the product. Hemlock, for example, is very natural—but it also is a poisonous plant that is deadly!

Which Comes First—Treatment or Prevention?

Although alternative treatments such as acupuncture to reduce nausea with pregnancy or chemotherapy, cranberry juice to help prevent urinary tract infections, or meditation to reduce blood pressure may have scientific backing, alternative medicine is not recommended to replace conventional medical care in any circumstances.

Traditional medicine is crucial, especially for important preventive tests, lifesaving surgery to remove an existing malignant tumor, or coronary artery bypass surgery for serious heart disease. Laetrile, the extract of apricot pits, was touted as a miracle cancer treatment in the 1970s. Many terminally ill patients, without any scientific substantiation, opted to take this alternative treatment instead of chemotherapy or radiation. Ultimately, it was proven useless. No matter what advertisers claim, it is not advisable to think that a coffee enema will resolve an acute asthma attack, that meditation can stop the warning signs of a heart attack, or that green algae pills will ward off a diabetic coma. Call your medical doctor immediately for any serious condition or new symptoms. Alternative therapies, however, may allow you to delay or even prevent chronic or terminal conditions. If you do not have heart disease, for example, following a regular regime of a low-fat diet, regular aerobic exercise, and alternative stress-reduction techniques such as guided imagery or meditation could help prevent a heart attack from happening altogether. If you do have heart disease, this regime possibly could start to unclog blocked arteries and significantly extend your life. Likewise, if you do not have diabetes, following a healthful diet, exercising regularly, and keeping life's stressors at bay may help keep your body well. If you do have diabetes, preliminary studies show that the mineral chromium picolinate, when used with conventional medical treatments, may help keep blood-sugar levels even. In addition, a low-fat diet with plenty of fruits and vegetables may help you keep your blood pressure, cholesterol, and weight at a normal level, and you might even avoid some types of cancer.

Getting Back in Control

If some nonstandard treatments sound too good to be true, they probably are. The Food and Drug Administration estimates that 38 million Americans have used a fraudulent health product or treatment, spending billions of dollars annually. Because responses to treatments for many ailments are highly individualized, it is important to be a savvy consumer and to check out all the facts about a treatment prior to using it. Before you believe everything you read, investigate the treatment or product. Talk to your medical doctor or pharmacist and ask about side effects. What may be safe for your neighbor may not be appropriate for you. Remember, you only get one body, and you must govern what goes into it!

Today, thanks to ongoing research in both the medical and alternative medicine fields, doctors have a better understanding of what it takes to keep us healthy. Most will acknowledge that health is not constant; it is an ongoing process. Being born healthy does not mean you are going to stay that way. Believers in alternative medicine tout that only through responsibility and persistence by the patient—not the doctor—can they ultimately experience optimal health and healing. This is not to say that medicine should be ignored; however, you must understand that conventional medicine emphasizes crisis intervention rather than personal responsibility for wellness.

Simply stated, alternative medicine may put you back in control of your health, or it may make you ill. In this light, we must look at healing as an investment portfolio. Be discerning, study the facts, and ask many questions, but be wary of putting all your money in one fund. The safest approach to staying well is to rely on your conventional medical doctor. Then invest in your total health—mind, body, and spirit—with a wellness portfolio that blends conventional modes of therapy with safe, alternative treatments, thus providing the best of both worlds.

The Lowdown on Alternative Medicine

GET THE SCOOP ON...
Why blending conventional and unconventional treatment
will allow you to have the best of both worlds ▪ Why a
medical doctor should be your primary care physician ▪
Important factors to consider when selecting an alternative practitioner ▪ What you need to know before taking
any alternative treatments

PART I

Allopath, Alternative, or Both?

I n this era of health care choices, the options for healing seem endless. A host of new medical and alternative treatments are touted almost daily. How do you know which one to choose? Are there specific signs that indicate when you should seek conventional medical treatment for a physical or emotional problem? What cues indicate that it is safe to rely on alternative or complementary treatment? Remember, alternative therapies can range from those that are grounded in long traditions of scientific studies or cultural healing to those that are outright ridiculous and potentially harmful. To know which health problems can be entrusted to an alternative practitioner and which problems mandate medical care, it is important to become an expert in both fields.

The major difference between the two modes of health care is that only conventional medicine has the stamp of scientifically substantiated research to validate its claims. Fixing a broken bone, treating bacterial pneumonia, running a blood glucose test, and checking out an unusual lump or bleeding mole still safely falls within the arena of your conventional medical doctor. By contrast, if a medical problem related to your lifestyle interferes with your quality of life, you might consider talking with an alternative medicine specialist. Emotional stressors complicate the management of many medical problems. Common illnesses such as asthma, headaches, and hypertension often have a psychological component and respond well to a combination of medical and alternative therapies. In fact, nonphysical treatments such as meditation, guided imagery, and progressive muscle relaxation have been effective in controlled scientific studies for the following:

- Alcoholism
- Anxiety
- Arthritis
- Asthma
- Cardiac pain
- Colds
- Depression
- Diabetes
- Fever
- High blood pressure
- Insomnia
- Irritable bowel syndrome (IBS)

Check out the options
The first step in deciding whether you need allopathic (conventional), alternative (complementary),

or both types of treatment is to evaluate your options. Let's take a look at 42-year-old Jim, a weekend warrior who injured his back playing in a company softball tournament. After Jim slid into first base and felt something in his lower back that "burned like a blow torch," he immediately went to the walk-in medical clinic near his home. The doctor evaluated Jim's symptoms, such as shooting pain in his back that traveled down the back of his right leg and his inability to extend the big toe on his right foot. He took Jim's medical history, did a thorough physical examination and a series of laboratory tests, and concluded that our middle-aged warrior could possibly have a bulging disc in his back. Explaining that bulging discs do not show up on an X-ray, the doctor made an appointment for Jim to have an MRI, which is considered to be a reliable, noninvasive tool for detecting abnormal discs in the lower (lumbar) spine. For an MRI, the patient is placed in a long nonmagnetic tube. This tube is surrounded by a huge doughnut-shaped magnet that helps to produce an image of an area in the body. The entire procedure lasts between 30 and 90 minutes.

Based on Jim's experience, it seems as if there is only one answer to back pain—conventional medical treatment, expensive tests for diagnosis, and possible surgery. But let's be honest. Wouldn't you opt for a deep muscle massage over a surgical procedure if you knew it could stop the back pain and heal your injury? In that light, let's do an instant replay, only with Jim deciding to choose an alternative therapy instead of medical treatment. Where would he turn?

- He might try a practitioner who does *acupuncture.* This alternative form of treatment is based

Watch Out!
Ninety percent of patients with a ruptured or herniated disc improve within one year when using conservative, nonoperative measures to resolve symptoms.
A knowledgeable consultation with your doctor, or even a second medical opinion, is important.

on the premise that the body is a complex bio-electric system with a main life force circulating throughout. When this life force, or *qi* (pronounced *chee*), gets blocked, disease and distress result. The practitioner takes a thorough medical history, places hair-thin needles into Jim's body at specific places, and then manipulates the needles to stimulate nerve cells to release *endorphins* and end Jim's pain. *Endorphins* are the body's "happy hormones," natural biochemicals produced in the brain that help relieve pain and make you feel good.

- *Chiropractic* treatment is a likely alternative Jim could consider for back pain. In this, the second largest primary health care profession, a practitioner manipulates Jim's spine to restore normal nerve function and to ease the pain.

- *Massage therapy* also could alleviate Jim's aching back. Studies show that the benefits of massage include heightened alertness, relief from depression and anxiety, an increase in the number of natural "killer cells" in the immune system, lower levels of the stress hormone cortisol, and reduced difficulty in getting to sleep.

- Jim could choose *Ayurveda*, in which the practitioner carefully assesses his back problem and then uses herbal therapy, animal and mineral ingredients, steam baths, or even oil massages to help bring his body back into balance.

- With *biofeedback*, a therapist treats Jim's pain by connecting him to a machine and placing sensors over specific muscle sites. The practitioner reads the tension in Jim's muscles, the amount of sweat produced, or the measurement of finger temperature and teaches Jim to make a direct connection between his thoughts, his level of nervous-system arousal, muscular tension, and eventually, his pain level.

▪ Jim also could choose *hypnosis* as a way to control his back pain. During a session, the therapist makes suggestions to Jim that allows him to decrease the intensity of the pain, to move the pain to another area, or to try to build a feeling of separation from the pain. Although hypnosis comes from the Greek word meaning "sleep," it actually is an intense state of focused concentration. Many hypnotherapy patients report better outcomes with respect to their pain experience, fatigue on awakening, and sleep patterns compared to patients receiving physical therapy.

▪ A *naturopath* might be able to solve Jim's back pain by placing an emphasis on hydrotherapy (warm whirlpool baths), massage, and nutritional and herbal treatments. Naturopaths prefer to avoid drugs and surgery and try to rely on the body's natural healing capacity.

▪ Instead of getting a second opinion from a surgeon, Jim might go to an *osteopathic physician*, a doctor who views the body as a whole made up of interrelated parts. The Doctor of Osteopathy (D.O.) tries to find the underlying causes of Jim's pain and remedy them with manual adjustments of the muscles, joints, and spine before using drugs and surgery.

Get the best of both worlds

So there you have it—and these represent only a few of the health care alternatives Jim could take. As you can see, the choices we have for excellence in

> 66
> After having unsuccessful back surgery for a herniated disc, I finally found the best pain relief by using a combination of bodywork (massage), chiropractic (spinal manipulation and adjustment), and hydrotherapy (warm whirlpool spas).
> —Tomas, 29, professional soccer player
> 99

medical care are mind-boggling. In years past, most of us used the treatment methods passed down from our parents and grandparents and relied on a family doctor who treated us from conception to birth to death. Yet medicine has changed dramatically in the past few decades. The family doctor used to be the main medical care provider, but now the traditional, autocratic role of doctors is being challenged by millions. People today want to make informed choices regarding their bodies and prevention and treatment of illness.

If you are like most Americans, your choice for health care includes both conventional and alternative practitioners. Nonetheless, be aware that problems may occur when you have more than one specialist administering treatment. According to a study in the *New England Journal of Medicine*, more than 80 percent of the people who use alternative therapies also use conventional medicine at the same time, but many do not tell their doctors about these alternative treatments.

Unless effective communication takes place between you and your health care professionals, you might find yourself in a precarious situation with your health. Your primary care physician, for example, may prescribe strong antibiotics to help stop a respiratory infection. Your naturopath might suggest that you try several herbal products for the same infection. This combination of medication and herbs could potentially be toxic and cause other serious health problems. You might then see an acupuncturist who suggests you quit taking all medications and herbs, and instead undergo a series of fine-needle treatments.

Even though, in good faith, all these professionals are using their knowledge and skills to help get you well, it is important for you to inform *each* practitioner you see—whether alternative or conventional or both—all about you: your medical and family history, your symptoms, your treatment plan, and the specific medications or herbs you are taking. It must be emphasized that knowledgeable patients who reports these details, including changes in medications or alternative therapies, to each doctor or practitioner will help themselves.

Start with a medical doctor

It's important to find a primary care physician you like because he or she will play a significant role as you seek to stay well. This family practitioner or internal medicine specialist, who has completed three to seven years of training by medical school graduation, should be board certified. This means she has passed a comprehensive examination given by a governing board in her specific discipline. Not only does she serve as a person who can make an accurate, scientific diagnosis and can prescribe medical treatment for an acute, chronic, or serious problem, this medical doctor may become a close, dependable friend you can talk to when concerns turn into ongoing worries and anxieties.

Before you choose your primary care physician, contact your health insurer and ask for a directory of affiliated physicians. If you are enrolled in a managed care health plan—such as a Health Maintenance Organization (HMO) or a Preferred Provider Organization (PPO)—you need to choose a physician who is a member of that plan's network. Questions to consider include:

Unofficially...
Senator Tom Harkin (D-IA) has launched a major effort to get the federal government to research non-traditional approaches to prevention and treatment of diseases. Harkin wants to combine the two National Institute of Health (NIH) offices that deal with alternative medicine and dietary supplements. He also wants to expand the center to include the spiritual side of healing.

Bright Idea
You can call
800-358-9295
for the free
booklet *Questions
to Ask your Doctor
Before You Have
Surgery*. For a
list of physicians
who also use
alternative
therapies, write
to the American
Holistic Medical
Association,
4101 Lake Boone
Trail, Suite 201,
Raleigh, NC
27607.

- Is the doctor a good communicator, answering questions and using words you understand?

- Is the doctor interested in your total health— mind and body—and not just the physical problem you present?

- Is he a licensed medical doctor (M.D.) or doctor of osteopathy (D.O.) from an accredited medical school?

- Did she pass special boards for certification?

- Are the office hours convenient?

- With what hospitals is the doctor affiliated?

- Do other doctors take calls after hours, or is this doctor the one you will always see?

- Will his office bill your insurer or must you pay at each visit?

- What are her views on alternative treatments?

Conventional medical doctors provide the necessary screening tests to prevent major diseases. But just because your medical doctor does preventive tests such as blood pressure and cholesterol screenings, colon cancer screenings, and gender-specific cancer screenings, do not assume she will be thumbs down on alternative therapies. A national survey published in 1994 found that 60 percent of medical doctors had, at some time, referred patients to practitioners of alternative medicine.

Add an alternative practitioner

While medical doctors use sophisticated laboratory tests to make a conclusive diagnosis, the alternative practitioner may use a physical examination, a history-taking interview, or a questionnaire to find the source of your chronic problem. Ailments such as lower-back pain, gastrointestinal problems, migraines, chronic pain, and even depression can fare well from alternative forms of treatment.

Finding the right alternative medicine practitioner who is qualified to treat problems properly and cost-effectively is not always easy. One of the most important steps to take is to know yourself, including your personal likes and dislikes. Because you may spend more time talking with the alternative therapist than your medical doctor, it is important to choose someone with whom you feel comfortable. Consider the following:

- Do you feel more at ease with a man or woman?

- Should the practitioner be older than you, the same age, or younger?

- Do you have a preference as to educational background, certification, or licensing?

These questions are important to consider before making the first appointment. The following descriptions also should help you get a handle on who's who in the world of alternative medicine:

- **Ayurvedic** practitioners believe in an ancient Indian medical system that goes beyond treating disease and focuses on a complete-wellness approach to life.

- **Chinese medicine** practitioners use herbs, acupuncture, acupressure, and shiatsu. They believe the body has the potential to cure its own diseases if treated correctly.

- **Environmental medicine** practitioners focus on how factors in our environment (foods, chemical, water, air quality) affect us. Treatments range from environmental control to immunotherapy.

Timesaver
How do you find an alternative medicine practitioner in your area? Using the resources in Appendix B, call or write to specific governing organizations and ask for the names and credentials of alternative practitioners in your town. Ask your doctor or medical society for highly qualified practitioners or call a nearby medical school to see if it provides referrals. Check with friends or do a search on the Internet. As a last resort? Check your Yellow Pages under Holistic Practitioners.

- **Holistic medicine** practitioners emphasize the whole person—physical, mental, emotional, and spiritual—as well as personal responsibility and participation in one's own health care.

- **Homeopathic** practitioners strive to treat disease by stimulating the body's own defense and repair systems with highly diluted doses of medication.

- **Naturopathic** practitioners believe in the healing power of nature and use a variety of approaches (Chinese medicine, physical, homeopathic, botanical, and herbal, among others) to help the body heal itself.

- **Nutritionists** believe that diet and food can be used to keep you well and to prevent disease.

Doing a background check

Ask your medical doctor, trusted friends, or coworkers to recommend a credible alternative practitioner. Call a local university's medical school and ask for recommendations. Follow up on these doctors or practitioners with a background check of the person's credentials. Call governing boards for referrals (see Appendix B) and ask for client references. While all states license chiropractors, licensing of naturopaths, homeopaths, acupuncturists, and practitioners of Chinese medicine is varied or even nonexistent, depending on the therapy and the location. This means you cannot be sure the practitioner you choose is qualified to treat you. Until recently, most alternative practitioners did not have medical degrees. The good news is that, today, your alternative practitioner might also be a medical doctor (M.D.), a doctor of osteopathy (D.O.), a doctor of chiropractic (D.C.), or have other degrees depending on the schools he attended.

Keeping costs in mind

Alternative does not necessarily mean cheap. Americans spend more than $13 billion each year on alternative therapies and most are out-of-pocket expenses. Even if your alternative practitioner says he will not give you expensive drugs, supplements can become extremely costly if taken over a period of time. In this age of managed care, it is wise to check the list of practitioners who will accept your insurance provider. In some cases, if you are referred to an alternative practitioner from your primary care physician, your insurance company will pay the bill.

Planning an initial consultation

Get to know the alternative practitioner during an initial consultation. Instead of a conventional doctor's complete physical examination and laboratory tests, most alternative practitioners do a detailed interview that focuses on symptoms, lifestyle habits, and past health problems. An Ayurvedic practitioner may check your pulse to help obtain a diagnosis, while an osteopath will evaluate the condition of your musculoskeletal system, including range-of-motion and flexibility.

Open communication during this consultation is important so you receive the highest quality of care and the comfort needed during anxious moments.

During this interview, use the following questions to determine whether this person will meet your needs:

- What tests are used in forming a diagnosis?

- What is the preferred method of treatment and are these methods current?

Timesaver
Before you go to a new doctor, ask your current physician and any previous physicians for a copy of your medical records. Take this file with you to save time during the visit. If the doctors balk at this request, don't back down. Most states grant the legal right to patient access to medical records.

- Does the practitioner appear to relate well to you and to staff members?

- Is he accessible? (When you are ill, popularity is not important but availability is.)

- Is he extremely competent in his field?

- Does the practitioner spend ample time with you so that your questions are clearly answered?

During your initial consultation, check on office hours to be sure they fit your daily schedule. How is payment made? What insurance providers are accepted? Ask for information about emergency availability and charges. Even the receptionist's responses might set the tone and help you decide whether this is the right office.

Once you have narrowed down your practitioner choices, use the following questions to find the key person who will serve to keep you well:

- Are you certified? (This means the practitioner has passed a standard exam given by the governing board in her specialty.)

- Are you licensed in your field?

- What are your specializations?

- What special training do you have, or what school did you attend?

- How long have you been practicing alternative medicine?

- Are you a member of any governing organization?

- What insurance do you take? Do you accept Medicare/Medicaid?

- Do you file insurance?

- Do you take worker's compensation?

- Are you involved in any academic pursuits such as teaching, writing, or research? (This person may be more up-to-date in the latest developments in her field.)
- What is your philosophy of healing?

Natural remedy or lethal weapon?

Once you have chosen your alternative health care practitioner, it is important to ask questions about the safety of the recommended treatment. Just as medical doctors frequently prescribe antibiotics for illnesses that do not require them, alternative practitioners may give you samples of herbs or tonics, claiming they will cure your ills. Before you pop any substance into your mouth, become *medwise*. It may be hard to tell whether a new medication, herbal therapy, or amazing tonic is the great breakthrough we all have been waiting for or a dangerous treatment that doesn't work and may even cause harm.

Reading between the lines

Press reports may unintentionally make a new treatment seem better than it really is, especially after long-term use. After reading in a magazine advertisement about the benefits of a new liniment for arthritis, 57-year-old Sam sent away for this "miracle" cream. Just as the package label suggested, he diligently applied this cream to his knees and ankles three times a day. After two weeks of using the cream, Sam had experienced no relief at all and wondered why he was losing hair on these body parts. After comparing the active ingredients in the "miracle" cream with the ingredients in his wife's hair remover, he discovered that all he had put on his knees and ankles was hair remover. Not only was he out $39.95, he had no pain relief . . . and no hair.

The lesson? Don't believe everything you are told or that you read; be a discerning consumer. If an alternative practitioner makes the promise that a product will give you a quick, painless, and guaranteed cure, be wary of the product as well as the spokesperson. Get the facts and then make an intelligent decision after weighing the pros and cons.

If it sounds too good to be true, it might be

When you meet with your alternative practitioner, ask the following questions about any treatment, especially one that is new or makes promises that seem too good to be true:

- How old is the treatment? If it is new, find out the facts before you use it. Many health sites on the Internet give detailed, factual information about herbs and other alternative therapies.

- Is it approved by the Food and Drug Administration? The FDA requires extensive testing for drugs. It is not perfect, however, because herbal treatments are not regulated. But it does provide some reassurance if the treatment has been formally approved after scientific trials.

- What are the ingredients? Make a list of the contents and dosages, and ask your pharmacist whether he or she knows about the treatment's safety.

- What are the side effects? Just like prescription medications, some nonstandard treatments have dangerous side effects; others do not.

- What are the chances for improvement? If the practitioner claims this is a "miracle" cure, it is best to walk away. Real miraculous breakthroughs are few and far between, and a responsible scientist would not use the word "miracle."

- How much does it cost? Some alternative treatments will not be reimbursed by your health insurance provider.

- Can it be taken with traditional medical treatment? Avoid treatments that require you to stop any medication your conventional doctor has prescribed for you.

Buyer beware!

In 1994, Congress passed the Dietary Supplement Health and Education Act, which did away with regulations on alternative medicines that claim to be foods or dietary supplements. Herbs or vitamins can claim to cure diseases in magazine advertisements, books, or signs, as long as this information is not on the product label. But buyer beware when you purchase supplements because you may get a bottle of nothing. *Consumer Reports* tested 10 ginseng products last year, and one contained almost none of the active ingredients listed. The other nine products varied in concentration by 1,000 percent.

You *can* have it all

Whatever treatment you choose, remember that it's your body. You have the right (and the responsibility) to become an informed, educated, and active participant in your own wellness. You also have the right to get a second opinion, to change physicians, and to ask pertinent questions regarding medical or alternative procedures. Working in partnership with conventional and complementary practitioners, you can choose the safest and most effective treatments that will work with your body's own healing power so you will experience the pinnacle of optimum health.

Watch Out!
Attempting to counter illness using megadoses of vitamin supplements might backfire. Researchers from the Lauder Breast Cancer Center at the Memorial Sloan-Kettering Cancer Center in Manhattan found that large doses of vitamin C could blunt the beneficial effects of chemotherapy for breast cancer. Breast cancer cells were found to have large numbers of receptors for vitamin C, and this vitamin may act like a growth booster for cancer cells.

Just the facts

- You can take responsibility for your own health by choosing healing alternatives that are safe.

- A conventional medical doctor is best for doing preventive tests and for diagnosing and treating serious illness.

- An alternative practitioner can help with stress-related ailments and healthy-lifestyle education.

- Be a discerning consumer before you take any medication or treatment, especially one that has not been scientifically substantiated as safe and effective.

- Pick the best of both worlds—conventional and alternative treatments—to experience optimum wellness.

Body Makeover: Taking the Path to Optimal Health

F or years, most of us have trusted science to determine our longevity. Although many factors influence our health and life span, it seemed to be etched in stone that women outlived men and, if your parents died at an early age, you would too. While 66 years was the average life span in 1950, 75 years is the average today. If you live past that age, you are said to be living on borrowed time.

Today's scientists are rewriting the rules of aging. The prevalent thought now is that, if a Galapagos turtle can live to be 152 years old, maybe we can, too. Many researchers are starting to doubt that we have a definite limit to our life span. They suggest that, by taking responsibility for our health and lifestyle, we may slow down the aging process and push the life span boundaries forward. New breakthroughs in aging research may lead to innovative medical therapies to stave off age-related degenerative diseases,

Chapter 2

treatments for conditions ranging from heart disease and dementia to arthritis and wrinkles, and yes, perhaps even extending the human life span.

But enough talk about longevity—what is the point of living to be 100 if you aren't healthy? The fact that you are reading this book is an indication that good health, prevention of disease, and quality of life are important to you. Because of new breakthroughs in the early diagnosis and treatment of once-terminal diseases, the outlook for health in later years is remarkably better than in the past. In fact, most of us can coast to our mid-30s with the luck of good genes.

But then our luck will come to a screeching halt. You see, there is a guaranteed time of awakening—usually mid-life—when genetics subside and lifestyle factors take over. Surprisingly, research concludes that only about 30 percent of the characteristics of aging are genetically based; the remaining 70 percent are not. In fact, study after study now confirms that more than 85 percent of deaths are due to chronic conditions that can be prevented or alleviated by lifestyle changes.

Prevention as part of the cure

Since the turn of the century, our nation has focused on treating diseases using the best drug or surgical interventions available. Think about it: National health organizations have made it a priority to familiarize us with the warning signs of cancer, diabetes, and heart disease. Contrary to this focus, alternative or complementary practitioners tell us that we can actually make a difference in staying healthy—if we make important lifestyle changes to prevent cancer, diabetes, and heart disease altogether.

Although treating disease is critical, especially in the early stages when treatment works best, a compelling case can be made that is supported by a host of scientific data—prevention of chronic and terminal illness should be the utmost goal.

If what current research indicates is true, preventive measures such as health screenings and individual lifestyle changes could eliminate an estimated 45 percent of cardiovascular disease deaths, 23 percent of cancer deaths, and more than 50 percent of the serious complications of diabetes. Controlling such risk factors as poor diet, infrequent exercise, use of tobacco and drugs, and abuse of alcohol could prevent between 40 and 70 percent of all premature deaths, one-third of all acute disability cases, and two-thirds of all chronic disability cases.

Take heart disease, for example. Using a holistic program of nutritional therapy, exercise, stress-reduction techniques, and medications (if necessary) to treat hypertension or high cholesterol can help prevent this degenerative disease. Statistics show, however, that as a nation we are spending almost $9 billion annually for treatment with 300,000 coronary artery bypass graft surgeries. In this light, a fundamental principle of alternative medicine could deter or solve this health problem before it occurs.

Because prevention has become the prime word associated with alternative medicine, it is ironic how few people are willing to pay the price to stay well and to stay out of the doctor's office. Considering that Americans make about 1.5 billion doctors visits every year for preventable problems such as colds, hypertension, migraines, backaches, gastrointestinal

66

An ounce of prevention is worth a pound of cure."
—Benjamin Franklin

99

Moneysaver
Research has shown that for every $1 we spend on prevention today, we will save $30 on treatment tomorrow.

Bright Idea
Take time to laugh frequently throughout your day; it just may help you live longer. Studies show that a real belly laugh can increase antibodies that fight infection and can decrease cortisol, a stress hormone that suppresses the immune system.

complaints, unexplained fatigue, and obesity, the annual cost of staying well is a mere pittance compared to the annual cost of getting well (as shown in Table 2.1).

TABLE 2.1

The Annual Cost of Staying Well		The Annual Cost of Getting Well	
Daily walking	free	Coronary-bypass surgery	$40,000+
Electrocardiogram	$65	Hospitalization—heart attack	$18,200
Quitting cigarettes	free	Lung-cancer treatment	$34,000+
P.S.A. test	$60	Prostate-cancer surgery	$21,000+
Yearly mammogram	$110	Breast cancer/mastectomy	$7,500+
Preventive dental care	$150	Gum disease surgery	$1,500+
Sunscreen	$126	Skin-cancer treatment	$6,000+
Bone-density scan	$125	Hospitalization—broken hip	$16,871
Latex condoms	$115	AIDS (experimental medications and hospitalization)	$50,000+
Meditation, exercise	free	Medication for hypertension	$1,300
Social support	free	Weekly psychotherapy	$5,400+
Volunteering	free	Prozac (or other meds)	$500+

The facts speak for themselves. If you want to stay healthy for the rest of your life, it is cheaper (and wiser) to make prevention of disease a priority than to risk disrupting your body's healing system. Enter alternative medicine.

Before you delve into Part 2 of this book, which contains a myriad of alternative therapies that can reduce your stress, boost your immune function, and help keep you disease-free, it is important to first assess your lifestyle to see whether any key changes need to be made. Let the following unofficial tips be your challenge as you start the simple path to optimal health.

Unofficial tip #1: detox your body— kick the habit

How many times have you heard, "Don't smoke," "Smoking will shorten your life," or "Smoking causes cancer"? Well . . . believe it.

- Each year more than 390,000 people die from the direct effects of cigarette smoking.

- America spends more than $50 billion each year on health care costs for ailments attributable to smoking: cancer, heart disease, atherosclerosis, stroke, lung disease, diabetes, peptic ulcer, and many others.

- According to the American Lung Association, current male smokers over the age of 35 are 10 times more likely to die of chronic obstructive pulmonary disease (COPD) and are 22 times more likely to die of lung cancer than nonsmoking males.

- In women, lung cancer has now surpassed breast cancer as the leading cause of cancer deaths.

Watch Out!
More than *one-third* of all high school students smoke cigarettes at this time.

Stimulating the brain to feel good

Once in the body, nicotine hits brain cell receptors and stimulates the release of neurotransmitters—the brain's chemical messengers. These messengers—acetylcholine, dopamine, serotonin, and beta-endorphin—affect how we pay attention, think, eat, deal with stress, and feel pleasure. Perhaps that is why some people reach for a cigarette whenever they need to feel alert, to be productive, or to cope with daily anxiety and tension.

Quitting is not easy

Although smoking increases the risk of serious health problems, it is one important lifestyle habit you have control over. That is the premise of alternative treatments; they put you in control of your self-care. You can use nonprescription nicotine patches worn on the skin, nicotine gum, or other medications—both prescription and non—to get through the difficult period of withdrawal. Talk to your doctor or call the local chapter of the American Lung Association or the American Cancer Society for solutions in how to stop smoking. Then enjoy the rewards of better health (see Table 2.2). Check the Yellow Pages for the phone numbers in your city.

Within 20 minutes of smoking your last cigarette, the body begins a series of changes that continues for years.

Watch Out!
It is easy to have a relapse when you try to kick the habit. You have to fight the urge to smoke one day at a time. A cigarette craving may last one to two minutes and then subside. Chew gum or carrot sticks if you are tempted to give in.

TABLE 2.2   WHEN SMOKERS QUIT

20 Minutes

- Blood pressure drops to normal
- Pulse rate drops to normal
- Body temperature of hands and feet increases to normal

8 Hours

- Carbon monoxide level in blood drops to normal
- Oxygen level in blood increases to normal

24 Hours

- Chance of heart attack decreases

48 Hours

- Nerve endings start regrowing
- Ability to smell and taste is enhanced

2 Weeks to 3 Months

- Circulation improves
- Walking becomes easier
- Lung function increases up to 30 percent

1 to 9 Months

- Coughing, sinus congestion, fatigue, and shortness of breath decrease
- Cilia regrow in the lungs, increasing ability to handle mucus, to clean the lungs, and to reduce infection
- Body's overall energy increases

1 Year

- Excess risk of coronary heart disease is half that of a smoker

5 Years

- Lung cancer death rate for average former smoker (one pack a day) decreases by almost half
- Stroke risk is reduced to that of a nonsmoker 5 to 15 years after quitting
- Risk of cancer in the mouth, throat, and esophagus decreases to half that of a smoker

10 Years

- Lung cancer death rate similar to that of nonsmokers
- Precancerous cells are replaced
- Risk of cancer to mouth, throat, esophagus, bladder, kidney, and pancreas decreases

15 Years

- Risk of coronary heart disease is equal to that of a nonsmoker

(Source: American Cancer Society and the National Centers for Disease Control and Prevention)

Bright Idea
Ear acupuncture, or auricular therapy, is one alternative treatment that may help moderate to heavy (two or more packs daily) smokers. Although there are no scientific studies to prove it works, experts believe that stimulating certain points on the ear releases endorphins—the body's feel-good hormones—which help to relieve nicotine cravings.

Unofficial tip #2: make food your medicine

Many smokers claim, "If I stop smoking cigarettes, I'll eat everything in sight and become obese." Not if you binge on the right foods. Part 2 goes into more depth about nutritional therapy; for now, however, you need to know that nutrition plays a starring role in optimal health. New studies show that eating a variety of foods can provide hundreds of nutrient and nonnutrient compounds that can help your body defend itself against damage, just as they help plants defend themselves against sunlight and extreme weather conditions.

Cutting the risk of illness

Let's face it. If you are as busy as I am, you don't have time to get sick. Deep down, your immune system craves attention—the healthy attention you can give it with healing food. Yes, food is medicine! In fact, the term *nutraceutical* means "food medicine." This category includes favorites such as broccoli, garlic, onions, and carrots—each with their own specific healing power (see Chapter 9).

What you eat—or don't eat—will determine how your body protects you from illness, no matter what state your present health is in. Eating a healthful diet with a variety of foods such as broccoli, yogurt, fish, garlic, grapes and grape juice, soybeans, spinach, tomatoes, nuts, and whole-grain bread boosts your immunity.

Anyone who watches what they eat will tell you there are certain things you are better off without, such as too much saturated fat and too much sodium. For example, a diet high in sodium can raise blood pressure levels. A diet low in complex carbohydrates, such as fruits and vegetables, can affect the gastrointestinal tract. And a diet high in saturated fat (found in meat and dairy products) and trans-fatty acids (found in margarine, snacks and fast-food products, crackers, pastries, and many processed foods) can lead to many types of cancer, obesity, and even heart disease.

According to findings from the Harvard School of Public Health reported in *The New England Journal of Medicine* (1998), women with diets high in saturated fat and trans-fatty acids were more likely to develop heart disease than women who consumed less of these fats. The researchers estimated that replacing 5 percent of the total daily calories from saturated fat with unsaturated fat could reduce a woman's risk of heart disease by an estimated 42 percent. Replacing 2 percent of the daily calories from trans-fatty acids with unhydrogenated, unsaturated fat may reduce a woman's risk of heart disease by an estimated 53 percent. In a study at the University of North Carolina at Chapel Hill of 700 postmenopausal women, those with the highest levels of trans-fats in their fat cells were 40 percent more likely to develop breast cancer than those with lower levels.

Balancing hormones

Food also can affect fluctuating hormones. It may surprise you that, in Japan, there is no word for "hot flashes." Recent reports have found that, because of a diet high in soy products, the phytoestrogen level in Japanese women's blood is 10 to 40 times higher than in their Western peers. (*Phytoestrogens* are plant hormones that mimic estrogen without the deleterious side effects.) In fact, breast and prostate cancer rates for the Japanese are four times lower than in the United States. As you will learn on page 188,

Moneysaver
Want to save money on medical bills this year? Then make sure you get five to nine servings of fruits and vegetables each day. These low-cost, nutrient-dense, complex carbohydrates are filled with healing antioxidants and phytochemicals (pages 173–80). They can protect you from cancer, heart disease, and a host of other debilitating illnesses.

isoflavone-rich soy products greatly alleviate meno-pausal symptoms, such as hot flashes, while acting as a natural hormonal supplement.

Losing excess weight—winning optimum health

The good news is that certain foods can improve your health and increase your life span. The bad news is that, according to a Louis Harris and Associates survey in 1997, Americans are fatter than ever before. Seventy-four percent of Americans 25 or older are overweight, up from 71 percent in 1996, 69 percent in 1994, 66 percent in 1992, and only 59 percent 10 years ago.

Don't close the book—there is hope! According to Harvard researchers, gaining weight can increase the chance of conditions such as hypertension, but losing weight will reduce that risk. These findings are from the Nurses' Health Study, an ongoing study of 82,473 United States female nurses started in 1976 and reported in the *Annals of Internal Medicine* (1998). Those who reduced their risk of hypertension consequently reduced their risk of heart disease—the number-one killer of women today in the U.S.

Getting off the diet roller coaster

You may think it's time to get back on a diet, but that isn't necessarily the answer. In the past five years, comprehensive scientific studies have shed light on how deprivation diets impact weight loss, and the findings have consistently held true: *Dieting without excercise doesn't work*. Studies show that approximately 95 percent of people who go on weight-loss diets will gain all or some of it back within one year. In fact, some studies have found that, after a period of five

Watch Out!
Weighing as little as 10 or 15 pounds over your desired weight can exacerbate a heart condition, can elevate blood pressure and cholesterol, and can even increase your risk of certain cancers.

"

"After going on every diet imaginable—from the low carbohydrate diet to the liquid diet to Weight Watchers to Jenny Craig—I believe that the first three letters of the word *diet* describe exactly how you feel when you deprive your body of food."
—Linda, 38, teacher

"

years, not one advertised diet program was successful in keeping the weight off. The best way to maintain or reach an ideal weight is to burn more calories than you take in with exercise and activity. For example, you can either jog two miles in 20 minutes or jog one mile in the morning and one mile at night, and you will still burn the same 200 calories.

How much should you weigh? Although height/weight charts can provide a fairly accurate range, your body mass index (BMI) seems to give a more accurate picture of health. Using the BMI chart (see Figure 2.1), locate your height along the left-hand column and slide your finger to the right until you come to the number nearest your weight. For example, if you are 5'3" and weigh 125 pounds, your BMI is 22, which is in a healthy range. If you are 5' 5" and weigh 155 pounds, your BMI is 26, which is considered overweight. Keep in mind that each of us is different. Your weight can depend on many variables including your age, bone structure, and weight-cycling history (meaning, have you been gaining and losing the same 10 to 20 pounds?).

If necessary, begin a healthful weight-reduction program using the Food Guide Pyramid shown in Figure 2.2. The foundation of your diet, like the pyramid, should be built on plant foods—fruit, vegetable, and grain products. This does not mean you should eliminate the milk and meat or meat-substitute groups. Instead, use low-fat versions of these foods to complement the rest of the plant-based diet.

Watch Out!
The diet drug combination of fenfluramine and phentermine (fen-phen) helped millions of people lose weight—but not without dangerous side effects. In 1997, after finding a link between the drugs and heart valve abnormalities, the Food and Drug Administration (FDA) pulled *Redux* and *Pondimin* (the fen in *fen-phen*) off the shelves.

Weight / Height	100	105	110	115	120	125	130	135	140	145	150	155	160	165	170	175	180	185	190	195	200	205	210	215	220
5'0"	20	21	21	22	23	24	25	26	27	28	29	30	31	32	33	34	35	36	37	38	39	40	41	42	43
5'1"	19	20	21	22	23	24	25	26	27	27	28	29	30	31	32	33	34	35	36	37	38	39	40	41	42
5'2"	18	19	20	21	22	23	24	25	26	27	27	28	29	30	31	32	33	34	35	36	37	38	38	39	40
5'3"	18	19	19	20	21	22	23	24	25	26	27	27	28	29	30	31	32	33	34	35	36	37	38	39	40
5'4"	17	18	19	20	21	21	22	23	24	25	26	27	27	28	29	30	31	32	33	33	34	35	36	37	38
5'5"	17	17	18	19	20	21	22	22	23	24	25	26	27	27	28	29	30	31	32	32	33	34	35	36	37
5'6"	16	17	18	18	19	20	21	22	23	23	24	25	26	26	27	28	29	30	31	31	32	33	34	35	36
5'7"	16	16	17	18	19	20	20	21	22	23	23	24	25	26	27	27	28	29	30	31	31	32	33	34	34
5'8"	15	16	17	17	18	19	20	21	21	22	23	24	24	25	26	27	27	28	29	30	30	31	32	33	33
5'9"	15	16	16	17	18	18	19	20	21	21	22	23	24	24	25	26	27	27	28	29	30	30	31	32	32
5'10"	14	15	16	17	17	18	19	19	20	21	22	22	23	24	24	25	26	27	27	28	29	29	30	31	32
5'11"	14	15	15	16	17	17	18	19	20	20	21	22	22	23	24	24	25	26	26	27	28	29	29	30	31
6'0"	14	14	15	16	16	17	18	18	19	20	20	21	22	22	23	24	24	25	26	26	27	28	28	29	30
6'1"	13	14	15	15	16	17	17	18	18	19	20	20	21	22	22	23	24	24	25	26	26	27	28	28	29
6'2"	13	14	14	15	16	16	17	17	18	19	19	20	21	21	22	23	23	24	24	25	26	26	27	28	28
6'3"	12	13	14	14	15	16	16	17	17	18	19	19	20	21	21	22	22	23	24	24	25	26	26	27	27
6'4"	12	13	13	14	15	15	16	16	17	18	18	19	19	20	21	21	22	23	23	24	24	25	26	26	27

Figure 2.1: Body Mass Index.

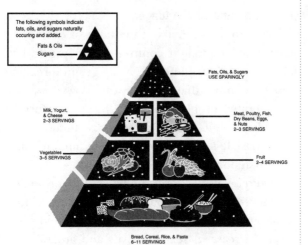

Figure 2.2:
Food Guide
Pyramid.

Unofficial tip #3: rev up with exercise

If statistics ring true, America is in trouble when it comes to aerobicizing. Government statistics show that 60 percent of all Americans get no regular exercise, a statistic that has remained steady for the last two decades. Additionally, about $5.7 billion is spent each year in the United States on medical costs and lost productivity of people who could have fought off heart disease with a little exercise. Compare this with the $30 billion spent on diet foods and diet programs each year by the American public.

It's not news that most of us slow down with age. According to the Centers for Disease Control and Prevention (CDC), 56 percent of men and 44 percent of women between ages 18 and 29 exercise regularly. These numbers drop to 44 percent and 40 percent, respectively, among people 30 to 44 years old. Aerobic exercise, however, is vital to stay at a normal weight; to improve erratic sleep symptoms; to restore fitness to stiff, inflexible bodies; and to prevent the muscle aches and pains associated with aging.

Moving around to live longer

There's no question about the value of exercise or movement for weight control, disease prevention, and health in general. New groundbreaking research shows that exercise can slow down the degenerative problems of aging. Studies performed on elderly adults reveal that senior endurance exercisers have less age-related decline in immune function than nonexercising senior adults.

Exercise also restores the body's neurochemical balance, which affects our emotional state. A study performed on one group of women reported a dramatic increase in sexual activity and arousal after beginning a regular exercise program. Not only were they more physically fit, their stress levels were greatly reduced, which helped to enhance their sex life. Could exercise be an aerobic aphrodisiac? This also could be the result of increased confidence in body image. People that exercise tend to feel more confident about their bodies.

Moving around more can help you reduce anxiety because exercise acts as a displacement defense mechanism. The more active you are, the more you can gain hopeful feelings about yourself. Isn't it difficult to worry about daily problems when you are working hard physically? All that is on your mind is getting through the routine . . . *not* the problems you face each day.

Amazing benefits in just 30 minutes a day

You don't have to run a marathon to reap the amazing benefits of exercise. According to experts from the American College of Sports Medicine (ACSM) and the Centers for Disease Control and Prevention, the "no pain, no gain" theory is out. Experts emphasize that we should strive to accumulate 30 minutes of moderately intense physical activity every day of the week or enough to burn about 200 calories (equal to a brisk 2-mile walk). Not only will this exercise burn fat, it also will lower your cholesterol level, build muscle and bone, and improve your mental health.

So what type of exercise do you enjoy? The chart on page 35 shows popular exercises and the average number of calories they burn per hour. Of course, this amount varies depending on your weight and how hard you work out. Each of these exercises can fit into one or more of the following three categories:

- **Range-of-motion or stretching exercises.** These exercises involve moving a joint as far as it will go (without pain) or through its full range-of-motion.

- **Endurance or conditioning exercises.** These exercises involve cardiovascular forms of exercise such as walking, running, biking, swimming, rowing, or aerobics.

- **Strengthening exercises.** These exercises help build the strong muscles, ligaments, and tendons needed to support your body.

In addition to picking out an exercise you like, look at these categories to help pinpoint what you want to accomplish. In addition to improving your overall health, do you want to improve your endurance? Do you wish you were a little stronger? Would you simply like to be able to touch your toes? As long as you keep your goals realistic, anything is attainable.

Making it fun

Using the suggestions in Table 2.3, find the exercises and activities you enjoy . . . then do them!

Bright Idea
If you don't change what you eat and burn an additional 200 calories a day, you could lose about 20 pounds in one year. Now that's good news!

Choose pleasurable activities that you will stick with—and don't forget, housework and gardening are excellent forms of exercise if you really put your body in motion. Depending on your personal fitness level, vary the exercises to keep from getting bored. Doing the same exercise repeatedly is like having peanut butter and jelly sandwiches every day for lunch—it just gets old.

Don't let the change of seasons stop you from staying fit. If you enjoy walking outside during the summer, consider joining an indoor aerobics class during the winter. If you are passionate about beach volleyball, check out your local YMCA for the indoor volleyball schedule during cold months. If you thrive on swimming at the lake, continue this water sport in an indoor pool when it's too chilly outside for your bathing suit.

If you don't like to exercise outdoors or with a group of people, look at some popular exercise videos and do them in the comfort and privacy of your own home. Instructional videos exist for all levels of fitness and all types of exercise. Get up 15 minutes earlier in the morning, pop in the tape, and get moving—no excuses!

Although 30 consecutive minutes of moderately-intense exercise is optimal, newer studies report that you can get the same benefit from 10-minute segments of exercise done three to four times a day. Adding at least this much exercise to your daily routine not only will help you feel healthier, it will work to keep your cardiovascular and immune systems functioning properly, to keep your muscles and joints strong, and to boost a sagging metabolism by helping to burn calories. The list in Table 2.4 gives you an idea of how many calories you can burn if you move around a bit more each day.

Timesaver
It's easier than you think to add exercise to your life. You could do 10 minutes of aerobic exercise with your video before work, walk the stairs for 10 minutes during your coffee break, take a jog around the block with your dog after work, and then end your day with a 10 minute ride on your stationary bike while watching the news.

TABLE 2.3

Activities and Exercises to Keep You Healthy

Badminton	Karate	Stair climbing
Baseball	Kick boxing	Stationary cycling
Basketball	Jumping rope	Strength training
Biking	Low-impact aerobics	Swimming
Bowling	Mall walking	Tae kwon do
Dancing	Mowing the yard	Tai chi
Gardening	Rollerblading	Tennis
Golf	Roller skating	Vacuuming
Handball	Rowing	Walking
High-impact aerobics	Running	Washing windows
Hiking	Soccer	Water exercises
House cleaning	Softball	Yoga

TABLE 2.4   BURNING IT OFF*

Activity	Male	Female
Carpentry	270	195
Cycling (10 mph)	486	351
Dancing (disco)	468	338
Golf (walking)	411	299
Hiking (hilly)	648	468
Jumping rope	684	494
Mopping	306	221
Raking	270	195
Rowing machine	558	403
Skiing (cross country)	666	481
Snow shoveling (light)	702	502
Swimming (slow crawl)	630	455
Tennis (singles)	522	377
Trimming hedges	378	273
Walking (2–2.5 mph)	288	208
Weeding	360	260
Weight training	342	247
Window cleaning	288	208

*Calories per hour burned by various activities. Figures shown are for a 180-pound male and a 130-pound female.

Timesaver
No time to go to the gym? Consider building your own. Check the classified advertisements for used exercise equipment such as electronic treadmills or stationary bicycles, but be sure to use them for more than hanging clothes at the end of the day.

Watch Out!
If you are over
35 years old or
have a chronic
illness, get a
medical doctor's
consent before
engaging in any
exercise program.

Keeping track of your pulse

To make sure you are not overdoing it with exercise, keep track of your pulse. You can find a pulse by placing your index and middle fingers (never your thumb) on the artery on the side of your windpipe (your carotid pulse) or on the thumb side of the wrist.

Stop periodically during your workout and count your pulse rate for 15 seconds. Multiply this number by four to get your total pulse for one minute. Speed up or slow down your exercise pace to keep your heart within the target heart-rate range (see Table 2.5). Continue to check your pulse periodically to make sure you are not overdoing it (or going at a snail's pace).

Your target heart-rate zone will vary depending on your age and your fitness level. You can use Table 2.5 to compute your heart-rate zone. Subtract your age from 220 and multiply this number by 60 percent. This gives you the low end of your range. Now subtract your age from 220 and multiply this number by 80 percent to figure the high end of your range. It is important to keep your heart rate in this zone while exercising. Table 2.6 gives you an estimate of heart-rate zones according to age.

TABLE 2.5

Sample Target Heart-Rate Zone for Age 40

Low zone: $220 - 40 = 180 \times 60\% = 108$

High zone: $220 - 40 = 180 \times 80\% = 144$

Target heart-rate range: $108 - 144$

Use the following chart to find the low and high ends of target heart-rate ranges according to age.

TABLE 2.6	STAY ON TARGET	
Age	60%	80%
20	120	160
30	114	152
40	108	144
50	102	136
60	96	128
70	90	120
80	84	112
90	78	104

Unofficial tip #4: practice prevention

No matter how you look at it, it's up to you to choose the path to optimum health. What is the alternative? The annual worldwide statistics are frightening:

- More than 6 million people die from heart disease.
- Strokes take the life of more than 4 million people.
- Pneumonia and lower-respiratory-tract infections kill almost 5 million people.
- Lung, stomach, and breast cancer take the lives of more than 3 million people.

Detecting problems early leads to successful treatment

Early detection of medical problems enables you to receive treatment when it is easier and most effective. For example, a simple, painless test detects blood in the stool and allows early treatment of intestinal cancer long before it causes any other signs. A mammogram (a breast X-ray) may allow detection and treatment of breast cancer before any other signs are present. A blood test can tell whether your blood glucose is high, which could signal diabetes. A pneumonia or flu vaccine can prevent illness.

Although it is not practical to test for all possible medical problems, preventive efforts can be focused on the specific medical problems most likely to occur at your age or with your family history and lifestyle. This can allow you to maintain your current health or even improve it if you make the other important lifestyle changes.

Assessing the annual exam

An annual physical examination with a conventional medical doctor is recommended by most health care experts. During this exam, your doctor will take a complete medical history, which should include a discussion of any current or past medical problems. Laboratory tests may be conducted and can include:

- Complete blood count (CBC)
- Blood chemistries including cholesterol and glucose
- Urine testing
- Rectal exam and prostate
- Pelvic exam and PAP test (for women)
- Colon cancer screening
- Chest X-ray (if a smoker)
- Electrocardiogram
- Mammogram (for women)
- Prostate-specific antigen test (PSA, for men)
- Bone density test

Depending on your sex, age, and personal health history, your doctor will review risk factors for coronary heart disease, cancer, diabetes, and osteoporosis and will discuss removal or control of these risk factors. Hearing, eye, or dental examinations, a skin test for tuberculosis, and other tests also can be planned.

During your annual "well visit" to the doctor, ask about necessary immunizations. Adults need a tetanus booster every 10 years. Women of childbearing age who have no history of a rubella (German measles) vaccination may want to be tested for antibodies and receive this immunization. Other immunizations may include the hepatitis B series and a flu or pneumonia shot, if needed.

Unofficial tip #5: seek social support

According to comprehensive studies, depression, loneliness, and sadness are as great a risk factor for disease as smoking cigarettes or eating a high-fat diet. In fact, studies show that heart patients with a "type D"—for distressed—personality may have a greater risk of a second heart attack than people with a more cheerful disposition. Negative or anxious patients who had difficulty expressing their feelings were three times more likely to suffer another heart attack.

Laughing your way to optimum health

Optimism has a profound influence on immunity and, subsequently, on longevity. Take laughter, for example. The finding is disheartening, yet it may come as no surprise—the average adult only laughs about 17 times a day, while a 6-year-old laughs as many as 300 times. The results of a variety of studies now provide mounting evidence that laughter, general happiness, and a positive attitude may be key elements in our quest to extend longevity. These factors speed production of new immune cells and reduce the stress hormone cortisol.

Bright Idea
To make sure your doctor knows all your medications, vitamins, and supplements, pack them in a paper bag and take them to your next doctor's visit. This will help her make sure you will not have a drug-drug interaction. Also ask her to check the dates to make sure they are not expired.

Scientists have found that laughing can produce a state of positive stress, or what is called *eustress*. While studying laughter's effect on the immune system, researchers at Loma Linda University in California showed a video of a comedian. Blood samples drawn during and after the video showed significant increases in various measures of immune function, particularly T-cells and NK (natural killer) cells. Interestingly, levels of the stress hormone cortisol, which suppresses the immune system, also were lower. The researchers concluded that laughter creates its own physiological state with positive changes in the immune system that are the opposite of negative stress, or distress.

Increasing your social network

Another vital key in staying well and increasing life span is social support. In fact, it is well documented that people who are happily married and/or have a large network of friends not only have a greater life expectancy compared with those people who do not, they also have fewer incidences of almost every type of disease. Close personal relationships give us a buffer in times of great stress and allow us to safely get our burdens off our chests. Dr. David Spiegel, a psychiatrist at Stanford University, documented what many scientists had speculated—that social support can be a significant factor in prolonging the lives of women with breast cancer. Spiegel reported through his studies that this simple intervention prolonged life expectancy by an average of 18 months.

Unfortunately, in our busy society, social support is limited for many people. If the thought of making time for friends adds to your stress level, consider getting a pet. Countless papers are published in the area of animal-human bonding that reveal the health benefits of social support. Even having a plant can be beneficial to your health. This was revealed in a study conducted at Yale University by Dr. Judy Rhodin. Rhodin found that, when people had a plant present in their rooms, they had speedier recoveries from illness compared with people who did not.

The variety of social contacts a person has also helps protect the immune system. According to a study from Carnegie Mellon University in Pittsburgh, when 276 health volunteers ages 18 to 55 were exposed to cold viruses, those with fewer links to family, friends, and community support were more likely to become ill. This study has been reinforced by other similar research such as studies done at Dartmouth-Hitchcock Medical Center in New Hampshire. In these studies, scientists reported that heart patients were 14 times as likely to survive surgery if they were socially active and if they found comfort in their religious faith. A groundbreaking study reported in the *Journal of the American Medical Association* (1997) revealed that people involved in a variety of activities—such as work, church, family, sports, or even barbershop quartets—get fewer colds than those who are exposed to the same number of people but only have a few things to occupy them. Researchers speculate that being happy and involved keeps our immune systems strong.

Your free Rx to optimum health

What does all this mean to you? If you are a relatively healthy person, moderation and balance appear to be the wisest prescription on the path to optimum health. Work on incorporating each of the five unofficial tips in your lifestyle. This means:

Watch Out!
The increasing resistance of pneumococcal bacteria to penicillin and other antibiotics makes flu and pneumonia vaccines crucial. This preventive treatment is particularly important for people over age 65 or younger adults and children with respiratory problems or chronic illness.

- Start a campaign to stop smoking; if necessary, seek support from your doctor, family members, and friends.

- Follow a diet low in saturated fat and rich in grains, fruits, and vegetables.

- Move around more—walk vigorously throughout your day, take the stairs instead of the elevator when you can, and enjoy recreational activities such as skiing, tennis, biking, and hiking with friends and family members.

- Make plans to get important preventive check-ups and immunizations; volunteer to help someone.

- Most importantly, smile—you'll attract more friends, which can make all the difference in the world!

Emergency first aid kit

Keep the following treatments on hand in case you have a home accident or illness. Be sure to keep them out of the reach of young children.

- 3×3–inch sterile gauze dressings
- Box of plastic strips in an assortment of sizes
- Roll of $1/2$-inch adhesive tape
- Antibiotic cream, ointment, or other antiseptic
- Box of baking soda or Adolph's unseasoned meat tenderizer for bee and other insect stings
- Hydrocortisone cream for rashes
- Syrup of ipecac to induce vomiting in case of poisoning (Call Poison Control before using)
- Calamine lotion for rashes
- Alcohol or peroxide to clean wounds
- Antibiotic cream
- Petroleum jelly

- Over-the-counter vaginal cream for mild yeast infections
- Thermometer
- Ice bag
- Nonaspirin pain reliever for children
- Benadryl or another antihistamine for swelling in case of allergic reactions
- Tweezers for taking out splinters or pieces of glass
- Blunt scissors

Just the facts

- Making crucial lifestyle changes may increase our life span.
- Smoking is one disease risk factor you can control.
- Healing foods filled with nutrients are like natural medicine to keep you well and to prevent disease.
- Exercise and activity can help ward off anxiety and depression and can act as an aerobic aphrodisiac.
- Your conventional medical doctor can run certain preventive tests that are crucial for optimum health.
- As you increase social support with cultural outings, gatherings with friends, and volunteering, you are more apt to increase your longevity.

A Guide to Alternative Treatments

GET THE SCOOP ON...
Why Ayurvedic practitioners believe that stress or imbalance in a person's consciousness causes disease ▪
The National Institutes of Health's latest findings regarding acupuncture and pain ▪ How tai chi can help reduce stress in the general population and increase balance in the elderly

PART II

Ancient Systems of Healing

I f you are just now becoming aware of alternative medicine, it's important to know that this type of treatment is not new. In fact, alternative treatments based on herbs, massage, spiritual healing, and diet have been used for thousands of years. Ayurvedic treatments and traditional Chinese medicine are considered to be the grandfathers of alternative treatments, and both date back as far as 4,000 to 5,000 years in history. Today, 80 percent of the world's population still depends on holistic or alternative medicine as opposed to Western or conventional medicine, which is used in the United States and Europe.

Ayurvedic medicine

Ayurveda is a holistic healing science that focuses on preventive health care using natural therapies. The theory behind Ayurvedic is that diseases begin with an imbalance or stress in a person's consciousness. This imbalance is treated with lifestyle interventions that take into account your inherited tendencies, environment, diet, work, and family. Ayurveda is the oldest system of medicine in the world, tracing its roots to the Vedic period in ancient India. Its origin is traceable to four Sanskrit books called the Vedas—the oldest and most important scriptures of India. These books attributed most disease and bad luck to demons, devils, and the influence of stars and planets. In 16th-century Europe, Paracelsus, who is known as the father of modern Western medicine, practiced and publicized a system of medicine that borrowed heavily from Ayurveda.

How it works

According to Ayurvedic belief, health is the state of balance, and disease is the state of imbalance. Ayurveda's premise is that the body's functions are composed of combinations of five elements: air, fire, ether, water, and earth. There are three other physiological forces called *doshas* (vata, pitta, and kapha), in which the five elements are manifest. All of us are composed of a combination of *doshas* that give us a particular metabolic type, yet each of us has one dosha that dominates. *Vata* people are thin and energetic, *pittas* are hot tempered, and *kaphas* are slow and solid. To determine the imbalance in your body, the Ayurvedic practitioner will feel your wrist pulse. Using such therapies as meditation, detoxification, breathing, herbal and mineral preparations, exercise, and dietary advice based on your particular mind-body type, the Ayurvedic practitioner will help you to achieve balance or wellness.

There is a growing body of evidence that Ayurvedic therapies might be potentially beneficial for disease prevention and treatment. Published scientific studies have documented reductions in

Watch Out!
You may be hard pressed to find qualified practitioners in the United States because there are no schools here and no licensing is required. In addition, Ayurvedic treatment is not covered by insurance unless the services are provided by a licensed medical doctor.

cardiovascular disease risk factors, lowered blood pressure and cholesterol, and reduced stress in people who practice Ayurvedic methods. Transcendental meditation (TM), for example, is an Ayurvedic technique in which you sit comfortably with your eyes closed and mentally repeat a Sanskrit word or sound (a mantra) for 15 to 20 minutes, twice a day. It allegedly helps people think more clearly, improve their memory, recover from stress, reverse the aging process, and appreciate life more fully. In a study reported in the journal *Hypertension* (1996), TM was found to surpass other forms of relaxation therapies at lowering blood pressure. In this study, 111 African-American men and women aged 55 to 85 were assigned to practice TM daily. The blood pressure reductions they reported were similar to those commonly achieved with antihypertensive medicines. In long-term drug studies, such reductions have been associated with about 35 percent fewer strokes and heart attacks.

What it does

Clinical studies have found some Ayurvedic herbal treatments and therapies to be useful for promoting good health, preventing and treating some cancers and infectious diseases, and stopping degenerative diseases associated with aging. Specific conditions that may respond to Ayurvedic medicine include allergies, anxiety, depression, digestive disorders, headaches, high blood pressure, insomnia, respiratory problems, and stress. You may have heard some hype, however, about using the wrist pulse to detect diabetes, cancer, musculoskeletal disease, asthma, and imbalances at early stages when there may be no other clinical signs or when mild forms of intervention may suffice. The truth is there are

Watch Out!
Although Ayurveda can provide healing benefits when combined with conventional treatments, avoid taking any Ayurvedic herbs along with prescription drugs. You may have a negative interaction, or the herbs may reduce the potency of medications. Discuss Ayurvedic therapies with your medical doctor.

no scientifically substantiated studies suggesting that conventional medical diagnostic measures should be replaced with the Ayurvedic practice of feeling the wrist pulse. As I said before, you shouldn't entirely abandon conventional medicine; instead, use conventional medicine and alternative forms together to get the best possible health results.

Bright Idea
Need a quick immune booster? Eating a daily spoonful of *amla,* a gooseberry jam found in Indian import stores that may help increase immune function and promote well-being.

The basics

1. *How often should it be done?* Because Ayurveda focuses on lifestyle, the many practices are incorporated into your daily routine. If you decide to see an Ayurvedic practitioner for treatment or consultation, your particular condition may respond within three to five visits.

2. *How much does it cost?* The cost of Ayurvedic medicine can vary depending on the treatments you are using. An initial consultation may cost from $50 to $225. Some Ayurvedic treatments cost several hundred dollars, while others can run into the thousands.

3. *How long until it works?* How quickly the treatments take effect greatly depends on the nature of your imbalance. If you want to further investigate Ayurveda, the following clinics may be good sources of information:

   - Maharashi Ayurveda Clinics, multiple locations: 800-843-8332

   - Ayurveda Holistic Center, New York City, NY: 212-924-4933

   - The Ayurvedic Institute, Albuquerque, NM: 505-291-9698

   - Ayurveda Health Center, Albuquerque, NM: 505-296-6522

- The Chopra Center for Well-Being, La Jolla, CA: 619-551-7788

- The American Institute of Vedic Studies, Albuquerque, NM: 505-983-9385

- The Himalayan Institute, Honesdale, PA: 717-253-5551

Yoga

Ayurvedic practitioners use yoga as one form of treatment. Yoga is a classical Indian practice built on the foundation of ethics (*yama*) and personal discipline (*niyama*). It is used to relieve stress, to achieve mind/body connection, and to heal the body. The postures or movements are structured to stretch the mind and body beyond their normal limits and then make them act in unison again. Using deep breathing, concentration techniques, and body poses, you learn to calm your mind and to increase flexibility and strength. The term *yoga* comes from a Sanskrit word meaning *union* and goes back as far as 5,000 years. While yoga is an Eastern philosophy, Westerners are more accustomed to *hatha yoga*, which focuses on fitness. With the latter, yoga postures can relieve mild aches and pains, menstrual cramps, and lower-back pain. It also can increase flexibility and coordination, can reduce stress, and can promote deep relaxation. Breath exercises done with different yoga positions can increase blood circulation.

How it works

Cardiologist and author Dean Ornish, M.D., recommends yoga to people with coronary heart disease as a way to relax. Yoga also may be helpful with some respiratory problems. It not only provides the benefit of relaxing your body, the various positions can

Unofficially...
Author and lecturer Deepak Chopra, M.D., is associated with The Center for Mind/Body Medicine in La Jolla, California. This Ayurveda-based medical center provides education and training programs for health care professionals and lay people. It also offers both residential and outpatient programs. For information, write to P.O. Box 1048, La Jolla, CA 92038 or call 619-794-2425.

help to improve your breathing and to ease the expectoration of mucus.

The basics

1. *How often should it be done?* To experience optimum results, yoga should be practiced daily in the form of meditation and postures.

2. *How much does it cost?* Because the equipment for yoga is your own body, learning it can cost as little as $10 to purchase a how-to book or an instructional video. Another option is to join a yoga class at your local health club or YMCA for a monthly rate (which is, of course, variable depending on facility and location).

3. *How long until it works?* Some people feel more relaxed after the first session. Give it at least three weeks to see if it makes a difference in how you feel.

If you are looking for a nonimpact fitness program that can increase coordination and flexibility, can help you feel relaxed, and can reduce the chances of injury, yoga fits the bill.

Chinese medicine

Chinese medicine is a complete health system consisting of acupuncture, exercise, herbal medicine, massage, nutrition, and healthy living. Unlike Western medicine, which relies on aggressive and invasive surgery or modern drugs, Chinese medicine tries to diagnose disturbances of qi, or vital energy, in health and disease. Practitioners correct this disharmony in the body using acupuncture, herbal medicine, massage, or qigong. Two other important therapies include:

1. **Acupressure.** A well-known ancient form of physical therapy using the same points as

acupuncture. It works by stimulating your body's main trigger points to release energy, or to unblock qi. Today, acupressure is practiced mainly in Asian countries such as India, China, Japan, and Korea. It is used to relieve everyday aches, pains, and stress as well as specific conditions such as sinus pressure, leg cramps, headaches, temporomandibular joint disorder (TMJ), and carpal tunnel syndrome.

2. **Shiatsu.** A type of therapy that draws on the Chinese notion of qi, or energy, which flows along meridians throughout the body. The sessions focus on relieving pain and helping the body rid itself of any toxins before they develop into illness. Firm, rhythmic pressure is applied for 3 to 10 seconds on specific points. This pressure is given to wake up the meridians, or healing channels, of the body. The pressure may help by stimulating the body's endorphins to produce a tranquilizing effect or by loosening up muscles and improving blood circulation. Shiatsu is said to help ease or eliminate back pain, digestive problems, headaches, insomnia, leg and menstrual cramps, respiratory problems, and shoulder stiffness.

How it works

Health is said to exist when qi (vital energy) and blood flow smoothly throughout all parts of the body. External factors such as climate, diet, emotions, and lifestyle factors can disrupt qi. The Chinese doctor interprets any symptoms as an imbalance within the entire system of the body and uses the holistic therapies to remove the blockage.

What it does

According to studies done in China and Japan, traditional Chinese medicine may have therapeutic value in the following areas:

- Chronic hepatitis
- Rheumatoid arthritis
- Headaches
- Menstrual cramps
- Lower-back and neck pain
- Substance abuse
- Hypertension
- Atopic eczema
- Immunologic disorders
- Acquired immunodeficiency syndrome (AIDS)
- Some cancers

Bright Idea
Looking for a reputable Chinese medicine practitioner? Try New Mexico. In the United States, the legal sanctioning of Chinese medical practice is most prevalent in that state.

There has been some hype that Chinese medicine is more effective than conventional medicine because it deals with the whole person, focusing on removing energy blocks that lead to illness.

The fact is, Chinese medicine uses more than 5,000 different plant and animal agents for healing, but they are not regulated for safety, potency, or effectiveness. There also is the risk, for example, that an acupuncturist whose approach to diagnosis is not based on scientific concepts will fail to diagnose a more serious condition such as cancer. Although some studies are finding that acupuncture and some herbs may have medicinal value, most Chinese therapies still need to be studied in the United States using the highest research criteria.

The basics

1. *How often should it be done?* Much of Chinese medicine can be incorporated into your daily

life. Lifestyle therapies such as acupressure or shiatsu treatments may be done once or twice a week for optimum effect.

2. *How much does it cost?* Cost depends on the specific type of treatment you choose. An initial visit with a practitioner may cost $75 to $150, with follow-up visits costing around $50 to $100. A session of Chinese acupressure may cost from $25 to $75, while Chinese herbal remedies range from $5 to $15 per bottle or about $20 to $50 a month (slightly more if you prefer to use the teas). Insurance coverage varies from state to state.

3. *How long until it works?* How quickly you'll start seeing results depends on the type of therapy and the specific problem you are trying to treat or cure.

Of the various types of traditional Chinese medicine therapies, stick with acupuncture if you want treatment proven to work. The NIH confirms that acupuncture works with ailments such as nausea during pregnancy, nausea from chemotherapy, and dental problems. Many American schools of acupuncture now are evolving into colleges that teach Asian medicine.

Acupuncture

With this alternative treatment, a specialist places very thin, stainless-steel sterilized needles into your skin at any of the 800 designated points on the body. Practitioners also may turn the needles or use heat, pressure, friction, suction, or electric or magnetic impulses to stimulate these points.

Acupuncture is the oldest known method for healing and has been practiced in China for more

Bright Idea
The Chinese immune-system tonifier *astragalus* (huang qi) may help to boost immune function and to prevent colds and flu. Make a tea by steeping dried astralgus sticks in water for 10 minutes. Drink one cup daily.

than 4,000 years. Although it came to the United States in the late 1800s, acupuncture has become increasingly popular in the past two decades. At this time, there are about 20,000 certified and licensed practitioners, more than 3,000 of which also are conventional medical doctors.

How it works

According to advocates, natural energy, or *qi* (pronounced *chee*), travels along 14 pathways (or meridians) in the body to keep your body nourished. These meridians are connected to specific organs and bodily functions. When qi is blocked or thrown off balance, illness or symptoms result. The acupuncturist stimulates the points along these meridian lines, using the needles to remove the energy block and to restore balance and flow of energy along the pathway. When one portion of the body is stimulated, an effect is obtained in the same or another portion of the body. It also is believed that acupuncture causes the body to release endorphins—your body's natural pain relievers—which explains the pain relief felt when the pin pricks occur. Acupuncture also may trigger the release of certain hormones such as *serotonin,* a chemical in the brain that makes you feel calm and serene, and the anti-inflammatory chemical known as *cortisol.*

With acupuncture, the practitioner places needles in various points and leaves them in place for 15 to 30 minutes, sometimes manually twisting them to get better results. Other elements of acupuncture include:

- **Electro-acupuncture,** in which the practitioner, once the needles are in place, hooks up small wires connected to very slight electrical currents. Heat (*moxibustion*), suction (*cupping*), and

Watch Out!
Be sure to go to a licensed acupuncture practitioner and insist on disposable needles.

massage (*acupressure*) also are used during this process.

- **Moxibustion,** which involves burning herbs, or *moxa*, at the specific acupuncture points to stimulate qi.

- **Cupping,** which involves applying suction to the points.

- **Acupressure,** which involves using finger pressure or massage on the points.

Practitioners also can perform a procedure without needles that is similar to acupuncture by using very sophisticated pieces of electronic equipment to detect the local acupuncture point and then treat it with electrical microcurrents.

What it does

Acupuncture is approved by the National Institutes of Health (NIH) for the following uses:

- Nausea during pregnancy
- Nausea and vomiting associated with surgery or chemotherapy
- Postoperative dental pain

The World Health Organization (WHO) of the United Nations has compiled the following list of ailments that may respond well to acupuncture:

- Arthritis
- Asthma
- Bladder dysfunction
- Bronchitis
- Cervicobrachial syndrome
- Colitis
- Constipation

Timesaver
Searching the Yellow Pages for a qualified acupuncturist? Write or call the American Academy of Medical Acupuncture (AAMA). This organization, formed in 1987, restricts membership to medical doctors (M.D.s) and doctors of osteopathy (D.O.s). Members have more than 220 hours of formal training and meet the board's stringent requirements. Write to 5820 Wilshire Blvd., Suite 500, Los Angeles, CA 90036 or call 213-937-5514.

- Diarrhea
- Duodenal and peptic ulcers
- Facial or Bell's palsy
- Frozen shoulder
- Gastric hyperacidity
- Gastritis
- Headaches and migraines
- Hiccups
- Hypertension
- Intercostal neuralgia
- Lower-back pain
- Nausea
- Meniere's disease
- Paralysis following a stroke
- Paralytic ileum
- Peripheral neuropathy
- Premenstrual syndrome (PMS) and irregular menstruation
- Rhinitis
- Sciatica
- Sinusitis
- Spasm of esophagus
- Tennis elbow
- Torticollis
- Trigeminal neuralgia

Although acupuncture has been touted as a treatment and possible cure for a myriad of ailments from pain to heart disease to cancer, the NIH only has approved it for the three previously mentioned specific medical problems.

There is evidence, however, that for certain types of pain or chronic problems, acupuncture might be useful in combination with conventional therapies. The existence of meridians, acupuncture points, or qi has never been scientifically validated. According to some new reports, acupuncture may reduce the severity of asthma attacks and the amount of medication asthma patients must take, but this is not yet proven. Some specialists are finding that receiving acupuncture along the external parts of the ear may help crack, alcohol, and cigarette addicts beat their drug and alcohol problems. Again, it's unproven; if it doesn't hurt, however, it's definitely worth a try.

The basics

1. *How often should it be done?* The average treatment takes between 20 minutes and one hour and is given either daily or one to three times a week. Clinical data shows that receiving three treatments per week may result in quicker healing. You may have to go through a series of at least 8 to 10 treatments before deciding whether this is effective for you.

2. *How much does it cost?* Initial sessions can range from $40 to $100 with a nonphysician. Expect to pay more with a physician or a medical doctor.

3. *How long until it works?* Improvement may be felt after the first visit, or it may take several weeks of treatment.

Acupuncture may work for you, or it may not work at all. It has very few contraindications, and the side effects are few, if any.

Qigong

Tagged as the mother of Chinese self-healing, *qigong* (pronounced *chee-gong*) is said to be one of

Watch Out!
Certain disorders such as easy bleeding or local infection may stop you from receiving acupuncture treatments. Make sure you discuss any medical conditions you have with a prospective acupuncturist ahead of time.

Moneysaver
Let your insurer pay the bill. In 1996, acupuncture needles were recognized as medical devices, which means many insurers are more likely to cover them. This may vary depending on state regulations, licensing, and medical supervision, so check it out ahead of time. The NIH consensus panel on acupuncture recommended that it be covered by Medicare.

the most powerful healing traditions ever developed in human history. It is a posture-related discipline that can easily be done anytime.

How it works

The Chinese believe that the primary mechanism triggered by the practice of qigong is a spontaneous balancing and enhancing of the natural healing resources in the human system. Actually, by adopting specific physical postures that dissolve tension, the practice of qigong triggers a wide array of physiological mechanisms that have profound healing benefits.

- It increases the delivery of oxygen to the tissues.

- It enhances the elimination of waste products and the transportation of immune cells through the lymph system.

- It shifts the chemistry of the brain and the nervous system. There are at least 1,000 varieties of qigong, all of which focus on getting qi, or energy, moving smoothly through the body. When qi is obstructed, you will have fatigue and illness.

If you break down the word qigong, it comes from *qi*, meaning energy or vitality, and *gong*, meaning to practice or cultivate. Its history dates back as far as 500 B.C. Both the health and spiritual applications of qigong are rapidly gaining popularity in both China and the Western world as people look for mind/body disciplines to gain peace of mind.

What it does

Qigong increases energy, decreases fatigue, and alleviates pain. Some proponents claim it heals back pain, carpal tunnel syndrome, circulatory problems,

Bright Idea
Start to experience qigong right now. Put this book aside, sit in an upright posture, take a deep breath using your lower abdomen, and relax your mind. Qigong will correct high-chested breathing if you focus on moving your lower abdomen instead of your upper chest and shoulders.

depression, high blood pressure, insomnia, meno-pause, neuralgia, chronic pain, and TMJ syndrome.

People who use qigong faithfully need less med-ication and acupuncture, and they heal faster.

The basics

1. *How often should it be done?* Experts conclude that qi must be cultivated daily, so the rudimentary exercises should be done each morning to build qi.

2. *How much does it cost?* Initially, you may have to pay a practitioner to teach you qigong. Once you understand the positions, however, you can do this at any time at no cost.

3. *How long until it works?* Some people feel results instantaneously; for others, it may take days or weeks before a difference is noticed in mood, energy, and strength. It can't hurt you, and it may help! A few years ago, qigong treatment was recognized as a standard medical technique in Chinese hospitals. In addition, qigong and human—body-science programs have been inserted into the curriculum of major universi-ties in China. Find a practitioner or class, and take advantage of this mind/body technique.

Tai chi

Tai chi (or tai chi chuan, as it is known in China) is an ancient Chinese defensive martial art similar to shadow boxing. For centuries in China, tai chi was a secret heritage among the people and was taught from one generation to the next. It has become increasingly popular in the 20th century and is prac-ticed worldwide. With tai chi, you follow a series of slow, graceful movements that mimic the movements you do in daily life (as shown in Figure 3.1).

Figure 3.1: Tai chi requires you to move forward, backward, and from side to side in a carefully coordinated manner—flowing together in continuous harmony as though your body was doing one continuous movement.

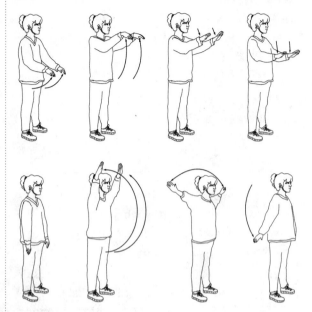

How it works

Tai chi is based on the theory that continuous practice will help to train the body to respond quickly in a crisis. Since the movements emphasize complete relaxation and passive concentration, they can be compared with "meditation in motion," which is said to be healing to the nervous system. The gentle, graceful movements, along with deep breathing patterns, are said to lower blood pressure and heart rate.

What it does

Tai chi is said to speed healing, to improve circulation, to boost immune function, and to decrease stress. Dramatic, flowing movements are used instead of forceful actions. The exercise emphasizes deep abdominal breathing that could help to maintain better lung function. As a low-impact exercise, it is perfect for older people or for people who have severe breathing difficulties. It improves the heart rate and overall cardiovascular function.

According to clinical research, tai chi may provide the added benefit of warding off age-related breathing problems, especially in elderly people. In a study reported in the *Journal of the American Geriatrics Society* (1995), tai chi was found to help improve lung function in older people. Other studies have shown that practicing tai chi may help senior citizens improve their balance and reduce the number of times they fall. In one study, elderly participants who practiced regularly found that tai chi helped them achieve the ability to balance as well as someone 3 to 10 years younger. This study of 200 people 70 and older also appeared in the *Journal of the American Geriatrics Society* (1996). Those who took part in a 15-week tai chi program reduced their rate of falls by 47.5 percent.

The basics

1. *How often should it be done?* Many proponents of tai chi find that once a day, usually during the early morning, is adequate to receive its relaxing and toning benefits.

2. *How much does it cost?* You can hire a private tai chi instructor to learn this discipline at a cost of $25 to $50 an hour, or you can enjoy the company of doing tai chi with others at a local health spa or YMCA. The cost depends on the facility and its location. You also can purchase a book or video about tai chi, although it can be difficult to learn on your own without an instructor.

3. *How long until it works?* You may notice a difference in your stress level within days of performing tai

Timesaver
You can call the
Taoist Tai Chi
Society of
the U.S.A. at
904-224-5438 to
find classes in
your area.

chi. It can take weeks or months to feel more flexible, to see increased muscle tone, or to experience a respiratory benefit. Whatever your age or level of fitness, tai chi provides an excellent program of exercise and stress reduction.

Just the facts

- Ayurveda is the oldest system of medicine in the world. It includes a myriad of therapies such as meditation, detoxification or purification, herbal and mineral preparations, exercise, and dietary advice based on your particular body type, or dosha.

- Acupressure and shiatsu are similar to acupuncture except they rely on the hands for massage and touch instead of needles.

- Yoga is an effective mind/body treatment to reduce stress, to increase flexibility, and to tone muscles.

- In China, qigong is used to treat depression, chronic pain, insomnia, and a host of other stress-related illnesses.

GET THE SCOOP ON...
How chiropractors manipulate the spinal bones and muscles
to relieve pain and to bring the body back to health ▪ Why
naturopathic practitioners believe that illness or symptoms
are the body's way of trying to heal itself ▪ The many ways
in which hydrotherapy has been used to strengthen the
immune system ▪ The principle behind Osteopathic
Manipulation Treatment (OMT) and disease

Healing Systems from the 19th Century

Although many alternative systems and methods of healing are described in this book, chiropractic, naturopathy, and osteopathy all originated around the same time in the late 19th century. In some ways, these healing disciplines are similar in approach because each focuses on preventive care and healing the "whole" person. Though the means are varied, with each of these methods, the practitioner or doctor pays considerable attention to healthful lifestyle changes and to finding the underlying cause of disease.

Yet in the midst of trying to prevent disease, there are some key differences between these alternative systems of health care. For example, unlike chiropractic doctors or naturopath practitioners, osteopathic physicians are as well-trained as conventional medical doctors and are licensed in the United States. A Doctor of Osteopathy (D.O.) must complete four years of medical school at an accredited college of osteopathic medicine and must complete an internship. A D.O. can prescribe medicine and can perform surgery. Doctors of chiropractic also take premedical courses in college; they then undergo another four years of training at a chiropractic school. They also are licensed in all 50 states.

While traditional osteopaths focus more on the musculoskeletal system—manipulating muscles and joints to treat disease—and can prescribe medications, chiropractic doctors treat the spinal bones with adjustments or force. Naturopaths believe in natural herbs, diet, and spiritual healing methods to keep the person "in balance" and well.

Chiropractic medicine

This drug-free therapy is based on the theory that the body is a self-healing organism. Hippocrates, the father of medicine, used techniques involving spinal adjustment over 2,000 years ago. Modern chiropractic began as an organized profession in 1895, however, when its founder, D.D. Palmer, reported his first chiropractic success story. Reportedly, Palmer's father, a fish peddler, invented chiropractic medicine when he cured a man's deafness with a blow to his back. In 1963, the National Board of Chiropractic Examiners began requiring that chiropractic graduates pass a nationally uniform exam before they began practicing. Today, chiropractors receive impressive educational training and are licensed in all 50 states.

Instead of treating symptoms, such as lower-back pain, chiropractors focus on treating the spinal bones that are thought to lose their normal position and motion from stress, trauma, or other causes (see Figure 4.1). The doctor will administer an adjustment or a specific force in a precise direction to a joint that is restricted or not moving properly.

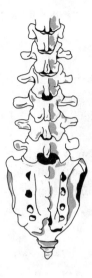

Figure 4.1:
Using manipula-
tion of the spine
and muscles, a
chiropractic doc-
tor will try to
find blockages in
the body and
eliminate them
to let it move
back to health.

How it works

According to doctors of chiropractic medicine, your
nervous system controls all functions in your body.
Messages must travel from your brain down your
spinal cord, out to the nerves at particular parts of
the body, back to the spinal cord, and then back up
the spinal cord to the brain. The theory is that
abnormal positions of the spinal bones may interfere with these messages and often are the underlying cause of many health problems.

Doctors of chiropractic correct the abnormal
positions of the spinal bones with spinal manipulation. Either the doctor's hands or a specially
designed instrument applies a brief and accurate
thrust to a joint. This form of manipulation or
adjustment is said to help return the bones to a more
normal position or motion, helping to relieve pain
and reduce ill health. The chiropractic doctor may
also recommend a program of rehabilitation for
your spine to stabilize and reduce joint involvement,

Timesaver
Even though
recent scientific
studies have
found that most
cases of lower-
back pain will
get better on
their own, the
Agency for
Health Care
Policy Research
agrees that
spinal manipula-
tion does indeed
help reduce
lower-back pain
(and speeds up
the healing
process).

to rehabilitate muscle ligament tissue, and to balance nerve impulses.

What it does

Chiropractic medicine is successfully used to treat back pain, chronic headaches, neck pain, and pain from musculoskeletal injuries. There also has been some hype that chiropractic physicians can treat serious problems such as tumors and heart disease and can provide overall preventive care. However, there is no scientific evidence to substantiate these claims.

The basics

1. *How often should it be done?* It can be done weekly or every two weeks initially or until improvement is seen.

2. *How long until it works?* Patients may see improvement in 8 to 10 visits or less and should be prepared to receive adjustments for at least one month.

3. *How much does it cost?* Chiropractic visits range from $25 to $75 per visit, depending on the severity of the problem, any special tests or X-rays needed, and geographic location. Chiropractors are licensed in every state, and many insurance plans, including Medicare and many Medicaid programs, cover this alternative treatment.

Chiropractic manipulation is not done when there is a fracture, infection, cancer, severe arthritis, or another condition that would contraindicate its use, especially injuries or problems in the neck. Your chiropractor will decide if manipulation is not safe, but if you are concerned about a procedure, discuss it with your practitioner first.

Watch Out!
While 90 percent of people see a chiropractor for musculoskeletal problems, be wary when a chiropractic doctor begins to take frequent X-rays to discover problems, tries to sell you a vitamin regimen, or wants to do spinal adjustments on children (the manipulation can be dangerous). If a tumor or fracture is present, chiropractic adjustments may cause severe injury.

Over the years many myths have circulated regarding the chiropractic lifestyle, but today's doctor of chiropractic medicine is well educated and must complete premed undergraduate studies and an additional four-year program at a chiropractic college. They meet stringent licensing requirements in 50 states and the District of Columbia, follow a strict code of ethics, and are approved by governmental agencies.

Naturopathic medicine

Naturopathy is based on the belief that diseases are a violation of nature's laws. Naturopathy's roots stem from the 19th century, when some physicians retaliated against the popular bleedings and purgings of prescientific medicine. Benedict Lusk, a German physician who immigrated to the United States in 1892, is credited for bringing homeopathy to the United States. Lusk opened his own water-cure facility in New York City and, by 1902, was operating a school of massage, chiropractic, and naturopathy. In 1919, he founded the American Naturopathic Association.

Naturopathic doctors (N.D.) claim to remove the underlying causes of disease while also stimulating the body's natural healing processes. They believe that diseases are the body's effort to defend itself and that cures result from increasing the patient's "vital force" by ridding the body of waste products and toxins.

How it works

Naturopaths use a variety of therapies to balance the physical, mental, and spiritual roots of an illness. Using a combination of nutrition, botanical medicine, homeopathy, Chinese medicine, hydrotherapy, and naturopathic manipulative therapy, along with scientific medical diagnostic science and standards of care, the N.D. will help you rev up your immune system and, hopefully, end the illness.

Many naturopathic practitioners believe that all diseases—strokes, myocardial infarctions, cancers—are manifestations of the body's attempt to heal itself and that all a physician needs to do is assist this process. Consequently, there have been many documented cases in which people under the care of naturopaths were told, as they worsened, that they were actually getting better. The drawback is that an N.D. cannot prescribe pharmaceuticals, which are necessary for many infections and illnesses.

What it does

Naturopathic physicians provide natural childbirth care in an out-of-hospital setting. They believe the naturopathic approach strengthens healthy body functions so that complications associated with pregnancy may be prevented. The N.D. also handles psychological medicine, believing that mental attitudes and emotional states may influence, or even cause, physical illness such as digestive problems. Even minor surgery can be handled by a naturopathic physician, such as repair of wounds and removal of foreign bodies, cysts, and other superficial masses.

The basics

1. *How often should you do it?* Naturopathic therapies are intended to be incorporated into your lifestyle. You would then see a naturopathic practitioner as necessary for instruction or healing.

2. *How much does it cost?* Seeing a naturopathic practitioner costs from $25 to $150 per hour, depending on the geographic location.

3. *How long until it works?* If these methods improve your health problem, you will see results in two days to two weeks.

Although you may trust a naturopathic doctor for a stress-related ailment that can be treated naturally, be cautious when you are hit with serious ailments or diseases that might require strong medications to get well. Only 11 states license naturopathic doctors at this time, yet some insurance companies now are covering naturopathic services.

Hydrotherapy

One popular therapy naturopathic doctors use is hydrotherapy—the use of water in all forms, from ice to steam, to promote healing. You may have used hydrotherapy in ice packs for a sprained ankle, a hot compress for sinus pain, or a cold compress to reduce a fever. Other forms include sitz baths, spas, douches, whirlpools, colonic enemas, and steam.

Although hydrotherapy stems back to ancient times, it did not officially come to the United States until the 1800s, when natural healers used water treatments and spas to heal common ailments. Vincenz Priessnitz, an Austrian peasant and the founder of hydrotherapy, was greatly influenced by this natural remedy. Soon the "water cure" was used for a myriad of ailments.

How it works

Hydrotherapy acts to stimulate the body's own healing force. Cold compresses reduce swelling by constricting blood vessels that help to control minor internal bleeding.

In one type of hydrotherapy treatment used to boost the immune function and to help fight disease, you lie on a soft table while hot towels are

Watch Out!
As we age, our skin gets drier, leaving it flaky, bumpy, and less elastic. Yet the skin's moisture comes from inside the body. In addition to applying a moisturizer, be sure to increase fluid intake to keep aging skin hydrated.

applied over the upper torso. You then are wrapped in a sheet and covered with several layers of blankets. Once the skin is warmed, the heated towel is exchanged for a single cold one. The body reacts to this temperature change by greatly increasing blood flow to the skin and to the internal organs of the chest and abdomen.

What it does

Moist heating pads, whirlpools, or even a warm shower can reduce the soreness of aching joints or inflamed muscles. Even the simple act of running cool water over a wound can help get rid of dangerous bacteria and aid in healing. It's likely that you have felt the healing benefit of moist heat on a sore muscle.

Watch Out!
Be leery of some forms of hydrotherapy, such as colonics, because they deplete important electrolytes from the body. Steam baths also are dangerous for pregnant women, young children, the elderly, people with heart problems, and diabetics.

The basics

1. *How often should you do it?* The frequency of use depends on what you are treating. If you have a fever, applying a cold compress to the forehead can be done many times during the illness. If you are trying to soothe arthritic joints, applying ice packs or moist heat to your joints for 20 minutes, two or three times a day may be sufficient. For people who prefer to see a practitioner, hydrotherapy should be repeated three or four times per week for several weeks.

2. *How much does it cost?* The cost can range from pennies (water used at home) to hundreds of dollars (if you see a practitioner frequently for hydrotherapy treatments).

3. *How long until it works?* Ice can reduce swelling within a few hours, but some forms of hydrotherapy may take weeks or months to offer benefit, if any is offered at all.

As with all alternative treatments, be discerning. Don't agree to use water-based remedies that are not substantiated by research without finding out more information to substantiate their safety. Some therapies are downright dangerous, such as sweating to release toxins from the body. On the other hand, keep a moist heating pad or ice pack around for sprains, muscle soreness, or aching joints.

Osteopathic medicine

The term osteopathy is a combination of the words "bone" (osteo) and "suffer" (pathic) and is pronounced *AH-stee-AH-pah-thee*. Originally, osteopathic medicine was drugless medicine. Today, this type of treatment is a complete system of health care. Osteopathic doctors (D.O.s) can prescribe all forms of medication, can perform all manners of surgery, and can pursue all medical specialties. They receive identical training as M.D.s (with additional training in the musculoskeletal system) and work alongside their M.D. colleagues in most hospitals. Osteopathic medicine is governed by the American Osteopathic Association.

Osteopathy was founded in 1874 by an American named Andrew Taylor Still, M.D. Dr. Still was a physician who was disgusted with the medical treatment practiced by allopathic, or conventional, medical doctors. Dr. Still believed that proper structure of the body's musculoskeletal system, which could be maintained by occasional manipulation of the soft tissues, enabled the body to function properly and to resist disease by empowering the immune system. Not surprisingly, medications had no part in the early days of this philosophy. It was in the early 1900s that medication and surgery, now thoroughly

Bright Idea
Some common forms of hydrotherapy—ice and moist heat—are right at your fingertips. The next time you get an injury, immediately apply the R.I.C.E. theory—(Rest, Ice, Compression, and Elevation). Moist heat—a warm shower, a moist heating pad, a whirlpool spa, or even running warm water over the injury, sore muscle, or aching arthritic joint—can greatly alleviate pain and inflammation.

researched, became a permanent part of what is now known as osteopathic medicine.

How it works

The osteopathic profession now offers all modes of medical treatment in addition to osteopathic manipulation. an osteopathic physician may use *Osteopathic Manipulative Medicine (OMM)*, for example, a science and art that combines osteopathic philosophy, palpatory diagnostic skills, and Osteopathic Manipulative Treatment (OMT). *Osteopathic Manipulative Treatment (OMT)* is the therapeutic application of manually guided forces (similar to those of a chiropractor) by an osteopathic physician to improve physiological function and/or to support wellness. When properly applied, it can be curative for primary muscular and skeletal pain and can decrease symptoms (and possibly decrease the need for medications) in systemic diseases.

What it does

This type of medical care is good for most health problems. Today's osteopathic physicians deliver the same treatment as regular conventional doctors.

Because D.O.s have the same training as M.D.s, you can see an osteopath for any medical problem, and conventional laboratory tests are used. Doctors who believe in using specialized hands-on manipulation techniques for illness or musculoskeletal problems use this in combination with conventional medical treatment.

The basics

1. *How often should it be done?* It can be done once or twice a week if manipulation is performed.

2. *How much does it cost?* It costs an average of $50 to $125 per visit, depending on the treatment

needed and the geographic location. Insurance companies reimburse this expense.

3. *How long until it works?* With osteopathic manipulation, you should notice a difference in one to three visits.

Osteopaths receive training comparable to regular medical doctors with four years of osteopathic medical school, plus residency and internship. At this time, there are about 42,000 licensed D.O.s. They are licensed in all 50 states and the District of Columbia, and services are covered wherever conventional medical services are covered.

Just the facts

- Chiropractic has been proven to reduce lower-back pain in some scientific studies.

- Naturopathic practitioners believe emotional problems can influence disease and use psychological therapies to heal the patient.

- Moist heat or ice applied to an injury is one form of hydrotherapy with which most people are familiar.

- Osteopathic Manipulative Medicine (OMM) can be healing for primary muscular and skeletal pain and can decrease symptoms in some chronic diseases.

How massage can lower blood pressure, relax tight muscles, and even stimulate immune function to prevent disease ▪ The ancient art of reflexology ▪ Why some people believe that reflexology can release endorphins, or soothing hormones, into the body to enhance relaxation

Bodywork and Hands-On Therapy

For centuries, people have used massage and touch as a healing art. In fact, the first record dates back 4,000 years to ancient China. The word *massage* comes from the Arabic expression for "stroke." Throughout history, the phrase "laying on of hands" to enhance healing has been valued among spiritual traditions. In the past four decades, massage has become an integral part of health systems worldwide. In 1987, the National Association for Nurse Massage Therapists (NANMT) was started by nurses in Atlanta, Georgia, who believed in the medical benefits to therapeutic touch. An estimated 30,000 North American nurses now employ therapeutic touch or massage. The hands-on therapy of touch not only feels good, it is an excellent mind/body therapy. When you are very stressed and your muscles are tense, they build up lactic acid, which makes them even more tense. Massage can help to relieve this. Massage also stimulates the relaxation response (pages 153–54), which affects the entire body.

Chapter 5

77

66

Even Hippocrates, the father of medicine, included massage as a form of healing in his writings, saying, "The physician must be experienced in many things, but most assuredly in rubbing."

99

This form of drugless alternative therapy has been shown to increase circulation, to provide relief from musculoskeletal pain, to act as a mind/body form of stress release, and to increase flexibility and mobility. There are reports that patients who receive massage for pain-related ailments take fewer narcotics or sedatives for the pain—an important benefit for aging or aching Americans. People have reported decreased heart rate and blood pressure and even a reduced skin temperature after a partial or full-body massage because touch affects the body as a whole.

Bodywork

Bodywork is the umbrella term that describes the hands-on technique of massage, touch, and movement used to align the spine, muscles, and joints to promote the flow of energy. This alternative therapy promotes relaxation (especially with the musculoskeletal system), enhances the circulation of blood and lymph, and relieves muscle tension.

With more than 80 different varieties, massage is one of the most popular forms of alternative medicine. Although the therapist focuses on different muscles or trigger points on the body, the goal is to affect the body as a whole (see Figure 5.1). Massage acts as a mind/body form of stress release and increases flexibility and mobility. Other popular types of bodywork are explained in Table 5.1.

Several popular massage techniques include:

1. **General Swedish** is the foundation for all other types of massage; particular attention is paid to the back and the chest. The therapist uses a system of long strokes, kneading, and friction techniques on the more superficial layers of the

Timesaver
To quickly find a qualified practitioner, contact the American Massage Therapist Association for a copy of its membership directory. Write to AMTA, 820 Davis Street, Suite 100, Evanston, IL 60201-4444 or call 708-864-0123.

muscles. This is combined with active and passive movements of the joints. She will apply pressure and rub the muscles in the same direction as the flow of blood returning to the heart. Swedish massage is said to help flush the tissue of lactic and uric acids and other metabolic wastes and to improve circulation without increasing the load on the heart. Oil is used to help reduce friction of the hands on the body.

2. **Tapotement** involves a percussion-type movement that includes four types of short, quick strikes made with the hands or fingertips:

   - **Hacking:** Using the heel or ulnar border of the hand, it is used on muscles around nerve centers.

   - **Tapping:** Using the fingertips with light to brisk movements.

   - **Clapping:** Slapping and cupping performed with the palms or the flat surfaces of the hands and fingers.

   - **Beating:** Performed with a clenched hand, it generally is used on the buttocks and lower extremities.

3. **Trigger point** is a type of massage and pain-relief technique used to alleviate muscle spasms and cramping. The therapist will locate active and latent trigger points, and mild to moderate pressure is applied for a short time (about 7 to 10 seconds). The muscles then are gently stretched to help the relaxation process.

4. **Vibration** is a type of massage in which the therapist uses the heel of her right hand for vibration. The left hand is placed on top of the right for light compression.

Figure 5.1:
Trigger points
are localized
areas of tender-
ness around the
joints (not the
joints them-
selves) that hurt
when pressed
with a finger.

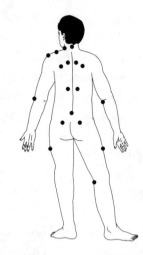

Figure 5.1:
Trigger points
are localized
areas of tender-
ness around the
joints (not the
joints them-
selves) that hurt
when pressed
with a finger.

Watch Out!
Check the cre-
dentials of the
massage thera-
pist you use to
make sure he is
certified and
licensed (L.M.T.)
by a state or
local govern-
ment. Better
still, try to find
someone who is
Nationally Cer-
tified in Thera-
peutic Massage
and Bodywork
(NCTMB). This
means the thera-
pist has passed a
national certifi-
cation exam.
Your medical doc-
tor also may be
able to refer you
to a qualified
professional.

Table 5.1   Other Popular Types of Bodywork

■ **Alexander technique.** This type of bodywork was developed in the late 1800s by Frederick Matthias Alexander, an actor who realized that the way he tensed his body negatively affected the relationship between his head, neck, and back and greatly affected his voice. These techniques are said to release painful muscle tension, to improve posture, and to reduce stress and fatigue through reeducation of the kinesthetic sense. Practitioners must complete a 1,600-hour instructional program at an approved school to be certified to teach the Alexander technique. Although there is no data to prove this technique works, one study has shown it may be helpful to healthy adults by enabling them to breathe more efficiently.

■ **Feldenkrais method.** Using functional integration (FI)—a type of subtle touch—practitioners of the Feldenkrais method help to improve the efficiency of the motor nervous system. A series of lessons will teach you how to improve your posture and become flexible and spontaneous. These subconscious holding patterns are brought to your awareness and then released to help you reclaim a mind-body connection.

▪ **Hellerwork.** Founded by Joseph Heller in 1978, Hellerwork is based on the assumption that every person is innately healthy. With this form of bodywork, a practitioner will combine hands-on massage, movement, and dialogue to help you release accumulated stress and rigidity. Rather than treating the symptom, Hellerwork focuses on rebalancing the entire body and returning it to a more aligned, relaxed, and youthful state. Hellerwork is effective for temporary pain or tension relief.

▪ **Polarity therapy.** This form of bodywork is based on the theory that energy fields exist everywhere in nature, including in the human body. Stress, tension, chronic pain, and environmental stimuli are among the many factors that can restrict this energy flow, causing disease. The therapist will use gentle body manipulation and hold pressure points to help restore natural energy flow. The practitioner also will educate you in exercise, nutrition, food combining, and maintaining a positive attitude to keep your energy fields balanced.

▪ **Reiki.** Based on the same energetic principles as tai chi and acupuncture, Reiki is neither invasive nor physical. Practitioners believe the vital energy of the universe is channeled through their hands to help energize you and promote your inner healing. Proponents claim that Reiki has a calming effect and can restore balance to

Bright Idea
You can use Reiki anytime to stop a headache. When a headache starts, sit in a comfortable position and put your hands on the painful area. Breathe slowly and deeply, and imagine healing energy flowing from your hands to your head. Do not think "pain or headache;" think "healing, sensation, pain free." By relabeling the pain and embracing it, you will feel release from tension and discomfort.

the body. During a Reiki session, you will stay clothed and lie on your back on a massage table. The Reiki healer will gently rest her hands on various parts of the body in patterns that include the head, abdomen, legs, back, and feet. You may feel a sensation of warmth during this treatment, which usually takes about an hour. You cannot receive too much Reiki energy; therefore, there is no limit to the number of Reiki sessions you may have. This form of bodywork is particularly effective if applied as soon as possible after a trauma occurs, whether it's a physical injury or a mental shock.

▪ **Rolfing/structural integration.** Based on the premise that most humans are significantly out of alignment with gravity, Rolfing promotes natural healing by realigning the body's underlying structure. The practitioner, or rolfer, uses fingers, knuckles, and elbows to sculpt the client's body into correct alignment. This deep pressure applied by the rolfer helps to stretch the muscles and *fascia*, the thick elastic connective tissue that envelops and supports muscles, tendons, and bones to make them more flexible. Although scientific studies do not show a benefit from rolfing, there have been many testimonials from people who believe it helps to reduce repetitive motion injuries (RMI).

▪ **Trager method.** The Trager method uses movements, stretching, and pressure to help you give up muscular and mental tension and sink into a feeling of deep relaxation. Practitioners claim that a Trager session can bring about a high-energy state beyond relaxation. Because pain—whether chronic (long-lasting) or acute (new, sharp)—causes tension in the body and in the mind, the Trager method works to ease these tensions by helping you to concentrate on peace and relaxation. There are more than 1,000 practitioners of Trager in the world today. These practitioners use the language of movement (gently rocking, swinging, stretching, and pressure) to help you focus on resolving conflict deep within the unconscious mind and to allow you to sink slowly into a very deep state of relaxation.

How it works

It's the constant but small annoyances in life that tend to cause symptoms of stress. When you are mentally stressed, your muscles become tense and build up lactic acid. Massage helps relieve this by sending a message to the brain to produce fewer stress hormones. It makes sense that, when you are less stressed, you will feel more alert and relaxed.

To see if life's interruptions cause you stress, read the list in Table 5.2. If you are more stressed than normal, some type of bodywork may help your situation.

What it does

For people with respiratory conditions, therapeutic touch is frequently suggested to help patients increase expectoration of mucus and to relax the back, shoulder, neck, and chest muscles for enhanced breathing (but don't forget your bronchodilator!). This form of bodywork is helpful for headache, TMJ, and sports injuries and can help to alleviate symptoms of muscle spasms, lower-back pain, and other common chronic pain. Unlike medications taken for these problems, massage has no

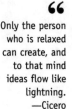

> Only the person
> who is relaxed
> can create, and
> to that mind
> ideas flow like
> lightning.
> —Cicero

TABLE 5.2   WHAT STRESSES YOU OUT?

_____ Waiting in long lines of traffic

_____ Inability to relax

_____ Fear of rejection from family and friends

_____ A telephone that rings constantly

_____ Not getting recognized for abilities at work or home

_____ Too much noise at home or work

_____ Prying neighbors, friends, or family members

_____ Decision making

_____ Out-of-control children

_____ Having to attend a party with strangers

_____ Difficulty with self-expression

_____ Lack of sleep

_____ Getting too much sleep and still feeling tired

_____ Meeting with the boss about a raise

_____ Social obligations

_____ An annoying friend

_____ Misplacing or losing things

_____ Inability to concentrate at work or at home

_____ Fear of confrontation with coworkers or family members

_____ Entertaining people at home

_____ Inability to get close to coworkers or friends

_____ Problems filling out forms

_____ Preparing for the holidays

_____ Dislike of preparing meals each day

_____ Redecorating the house

_____ Receiving a compliment from someone

_____ Having concerns about health

_____ Vacationing with family

_____ Completing the yard work

_____ Having no energy to do housework

_____ Not having enough money to make ends meet

_____ Too many medical bills, and insurance won't cover them all

_____ Having to wait in line anywhere

_____ Having to wait to see a doctor

_____ Having a doctor who does not listen

_____ Sexual problems with mate

_____ Marital or relationship problems

_____ Physical reaction to weather changes

_____ Not enough energy to keep up in life

_____ Declining physical abilities

negative side effects. In fact, studies released from the University of Miami School of Medicine's Touch Research Center found that the benefits of massage include heightened alertness, relief from depression and anxiety, an increase in the number of natural "killer cells" in the immune system, lower levels of the stress hormone cortisol, and reduced difficulty in getting to sleep.

You don't have to be an adult to benefit from theraputic touch. A study about premature newborns revealed that massage decreased the amount of time spent in the hospital. The infants were stroked for 15 minutes, three times daily for 10 days; on average, each infant's length of stay in the hospital was reduced by 6 days—a cost savings of $10,000 per infant. This could produce a savings of $4.7 billion annually if used on all premature babies in the U.S.

The basics

1. *How often should it be done?* For the maximum benefit, get a massage once a week; once a month is the minimum to get any type of benefit.

2. *How much does it cost?* Rates vary from $35 to $100 per session and depend on the type of massage, where you have it done, and the geographic location. If you have a home visit, you can expect to pay more.

3. *How long until it works?* You will reap the benefits of massage immediately. Although you can try to massage your own aching muscles and joints, a professional massage will offer a greater benefit. Massage therapy is licensed by more than half the states, and 85 percent of these licenses require a minimum of 500 hours of in-class

education. You can find massage therapists at spas and health clubs as well as at physicians' and chiropractic offices. Neuromuscular and sports/injury massage therapists specialize in relief of muscle pain and often work in medical settings.

Reflexology (zone therapy)

Reflexology, also called zone therapy, is a healing art based on the theory that reflex areas, or specific points, in the feet and hands correspond to all the glands and organs in the body. The term *reflex* refers to the fact that these points are responsive to stimuli.

Although ancient illustrations hint that the early Egyptians, Japanese, and Chinese worked on the feet and hands to promote better health, it was in the early 1900s that Dr. William Fitzgerald developed the zone therapy theory. This later became the basis for reflexology. In the early 1930s, physiotherapist Eunice Ingham studied the response of different areas of the body to zone therapy. The feet were found to have the greatest amount of sensitivity. Ingham probed the feet using precise thumb pressure on certain spots, and tender areas were discovered. Her methods equated these spots on the feet with the anatomy of the human body.

How it works

Practitioners believe that nerve pathways exist throughout the body. When any of these pathways are blocked, the body experiences discomfort. Reflexology will help to revive your energy flow and to bring your body back into homeostasis, or a state of balance. The zone therapy theory, from which reflexology was derived, states that there are 10

Watch Out!
A warning to people with high blood pressure: Ask your doctor before getting a massage. Some studies show that massage can cause a brief increase in blood pressure. Anyone with heart disease or circulatory problems also should check with their doctor before having a massage.

zones throughout the body—five zones on the right side and five on the left (see Table 5.5). Reflexes travel through the zones like the electrical wiring in your home. These zones are used to determine various locations of reflexes within the hands and the feet. All the body parts within any one zone are connected by the nerve pathways and are mirrored in the corresponding reflex zone on the hands and the feet.

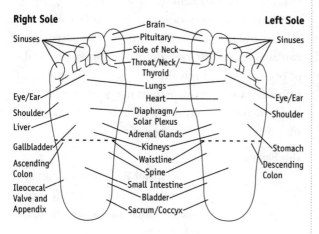

Right Sole ... **Left Sole**

Brain
Pituitary
Side of Neck
Throat/Neck/Thyroid
Lungs
Heart
Diaphragm/Solar Plexus
Adrenal Glands
Kidneys
Waistline
Spine
Small Intestine
Bladder
Sacrum/Coccyx

Sinuses — Sinuses
Eye/Ear — Eye/Ear
Shoulder — Shoulder
Liver
Gallbladder — Stomach
Ascending Colon — Descending Colon
Ileocecal Valve and Appendix

Figure 5.2: When pressure or massage is applied to specific points on the hands and feet, called reflex points, these points correspond to various organs or systems throughout the body.

TABLE 5.3

Reflex Point	Corresponding Body Zone
Metatarsal (balls of the feet)	Chest, lungs, and shoulder area
Toes	Head and neck
Upper arch	Diaphragm and upper abdominal organs
Lower arch	Pelvic and lower abdominal organs
Heel	Pelvic and sciatic nerve
Outer foot	Arm, shoulder, hip, leg, knee, and lower back
Inner foot	Spine
Ankle area	Reproductive organs and pelvic region

What it does

There are different theories regarding the uses of reflexology. Some people claim it releases pain-blocking endorphins into the bloodstream. Others say it relaxes the body and improves circulation. Although it is not scientifically proven, people have experienced relief from allergies, headaches, sinus problems, asthma, backaches, carpal tunnel syndrome, constipation, kidney stones, menstrual problems, prostate problems, and arthritis.

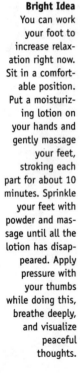

Bright Idea
You can work your foot to increase relaxation right now. Sit in a comfortable position. Put a moisturizing lotion on your hands and gently massage your feet, stroking each part for about 10 minutes. Sprinkle your feet with powder and massage until all the lotion has disappeared. Apply pressure with your thumbs while doing this, breathe deeply, and visualize peaceful thoughts.

Many practitioners claim foot reflexology can cleanse the body of toxins, can increase circulation, can assist in weight loss, and can improve the health of organs throughout the body. Some people claim reflexology is effective against many serious diseases. Keep in mind, however, that there is no scientific support for any of these assertions.

The basics

1. *How often should it be done?* Your partner can give you a loving foot rub each night, but most people see a reflexologist only once a week until the health problem is resolved.

2. *How much does it cost?* Expect to pay $35 to $100 for a session with a certified reflexologist.

3. *How long until it works?* You may feel more relaxed after just one session, but it usually takes 5 to 10 sessions to fully benefit from reflexology.

Although proponents claim health problems can be diagnosed by feeling the feet and that pressing each area can stimulate the healing of the corresponding body zone, these pathways in the body have not been anatomically demonstrated. A good foot rub might give you a soothing stress-free benefit, but stay in touch with your conventional medical doctor for serious problems.

Just the facts

- Swedish massage is used to flush lactic acid out of the body and to increase circulation.

- Massage is used successfully to stimulate growth and to increase immune function in premature infants.

- People with respiratory problems can benefit from massage therapy because it stimulates drainage of mucus from swollen airways.

- Reflexology is said to stimulate healing to different zones in the body, although it is not scientifically proven.

GET THE SCOOP ON...
Why increased liquids and sweating with exercise are two
safe methods of detoxification ▪ The problems that can
arise with invasive techniques such as colonic irrigation
and chelation ▪ Some actions you can take to detox your
home, ridding it of harmful and noxious substances

Detoxification and Purification

Chapter 6

In ancient biblical times, fasting was a common method of cleansing the body to remove harmful toxins. Today, a host of detoxification methods—from increasing liquids in the daily diet to not eating processed foods to avoiding industrial pollutants, herbicides, and chemicals—are used by millions. Other common forms of detoxing or purifying include increased exercise and the use of a sauna to sweat profusely, thus releasing toxins from the system. Environmental medicine, which focuses on the removal of harmful chemicals and toxins from your workplace or home, also is in keeping with the detoxification theory.

Although many methods of purifying the body and our environment are safe, healthful, and approved by the scientific community, there are some you need to approach with caution, including colonic irrigation and chelation therapy. Proponents claim these methods can cure you of many ills, but these invasive techniques have been associated with serious health problems. If you only learn one truth from this book, it should be this: If it sounds to good to be true . . . it probably is.

Detoxification and fasting

Whether from toxins in the air, food, or water or from other exposures such as mercury in dental fillings or aluminum in cookware and antiperspirants, we all are exposed to substances that can be irritating and harmful and can contribute to compromised immune function. Detoxification is one type of alternative treatment that cleanses these toxins from our bodies. *Fasting,* the avoidance of solid food, is one method of detoxification. *Colonic irrigation* also is a crucial part of this therapy. It usually is done by inserting a rubber tube into the rectum and then passing it for a distance of up to 20 or 30 inches. Warm water is gently pumped in and out through the tube a few pints at a time, typically using 18 to 22 or more gallons. Some practitioners add herbs, coffee, or other substances to the warm water. This procedure is said to detoxify the body.

How it works

Detoxification is centuries old, going back to early biblical times when fasting was used as a method of spiritual cleansing.

Today, detoxification is used to clear toxins from the body by neutralizing or transforming them, thus clearing excess mucus and congestion. The process also involves dietary and lifestyle changes that reduce the intake of toxins and improve elimination. Avoidance of chemicals in food, refined food, sugar, caffeine, alcohol, tobacco, and drugs helps minimize the toxic load. Drinking extra water (purified) and increasing fiber by including more fruits

Bright Idea
A CO detector, available at hardware and home-center stores for $30 to $50, can sense an unsafe level of carbon monoxide and sound a warning. A detector should be installed close to each bedroom.

and vegetables in the diet also are steps in the detoxification process. Some people use colonics or enemas to detoxify the body, while others prefer fasting or avoiding solid foods.

What it does

Detoxification can help clear out potential disease and can improve energy. Proponents believe that many common acute and chronic illnesses may be alleviated by a program of detoxification/cleansing. In fact, people with addictions to any substance may benefit from a detox program, even if it is only the temporary avoidance of the addictive agent or agents. Withdrawal symptoms—such as nervousness, sweating, sleeplessness, etc.—that commonly occur when a person stops using a substance—such as sugar, nicotine, caffeine, and over-the-counter medications—are accelerated by detoxification. Detox techniques are based on ancient naturopathic remedies; however, they have yet to be backed by conclusive scientific studies. For example, some proponents of detox feel that techniques such as body polishing (a rubdown with a dry loofah to stimulate circulation) and cleansing massages can flush out toxins and can nourish internal organs. While massage does flush lactic acid from the muscles, lactic acid is not a toxin. It is a normal byproduct of exercise and promptly passes out of the muscle without massage.

The basics

1. *How often should it be done?* Use detox procedures such as exercise, sweat, sauna, steam, increased fluid intake, vitamins, elimination diets, and getting more sleep any time you feel the need to cleanse and purify your system.

Watch Out!
Watch out for the following signs of toxicity:

Angina pectoris (chest pain)

Anorexia

Anxiety

Backaches

Bad breath

Circulatory deficits

Constipation

Cough

Depression

Dizziness

Environmental sensitivity

Fatigue

Fever

Frequent colds

Headaches

High blood cholesterol and triglycerides

Hives

Immune weakness

Indigestion

Insomnia

Irritated eyes

Itchy nose

Joint pains

Mood changes

Nausea

Nervousness

Runny nose

Sinus congestion

Skin rashes

Sleepiness

Sore throat

Stiff neck

Wheezing

2. *How much does it cost?* Detoxification costs range from free (drinking water or sweating from exercise) to $50 to $100 per session (therapeutic colon cleansing done by a holistic practitioner). The American Colon Therapy Association, which promotes colonic irrigation, reports that the number of practitioners has grown 50 percent in the past year in the United States, with about 500 now practicing.

3. *How long until it works?* You may notice relief within hours, but it often can take days or weeks to detect a difference in how you feel. Detoxification on a simple level makes practical sense if you follow a healthful cleansing routine of exercise and sweat, fresh fruits and vegetables, increased liquids with more frequent urination, or more sleep when under stress. The age-old theories behind colon cleansing or lengthy fasts are just that—ancient theories. In fact, these cleansing plans should not be done by expectant mothers, diabetics, and people who have chronic illnesses such as heart, kidney, or lung disease. Until research promotes these methods as safe and effective with substantial scientific evidence, stick to detox methods that you know to be safe. Ask your conventional doctor for more information.

Timesaver
If you are looking for detoxification treatment and education, call the Gerson Institute in Sedona, Arizona. This is the first U.S. alternative cancer-treatment center and is licensed by the Arizona Department of Health. Gerson therapy utilizes diet, detoxification, and therapeutic supplementation to reactivate and strengthen the immune system and to restore the body's essential defenses.

Chelation therapy

Although chelation (pronounced *key-lay-shen*) therapy has been used since the 1950s to help heart and blood vessel diseases, it remains controversial and relatively expensive. The regimen is said to help clear arteries clogged by atherosclerosis.

Chelation therapy was first used for treatment of lead poisoning. Doctors noted that patients with coronary artery disease and angina pectoris frequently reported a dramatic improvement in their conditions following this treatment.

How it works

Through a series of intravenous administrations, a chelating chemical (a synthetic amino acid—EDTA, or ethylene diamine tetra-acetic acid) is injected into the body to find toxins in the blood. The amino acid binds with, or chelates, certain minerals such as lead, calcium, and iron and removes them from the body through the urinary tract.

What it does

Practitioners in the United States use chelation as an additional therapy related to circulation in disorders such as cancer, arthritis, stroke, multiple sclerosis, and heart disease.

Although several studies worldwide strongly suggest that EDTA chelation therapy effectively reduces the symptoms of cardiovascular disease, use of chelation therapy for vascular disease has been condemned by The National Institutes of Health and every scientific medical organization that has reviewed it:

- The American Heart Association states that "there is no scientific evidence to demonstrate any benefit" from use of chelation in treating arterial disease.

- The California Medical Association warns, "Excessive use of EDTA can result in kidney damage and death."

- The U.S. Food and Drug Administration's *FDA Consumer* lists chelation therapy as one of the

Bright Idea
An easy cleansing fast that may fit your lifestyle includes brown rice, steamed fresh vegetables, and clear liquids or broths.

Watch Out!
The National Heart, Lung, and Blood Institute has documented many cases of kidney failure and death in people who have had chelation therapy as a treatment for heart disease.

country's top 10 health frauds. Among all this controversy, however, it is interesting to note that chelation therapy has been approved by the FDA since 1953 for the treatment of atherosclerosis.

The basics

1. *How often should it be done?* If you use chelation therapy, it is repeated daily for three to four weeks.

2. *How much does it cost?* The cost is well in excess of $3,000 per week, yet this can be much higher depending on your location.

3. *How long until it works?* This may vary depending on the severity of the disease, and it may not work at all. There is a red flag on chelation therapy. Although this alternative treatment is approved for hypercalcemia and heavy metal poisoning, there are no scientific reports of clinical trials in reputable health journals that confirm the benefits of chelation for diseases such as atherosclerosis. In 1953, however, it was FDA-approved for lead toxicity, hypercalcemia, and digitalis poisoning. Use this type of therapy with great caution; many researchers claim there are no reasonable theoretical grounds for effectiveness.

Environmental medicine

Environmental medicine is based on the concept that a myriad of physical and emotional symptoms are triggered by hypersensitivity to common foods, toxic substances, and chemicals. Proponents believe that the immune system is like a barrel that continually fills with chemicals until it overflows, indicating the presence of disease.

The roots of environmental medicine are traced to the practice of allergy treatment. In the 1940s, Dr. Theron Randolph identified a variety of common foods and chemicals that can trigger the onset of acute and chronic illness, even when exposure is at relatively low levels. With the increasing awareness of the environment and pollutants in the past three decades, research in this field has skyrocketed.

How it works

According to proponents of environmental medicine, illness can be caused by a wide range of toxic or harmful substances, including foods and chemicals found in the air, water, and food. Treatment focuses on eliminating the environmental hazardous sources we can control. You may be told to modify your diet and to avoid deleterious substances such as strong shampoos, aerosol deodorants, cigarette smoke, exhaust fumes, organic solvents and pesticides, plastics, paints, perfumes and colognes, medications, gas used for cooking and heating, building materials, synthetic fibers, and certain clothing.

What it does

Research studies support the use of environmental medicine for allergy, arthritis, asthma, chemical sensitivity, colitis, depression, panic attacks, reduced attention spans, eczema, fatigue, and hyperactivity. An example of the need to reduce environmental hazards is the association between lead and brain damage. The United States Public Health Service has called lead the most serious environmental hazard to young children and, along with The American Academy of Pediatrics, has recommended that all children under six years old be

Watch Out!
The rate of cancer in American children has risen over the past few decades, and many specialists believe increased exposure to toxic chemicals in the environment is a primary cause. According to experts, a newborn in the United States faces a 1 in 600 risk of contracting cancer by age 10. Although the exact causes are unknown, it is suspected that toxins in the air, food, dust, soil, and drinking water are key players.

tested for lead. Newly published findings suggest that lead damage in children's developing brains could mean the difference between being on the low end of normal intelligence and dropping below normal. The result, according to a report published in the journal *Epidemiology*, could be a tripling of the number of youngsters who need special education. Leaded paint in residential housing continues to be the overwhelming source of lead poisoning in children.

TABLE 6.1   CLEANING UP YOUR HOME

Go through your home or office and discover problem areas. Environmental triggers vary, but common triggers include:

Aerosols	Fresh paint
Chemical fumes	Humid air
Cigarette smoke	Mold and mildew
Cockroaches	Perfume and scented products
Cold air	Pet dander
Detergents	Pollen
Dust	Wood smoke

> **"**
> I suffered with allergy and asthma for most of my life, went through hours of painful allergy tests, and lived on decongestants, antihistamines, and bronchial inhalers—until I went away to a college about 300 miles away. Later, my allergist discovered that I was severely allergic to the allergens released into the air by the town's paper mill. Think about it! For 18 years I suffered because of polluted air.
> —Keith, 23, student
> **"**

Proponents of environmental medicine claim that an immune system breakdown can be triggered by a single serious episode of infection, stress, or chemical exposure (see Table 6.3). Practically everything encountered by modern humans can be a potential trigger, such as urban air, diesel exhaust, tobacco smoke, fresh paint or tar, household cleaners, rubbing alcohol, felt-tip pens, cedar closets, tap water, and electromagnetic forces.

Scientific studies, however, do not conclusively support the idea of environmental incidents causing all illnesses. But with such perplexing problems as sick building syndrome, Legionnaire's disease, and work-related asthma, environmental medicine offers a substantial theoretical basis for relieving or curing these problems altogether (see Table 6.2).

TABLE 6.2   COMMON OCCUPATIONS ASSOCIATED WITH ENVIRONMENTAL TOXINS

Animal breeders

Bakers

Detergent manufacturers

Dye workers

Epoxy resin, paint, and chemical workers

Farmers

Food processors

Food wrappers

Grain handlers

Hairdressers

Laboratory workers

Laxative manufacturers

Manufacturers

Metal workers, metal platers, welders

Nurses, hospital workers

Painters, printers, foam manufacturers

Pharmaceutical workers

Plastic workers

Printers

Textile workers

Woodworkers, carpenters

The basics

1. *How often should it be done?* This type of treatment can be ongoing as you reduce or eliminate hazardous chemicals, dietary additives, and nutritionally unbalanced foods from your lifestyle.

2. *How much does it cost?* Environmental treatment costs range from free (elimination of certain solvents, pollutants, or other harmful substances) to extremely expensive if you have to relocate your home or office due to unavoidable chemicals or toxic substances.

Watch Out!
Latex allergy is rapidly becoming a growing concern, especially for health care workers such as nurses and lab technicians. According to the American College of Allergy, Asthma, and Immunology, about 18 million Americans (64 in every 1,000) are affected by latex sensitivity. This is a dramatic increase from 1 in every 1,000 people in the early 1980s. Latex is used to make balloons, condoms, diaphragms, elastic for clothing, carpet backing, gloves, and toys. It also is an essential ingredient for many medical and dental tools and devices, including face masks and bandages.

3. *How long until it works?* You may notice a difference in the way you feel immediately, or it may take time, depending on how severe or debilitating your symptoms are. It makes sense that what we eat, breathe, wear, or sleep on can ultimately affect how we think, feel, act, and react. Environmental toxins, including processed foods and food additives, can tear down the body, resulting in poor emotional and psychological health. Removing the toxins you can control and focusing on natural foods and household cleaning products may help you to think clearer, to stay healthy, and even to regulate your moods.

TABLE 6.3   BEWARE OF THE AIR OUT THERE

What's in the air you breathe each day? Check out the following:

Ozone	Ozone is the major destructive ingredient in smog. It causes coughing, shortness of breath, and chest pain. It also boosts susceptibility to infection. At high concentrations, ozone can scar the lungs. People who exercise outdoors are particularly vulnerable to the effects of ozone.
Sulfur Dioxide	Sulfur dioxide, another component of smog, is created when sulfur-containing fuel is burned. It irritates the airways and constricts the air passages, causing asthma attacks. It also can suppress mucousal ciliary action and can set the stage for permanent lung damage.
Nitrogen Dioxide	Nitrogen dioxide contributes to ozone formation and is produced when fuel is burned, especially in motor vehicles and power plants. It causes bronchitis and, like ozone, increases susceptibility to infection. One study revealed that people who cook on gas stoves may be more prone to hay fever and asthma-related symptoms such as wheezing and breathlessness because of the released nitrogen dioxide.
Carbon Monoxide	This odorless, colorless gas mainly comes from automobiles and other combustion exhaust. It reduces oxygen levels in the blood, starving the body's cells. It is especially dangerous for people with heart disease and unborn or newborn children.

Just the facts

- Sometimes a modified fasting diet consisting of brown rice, steamed vegetables, and clear liquids can help rid the body of harmful toxins.

- Colonics or enemas are used to detoxify the body, as are fasting, avoidance of solid foods, and increasing fiber in the diet.

- Although chelation therapy is used for circulatory diseases, no clear-cut scientific proof exists to back its use. You should check with your doctor before starting this (or any) controversial therapy.

- Environmental factors can cause symptoms that mimic asthma (workplace asthma).

Herbs, Essences, Oils, and Tinctures

Chapter 7

If you've ever salivated when an aromatic whiff of Mom's homemade chocolate chip cookies drifted your way or felt alert even before you took that first sip of brewed java in the morning, you have successfully used aromatherapy. This pleasing form of alternative medicine is directly linked with Bach Flower therapy, herbal therapy, and homeopathy because most of these remedies are derived from plants. (About one-fourth of homeopathic remedies come from minerals, animal products, allergens, extracts of drugs, and noxious sources like snake venom.) While the nose or skin is the general point of distribution with aromatherapy, the mouth is the main site for other herbal, flower, and homeopathic remedies because you ingest them. No matter which type of treatment you prefer, proponents stand by its healing powers and claim it can positively affect psychological and physical well-being.

Aromatherapy

This type of nose-mind therapy involves the ancient art of using fragrances, or essential and absolute oils, and other substances for physical and psychological benefits (see Table 7.1). *Essential oil* is an extract or essence that's been distilled—usually by steam—from the seed, leaves, stem, flower, bark, root, or other parts of a plant; *absolute oil* is a very concentrated liquid taken from a plant extracted by alcohol. Essential oils often are diluted in a *carrier oil* such as sweet almond, grapeseed, olive, or canola oil before using with massage.

Each of the different aromas or oils has a specific healing power such as reducing stress, fighting infection, increasing productivity, or serving as an aphrodisiac. For example, lavender and spiced apples are said to increase the alpha-wave activity of the brain, leading to relaxation. On the other hand, increased beta activity in the front of the brain shows greater alertness and is said to occur with the smell of jasmine or lemon. Some research has found chamomile essential oil to be an anti-inflammatory, while clove oil is antimicrobial.

How it works

Exactly how aromatherapy works still remains a mystery, although everyone knows that odors you like can induce a positive mood. Researchers have discovered that, when you inhale aromatic molecules, they connect onto receptors and build electrical impulses that move up the olfactory nerves to the brain. The ultimate target is the limbic system where your emotions and memory are processed.

TABLE 7.1   USING ESSENTIAL OILS

- Inhale the oil by adding 5 to 10 drops to steaming water or to a humidifier.
- Mix one teaspoon oil with one pint carrier oil and use as a massage oil.
- Add 5 to 10 drops to warm bath water.
- Mix five drops with one cup warm water and mist into the air.
- Put one to two drops on a lit candle's melted wax, and inhale the warm scent.

Aromatherapy was used by ancient civilizations and is thought to be 6,000 years old. In fact, a medical papyri dating back to around 1555 B.C. contains remedies for illnesses with methods of application similar to the ones used in aromatherapy and herbal medicine today (see Table 7.2). Scientists in Europe and Great Britain began researching the effects of essential oils on bacteria in humans in the 19th century. In the early 1900s, French chemist René-Maurice Gattefossé burned his hand while working in a perfume laboratory. He applied lavender oil and found that, not only did the pain quickly heal, the wound healed without blisters or infections. Gattefossé went on to classify oils and their healing properties.

TABLE 7.2   AROMATHERAPY TIME LINE

- In ancient Egypt, frankincense was burned at sunrise as an offering to Ra, the sun god.
- The Greeks continued to use aromatic oils both medicinally and cosmetically.
- The Chinese used aromatic herbs and burned aromatic woods and incense to show respect to God.
- Lavender was used to perfume the baths of the Romans and for over 1,000 years in folk remedies.
- Traditional Indian medicine, known as Ayurveda (see Chapter 3), incorporates aromatic massage as one of its main aspects.
- The North American Indians used aromatic oils and produced their own herbal remedies.

Watch Out!
If swallowed, essential oils can be toxic. Keep them away from children. Essential oils often can be costly, and not all essential oils are pure; they may contain synthetic ingredients or vegetable oil. To determine whether the essential oil is pure, place a drop on a sheet of paper. Pure essential oil will evaporate without a trace; unpure oils will leave a mark.

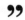

My grandmother used to rub my chest with Vicks VapoRub (Proctor & Gamble) when I had bronchitis or a cold, and I still use this today on my children. It works!
—Pamela, 34, homemaker

99

What it does

It's probably not news that certain scents such as eucalyptus make you breathe better. Perhaps this is why the over-the-counter cough drops and chest rubs have been popular for many generations. In Russia, eucalyptus oil has been said to cure a certain flu strain; in the United States and Japan, scientists are studying the effects of inhaled fragrances to relax claustrophobics. Other popular essential oils and their uses are described in Tables 7.3 and 7.4.

TABLE 7.3   COMMONLY USED ESSENTIAL OILS

Essential Oil	Common Uses
Anise (pimpinella anisum)	Used in soap to hide human odor
Basil (pimenta racemosa)	Increases alertness and concentration
Bay (Citrus bergamia)	Stimulates scalp and counteracts stress
Black pepper (Piper nigrum)	Loosens muscles and is an aphrodisiac
Cedarwood (Cedrus atlanticus)	Is an expectorant, a diuretic, and calms anxiety
Chamomile, German (Marticaria chamomilla)	Treats irritated skin
Chamomile, Russian (Anthemis Nobilis Organic)	Is a sedative and a pain reliever
Clove bud (Eugenia caryophyllata)	Stimulates mind, body, and memory
Cypress (Cupressus sempervirens)	Is an astringent and eases cramps
Eucalyptus (Eucalyptus globulus)	Fights viruses and eases muscle aches
Frankincense (Boswellia carterii)	Is an expectorant and calms anxiety
Geranium (Pelargonium graveolens)	Balances hormones and is a diuretic

Essential Oil	Common Uses
Ginger (Zingiber officinale)	Soothes aching joints and upset stomach
Grapefruit (Citrus paradisii)	Energizes and is uplifting
Juniper berry (Juniperus communis)	Is a diuretic and is uplifting
Lavender (Lavender vera lavender)	Is antifungal and antiviral
Lemon (Citrus lemon)	Is a germicide and an astringent
Mandarin (Citrus reticulata)	Is an antiseptic and has calming influence
Marjoram (Origanum marjorana)	Lowers high blood pressure
Myrrh (Commiphora myrrha)	Clears mucus and eases eczema
Orange (Citrus sinensis)	Refreshes and relaxes
Palma rosa (Cymbopogon martinii)	Releases anger and soothes grief
Patchouli (Pogostemon cablin)	Heals cracked or inflamed skin
Rosewood (Aniba rosaeodora)	Is an aphrodisiac and an antidepressant
Sage, Spanish (Salvia lavandulifolia)	Eases arthritis and painful muscles
Sandalwood (Santalum album)	Balances skin and lifts depression
Spruce, black (Picea Mariana Canada)	Stimulates and relieves anxiety
Tea tree (melaleuca alternifolia)	Is antifungal and antiviral
Thyme (trachyspermum copticum)	Is antibacterial and a fungicide
Yarrow (Achillea millefolium)	Balances skin and increases hair
Ylang-ylang (cananga odorata)	Is an antidepressant and an aphrodisiac

TABLE 7.4   ESSENTIAL OILS THAT RELIEVE STRESS

Essential Oils	Effect on the Body
Basil, rosemary, and lemon oil	Increases mental alertness
Lavender and chamomile	Relieves insomnia
Sandalwood and geranium	Improves sex drive
Frankincense and marjoram	Soothes raw nerves
Jasmine and rose	Increases confidence
Dill, ginger, lemon, and spearmint	Decreases appetite
Lavender, vanilla, and chamomile	Destresses
Basil, geranium, and orange oil	Combats depression
Peppermint and geranium	Boosts creativity
Orange, peppermint, and rosemary	Increases energy
Sandalwood and peppermint	Soothes upset stomach
Lavender and chamomile	For PMS and cramps

Moneysaver
If you are plagued with foot odor, but you hate spending money on another expensive product, make your own deodorizing spray. Mix four ounces of witch hazel with 40 drops of lavender, patchouli, or cypress essential oil. Put in a spritzer bottle, shake, and spray on your feet several times a day.

There is some hype that aromas can boost energy, productivity, and creativity, and can possibly provide relief from certain chronic illnesses. Few credible studies have been published in reputable scientific or medical journals, however, validating such claims as cures for chronic illnesses. One of the few, a report in the well-respected medical journal *The Lancet*, revealed that lavender oil was associated with reduced symptoms of insomnia in the elderly and, therefore, could reduce the need for hypnotic drugs. Except for the *Lancet* review, many scientists believe that anecdotal claims of mental and physical health effects are most likely due to the placebo effect. *Placebo* is a Latin term whose original meaning is "I shall please." It refers to the mysterious and uncharted mechanisms by which the power of suggestion can result in a physiological change. Critics complain that when the oil is taken out of a plant, chemical changes occur that may adversely affect the therapeutic value of the plant.

The basics

1. *How often should it be done?* There are no rules with essential oils, but if you find that an oil is causing inflammation or irritation with frequent use, stop using it. Most essential oils are not taken internally, and some can be toxic on the skin, so ask your doctor before using any unknown substance.

2. *How much does it cost?* Essential oils vary greatly in price, depending on the quality of the oil or the scarcity of the plant. You can buy a small bottle of oil for about $5 to $10 at natural food stores.

3. *How long until it works?* While some problems such as nasal congestion might respond immediately to inhaling an essential oil, sometimes it takes up to 10 sessions to find a positive effect.

Whether or not aromas can reduce stress, can act as an aphrodisiac, or can make your hair grow depends on your personal response. Some practitioners claim that herbs such as marjoram help migraines and that lavender and rosemary reduce the pain of other types of headaches. While there is no scientific proof for these claims, it may be worth trying. Keep in mind that fragrance allergy affects some people and that just because an oil is natural does not mean it is totally safe. Oils may be 100 times stronger than the dried versions of the plant. According to research, some essential oils can even be life-threatening and should be avoided during pregnancy or if you have epilepsy.

Bach Flower essences

Dr. Edward Bach, a noted British physician and immunologist, developed the Bach Flower Remedies in the l930s. The Bach system consists of essences made from 38 different flowers. Each remedy takes a specific action on a certain mental attitude.

How it works

A few of the diluted drops are placed on the tongue or rubbed on the body to gently help restore balance to the mind and body, to change your emotional and mental mood, and to stimulate the body's self-healing processes.

What it does

The remedies are said to change negative feelings such as anger, worry, jealousy, and fear into optimism, joy, and hopefulness (see Table 7.5). Problems such as digestive disorders, sleeplessness, stress, and skin problems may benefit from the Bach Flower Remedies.

TABLE 7.5   BACH FLOWER REMEDIES

Flower Essence	Condition
Gentian	Hopelessness, worry
Gorse	Despair, a sense of doom
Hornbeam	Mental fatigue
Mustard	Moody, gloomy
Sweet Chestnut	Overwhelmed, burned out

People who use Bach Flower Remedies claim they treat the real causes of mental disorders rather than covering them up as pharmaceuticals do. While this type of flower power may zap you out of a bad mood and have no known side effects, we continue to search long and hard for scientific studies of miraculous mental or emotional healing!

The basics

1. *How often should it be done?* To use these remedies, fill a one-ounce glass bottle with water and

add several drops of up to four essences, according to the condition you need to treat. Flower essences are taken several times a day for up to three weeks; you then stop taking the essences to see whether your condition has improved. You may benefit from two to three sessions with a herbal therapist to learn how to use these effectively.

2. *How much does it cost?* The essences cost from $6 to $10 per bottle, depending on the brand and your geographic location.

3. *How long until it works?* It may take one to three weeks to see improvement, if there is any.

Conditioned as we are to want quick fixes, don't give up your antidepressant quite yet. While the delightful fragrances may give you a lift, the scientific journals have yet to acknowledge that this treatment has any sound validity.

Herbal therapy

If you have ever downed a cup of hot coffee and realized that it allowed you to breathe better, you have tried herbal medicine. Herbal medicine uses natural compounds to treat ailments, such as ginger tea to fight off colds, St. John's wort to alter moods, or ginkgo biloba to increase concentration.

Since ancient times, all cultures have thrived on the use of plants and plant products for medicinal purposes. Traditional herbs are the backbone of Chinese medicine and are a common element in Ayurvedic, homeopathic, naturopathic, and Native American Indian medicine. According to the World Health Organization (WHO), about four billion people, or 80 percent of the earth's population, use herbal medicine to receive a desired benefit from the body.

Watch Out!
How do you know if a treatment really works or if it is your imagination? You might not. While the placebo effect is a positive healing effect resulting from your belief that a treatment will work, the *nocebo* effect is a negative outcome resulting from your belief that a treatment will not work. Your beliefs and expectations about a particular treatment are important for optimum healing, as are your health care providers' beliefs and expectations.

Moneysaver
Instead of buying expensive over-the-counter anti-gas medications for symptoms of an irritable bowel, make peppermint tea. Peppermint contains oils that can soothe the digestive track. Pour one cup of boiling water over one teaspoon of dried peppermint (or two teaspoons fresh peppermint) and steep for 15 minutes. Strain and drink to ease gas and cramping.

How it works

This alternative treatment is based on the actual therapeutic value that certain herbs are supposed to have. For example, slippery elm bark has been shown to soothe sore throats, saw palmetto may shrink enlarged prostates, and garlic may lower blood pressure and cholesterol. Some herbs also can revitalize hair (see Table 7.6).

TABLE 7.6   HERBAL INFUSIONS FOR HAIR CARE

For centuries, herbal infusions have been used as rinses to revitalize hair. To make your own infusion, steep 1/4 cup of one of the following fresh or dried herbs in three cups of water for 12 minutes. Cool, strain, and use as a final rinse.

- Chamomile adds gloss and highlights to light brown and blonde hair and can be used as an eye wash for tired eyes.
- Ginseng replenishes moisture, adds sheen, and gives hair flexibility.
- Lavender helps promote natural sleep and relieves headaches, depression, anxiety, and nervousness. It also renews your hair's shine and silkiness and can be applied to the skin to soothe stress-related skin rashes.
- Lemon grass conditions hair and makes it shine.
- Rosemary helps hair grow and controls dandruff.
- Yarrow helps make hair easy to manage.

Although some advocates claim that herbs can be used to cure any ailment from diabetes to AIDS to cancer, don't expect a guaranteed herbal cure for these serious diseases quite yet. Besides, you really do not know what you are getting when you purchase herbal remedies due to the lack of regulation. Qualities may vary, products often are misidentified, and some herbs are sold long after the shelf life has expired. In Europe, however, there have been many credible studies reporting the healing effects of herbs such as Ginkgo biloba (ginkgo), Silybum marianum (milk thistle), and Vaccinium myrtillus (bilberry extract). Ginseng and ginger have been studied extensively in China using acceptable scientific methods. Indian gooseberry, neem, and turmeric (common Ayurvedic herbs) have passed the scrutiny of scientific research in India. At this time, the NIH is studying St. John's wort and its possible use as an antidepressant. Because plants cannot be patented in the United States, most companies call herbs "foods" and market them that way. Although a few herbs are dangerous and should never be ingested or put on your skin (such as ma huang and chaparral), most herbs appear to be relatively safe.

The basics

1. *How often should it be done?* Because each herb has a different property and purpose, you need to read the label or ask a practitioner for proper dosing. It is advisable to buy herbal supplements from a reliable company and to make sure they have been standardized. This means the manufacturer has performed an analytical test to measure the amount of key ingredients in the batch. Whole herbs that are either organic or grown in the wild have the best chance of being safe. Remember, dosing is not exact with herbs and the potency can vary.

2. *How much does it cost?* Herbs are available in various forms. Some come in capsules, which are made from a whole herb or an extract, and are easy to store. Herbs also can come in liquid form, either a *tincture* (an alcohol/water extract made from the whole herb) or an *extract* (made from one of more parts of the herb). Liquids usually are diluted in another liquid and are more potent. The whole herb consists of the entire plant processed into liquid or capsule form. Herbs vary in price depending on where

> 66
> I tried dong quai because I read in a woman's magazine that it could ease menstrual cramps, yet instead it caused excessive menstrual bleeding, fever, and I ended up in bed for the weekend. Manufacturers should tell you all of the side effects—just in case of a problem like I experienced.
> —Keri, 29, graphic artist
> 99

they are purchased, how they are processed, and the strength of the herb. For example, a small bottle containing 60 capsules of St. John's wort can vary in price from $5.99 to $16.99, depending on the strength and the brand.

3. *How long until it works?* The length of time varies, depending on the herb you take and the condition for which you're taking it. If you drink a cup of valerian tea, you may begin to feel its effect within 30 minutes to two hours. It may take three or four weeks, however, to feel the mood-enhancing effect of St. John's wort. Herbs are natural substances, but they also can be strong medicines.

Most herbal products sold in the United States are not standardized. This means determining the exact amounts of ingredients can be difficult or impossible. Herbal preparations can affect your response to prescribed medication and can even be toxic to the liver. Check out the list of herbs that follows. If you decide to take herbal supplements, play it safe and talk to your doctor, pharmacist, certified nutritionist, or naturopath about side effects. Herbal therapies without supervision are not recommended for pregnant women, children, the elderly, or people with compromised immune systems.

Popular herbs

This section contains an alphabetical rundown of some of the more popular herbs and can be used as a reference.

Alfalfa

1. What it is good for:
   - Eases arthritis, allergies, morning sickness, stomach problems, and bad breath

Watch Out!
The FDA considers nine herbs to be unsafe: chaparral, comfrey, germander, jin bu huan, lobelia, magnolia, ma huang, stephania, and yohimbe.

- High in dietary fiber and can help eliminate body waste
- Use to boost the immune system, to help build strong muscles, and to gain weight
- Take for a rich source of vitamin B_{12}

2. How it is used: Available as herbs, seeds, supplements, and sprouts. Follow package directions.

3. Caution: May cause stomach distress due to high fiber content.

Aloe vera

1. What it is good for:

- Helps prevent scarring and reduces risk of skin infection
- Take internally to relieve constipation, gastritis, and stomach ulcers
- Use externally for skin irritations, minor burns, sunburn, cuts, skin irritations, rashes, canker sores, cold sores, ulcers, acne, frostbite, poison ivy, vaginal dryness, and skin abrasions

2. How it is used: Available as a powder, a gel, capsules, and a live plant. Follow package directions.

3. Caution: May cause intestinal cramps or allergic reaction.

Angelica (dong quai)

1. What it is good for:

- Relieves menstrual discomfort and minimizes symptoms of menopause
- Boosts production of red blood cells and treats weakness and fatigue

Bright Idea
If you are using fresh or dried herbs, you're in luck. Fresh herbs usually are higher in medicinal value, and dried herbs are available year-round. To make tea, use one teaspoon of dried herb (or one tablespoon of fresh herb) and one cup boiling water. Let steep for 10 minutes and then strain.

- Take to stimulate the immune system, to relieve colds and other respiratory problems, and to prevent arthritis

2. How it is used: Available as dried herbs, supplements, and a tincture. Follow package directions.

3. Caution: Angelica should not be used by pregnant women. It also can cause fever and excessive menstrual bleeding in some women.

Astragalus

Timesaver
Chop large dried plant parts such as roots, stems, leaves, and flowers into small pieces. Using a mortar and pestle (or a food processor), grind them until they are in powder form. Store in air-tight containers and have them available to add to drinks, salads, or soups.

1. What it is good for:

- Stimulates the immune system and boosts white blood cell activity
- Increases the production of interferon
- Take to promote urination, to speed healing of burns, and to bolster resistance to disease

2. How it is used: Available as dried herbs, capsules, and a tincture. Follow package directions.

3. Caution: May cause loose stools or abdominal bloating.

Bee pollen

1. What it is good for:

- Balances the endocrine system, helping to relieve menstrual or prostate problems
- Helps counteract the effects of aging and strengthens the body's natural immunity against illness
- Use as an antidote during allergy season to relieve bronchitis, sinusitis, and colds

2. How it is used: Available as bee pollen. Follow package directions.

3. Caution: Use cautiously if you have allergies. It may cause severe reactions in some people.

Black cohosh

1. What it is good for:

   - Acts similarly to estrogen, the female-produced chemical, and has been prescribed to women going through menopause

   - May help treat fatigue, sore throat, arthritis, and rattlesnake bites

   - Contracts the uterus and increases menstruation

   - Use as an astringent, an expectorant, a diuretic, a sedative, and an antispasmodic

   - Use as a poultice for inflammation

2. How it is used: Available as dried roots, capsules, and a tincture. Follow package directions.

3. Caution: Because of estrogenic effects, it should be avoided by pregnant women. Do not use if you have heart disease.

Borage

1. What it is good for:

   - Soothes the mucous membranes of your throat, sinuses, and mouth, and eases arthritis pain

   - Stimulates adrenal glands and helps restore energy

   - Use to treat bronchitis and digestive system upsets

2. How it is used: Available as seeds, leaves, flowers, a whole plant, and supplements. Follow package directions.

> **66**
> If you have any type of chronic illness, don't believe everything you read about natural cures. I saw an advertisement for bee pollen that said it would 'cure allergy and asthma.' Even though I'm severely allergic to bee pollen, I bought it and tried some. In about 30 minutes, I was sneezing, coughing, and wheezing and had to start oral steroids to get back in control. If in doubt, ask your doctor!
> —MaryAnn, 35, attorney
> **99**

Watch Out!
The bad news:
Pregnant women
who drink large
quantities of
coffee or other
caffeinated bev-
erages may be
putting their
infants at risk for
sudden infant
death syndrome
(SIDS). A New
Zealand study
found that moth-
ers who had con-
sumed 400
milligrams or
more of caffeine
a day—the equiv-
alent of four cups
or more of
coffee—while
pregnant
increased their
baby's risk of
SIDS by
65 percent.
The good news: A
preliminary test
has found that
heterocyclic
amines, a new
class of protec-
tive elements, are
found in both
caffeinated and
decaffeinated
coffee. These ele-
ments may work
like antioxidants
to protect against
diseases associ-
ated with aging,
cancer, and heart
disease.

3. Caution: Safe if used according to package directions.

Burdock root

1. What it is good for:

   - Promotes healthy kidney function and helps prevent water retention

   - Helps arthritis and rheumatism

   - Use as a blood purifier and cleanser or as a poultice to heal inflamed skin, eczema, and psoriasis

2. How it is used: Available as a dried powder, a tincture, and pieces of root. Follow package directions.

3. Caution: Should not be used by children or pregnant women without professional super-vision. It can stimulate the uterus.

Coffee

1. What it is good for:

   - Enhances the pain-relieving effects of aspirin

   - As a decongestant, helps ease congestion due to colds and flu

   - As a bronchodilator, helps prevent asthma attacks

   - Use to combat drowsiness and to temporar-ily boost athletic performance

2. How it is used: Available as dried whole beans, ground beans, a liquid, and in instant form. Follow package directions.

3. Caution: Coffee is addictive and can cause with-drawal symptoms, which can last several days. It can cause insomnia, increased anxiety, and irri-tation of the stomach lining.

Calendula

1. What it is good for:

   - Use for digestive and menstrual problems

   - As a topical remedy, use as a skin freshener and moisturizer or to heal skin irritations, cuts, bruises, sprains, burns, and hemorrhoids

2. How it is used: Available as dried leaves, flowers, roots, an ointment, and a tincture. Follow directions on package.

3. Caution: May cause irritation when applied to skin.

Capsicum

1. What it is good for:

   - Helps increase thermogenesis for weight loss (especially when combined with caffeine-type herbs) and increases heart action without increasing blood pressure

   - Take internally to cleanse the circulatory and digestive systems, to heal irritated mucous tissues, and to promote drainage.

   - Used externally as an over-the-counter cream or ointment, capsaicin is effective in treating muscle aches and arthritis pain; also may give relief in treating other painful areas such as leg pain

2. How it is used: Available as dried herbs, supplements, and ointments. To use creams, follow the label's directions and apply externally four or five times daily for at least four weeks. Cover with cotton flannel cloth.

3. Caution: May cause skin irritation. In large doses, can cause stomach upset, vomiting, and diarrhea.

Watch Out!
Be sure to wash your hands. Capsicum will severely sting and irritate eyes and mucous membranes.

Cat's claw

1. What it is good for:

    - Contains powerful antioxidants that fight free radicals, which set the stage for cancer and other diseases

    - Keeps blood platelets from clumping together and helps prevent strokes and heart attacks

    - Take to relieve joint pain and the inflammation of arthritis, bursitis, and other rheumatic diseases

2. How it is used: Available as dried roots, supplements, and a tincture. Follow package directions.

3. Caution: Cat's claw appears to be nontoxic, but pregnant women, children, and people with chronic diseases should not take it.

Chamomile

1. What it is good for:

    - Depresses the central nervous system and also may aid in boosting immune power

    - Increases relaxation and promotes quality sleep

    - Use to relieve nervousness, upset stomach, and menstrual cramps

2. How it is used: Available as dried herbs, supplements, and herbal tea.

3. Caution: Chamomile contains pollen, so it may cause problems for people allergic to ragweed (although there are no reports of toxicity).

Chapparal

1. What it is good for:

    - Calms nerves and improves appetite

Bright Idea
Add chamomile to a cool bath to help soothe the pain of sunburn or wind-chapped skin.

- Acts against free radicals and may be effective in preventing degenerative diseases associated with aging
- Use to clean and tone the digestive tract
- Take as a natural antibiotic for the body

2. How it is used: Available as dried leaves and supplements. Follow package directions.

3. Caution: Chaparral has been promoted as a cancer cure and as an acne treatment, but the FDA reports that it has been linked to cases of liver inflammation.

Chives

1. What it is good for:
   - Contains the phytochemical allicin, which has been found to lower blood pressure, to prevent certain types of cancer, and to reduce cholesterol
   - Use to increase your intake of vitamin C and for a mild antibiotic

2. How it is used: Available as dried herbs or live plants.

3. Caution: Has no apparent negative effect.

Cinnamon

1. What it is good for:
   - Calms the stomach and has an antifungal and antibacterial effect
   - Use to treat the discomfort of menopause and to stop excessive menstrual flow

2. How it is used: Available as dried bark, herbal tea, a spice, and supplements. Follow package directions.

3. Caution: Do not take cinnamon as a supplement if you are pregnant.

Comfrey

1. What it is good for:
   - Heals respiratory ailments
   - Aids digestion by promoting secretion of pepsin
   - Take to help regulate blood sugar levels

2. How it is used: Available as dried leaves and roots, herbal tea, and supplements. Follow package directions.

3. Caution: Comfrey has been linked to liver complications.

Dandelion

1. What it is good for:
   - Helps to support the body's potassium levels and to detoxify the system
   - Improves enamel of teeth when eaten as a food
   - Use the juice from the stem to treat acne, blisters, and corns

2. How it is used: Available as dried roots, fresh leaves, and seeds. Follow package directions.

3. Caution: Appears to be safe if used according to package directions.

Echinacea

1. What it is good for:
   - Stimulates the immune system and helps ward off colds or flu
   - Heals wounds and has an antiinflammatory, antiviral, and antibacterial effect in the body

2. How it is used: Available as supplements, a tincture, a liquid, and foods (cough drops). Follow package directions for correct dosage. It will take about one week before you notice a difference.

3. Caution: Take echinacea intermittently as the effectiveness wears off after eight weeks of continuous use. Echinacea may trigger allergic reactions in some people. It is not recommended for people with autoimmune diseases such as lupus. (Echinacea bolsters the immune system's white blood cells. Autoimmune diseases are caused by an overactive immune system.)

Elder flower

1. What it is good for:

   ▪ Use as an effective treatment for flu; eases fever, muscle aches, and other flu-like symptoms within 24 hours of starting supplements

2. How it is used: Available as aged bark, dried flowers, berries, leaves, and supplements.

3. Caution: None available.

Ephedra (ma huang)

1. What it is good for:

   ▪ Stimulates the adrenal glands and helps increase energy

   ▪ Use as a natural decongestant and antihistamine and to treat asthma and allergies

   ▪ Increases metabolism and body temperature; has been used to control weight and to help prevent sleep

2. How it is used: Available as a tincture, supplements and in over-the-counter weight-loss products. Follow package directions.

Watch Out!
The FDA recently proposed cracking down on the marketing of Herbal Ecstasy and other ephedra products, citing about 800 injuries and at least 17 deaths linked to the herbal stimulant. The proposals include limiting concentrations of the herb in any dietary supplement, requiring warning labels that its use can cause death, and banning claims that it can help people lose weight or build muscle. Some popular products containing ephedrine include Herbal Ecstasy, Ultimate Xphoria, and Herbal Phen-Fen. It also marketed as ma huang, Chinese ephedra, and epitonin.

3. Caution: Ephedrine is an amphetamine-like stimulant that can cause heart attacks, strokes, seizures, or death in people with heart disease, high blood pressure, or neurological disorders. It also can cause insomnia, dry mouth, uterine contractions, and early menstruation.

Eucalyptus

1. What it is good for:
   - Croup and chest congestion
   - Use healing steam to clear sinus congestion, bronchitis, and asthma
   - Acts as a powerful antiseptic and astringent
2. How it is used: Available as dried bark, seeds, leaves, and an oil. Follow package directions.
3. Caution: Do not use for long periods of time; it may cause kidney problems.

Evening primrose

1. What it is good for:
   - Contains gamma linolenic acid (GLA), an essential nutrient that creates substances called prostaglandins, which help keep your blood running smoothly
   - May help reduce appetite and promote weight loss
   - Take to reduce PMS symptoms such as cramping, bloating, and mood swings
   - Use to clear up skin allergies and eczema
   - May ease the pain of arthritis
2. How it is used: Available as capsules, supplements, and a tincture. Follow package directions.

3. Caution: Appears to be safe and nontoxic. Take this herb with at least 600 milligrams of vitamin C to enhance GLA absorption.

Feverfew

1. What it is good for:

   - May inhibit inflammation and fever, slow the blood vessel reaction to vasodilators like prostaglandins, and act similar to aspirin

   - Use to treat arthritis and chronic or migraine headaches

2. How to use it: Available as dried plants, tablets, or capsules. Take 125 milligrams daily to help with pain and inflammation, or make feverfew tea by steeping one teaspoon of dried plant in two cups of water for 15 minutes.

3. Caution: Anyone with a clotting disorder should consult their physician before taking feverfew.

Garlic

1. What it is good for:

   - Has antimicrobial and immunostimulating properties; may provide some relief from symptoms of colds or upper respiratory problems by stimulating the mucus-producing vagus nerve reflexes

   - Releases a powerful antibiotic called allicin

   - May help prevent some types of cancer

   - Lowers high blood pressure and prevents blood clots

   - Relieves pain resulting from insect bites and acts as an insect repellent

   - Can lower cholesterol

Bright Idea
Just remember the letter G for cold or flu relief. Goldenseal, garlic, ginseng, and ginger are powerful virus fighters. Use these in hot teas or as supplements for optimum relief.

2. How it is used: Available as dried cloves, a powder, an oil, supplements, and capsules. Take a dose of 4 grams of fresh garlic each day (equal to one clove). Garlic supplements may vary in potency, so follow package instructions.

3. Caution: Large amounts can reduce blood-clotting time and can be dangerous for people taking anticoagulants.

Ginger

1. What it is good for:

   - Stimulates mucus-producing vagus nerve reflexes

   - Has nearly a dozen antiviral compounds, including several called sesquiterpenes, which help fight cold viruses

   - Has an antioxidant and anti-inflammatory effect and stimulates the production of interferon

   - Helps fight nausea and improve digestion

2. How it is used: Available as dried roots, tea, an extract, tablets, and capsules. Follow package directions.

3. Caution: No reports of toxicity.

Ginkgo biloba

1. What it is good for:

   - Relaxes and opens up blood vessels

   - May increase male sexual performance and counteract male impotence

   - Protects cell membranes from free radical damage, improving concentration and memory, increasing blood flow, helping the symptoms of PMS, and aiding with depression.

- Helps people suffering from Alzheimer's and dementia with short-term memory loss, depression, and other problems of aging

2. How it is used: Available as supplements and tea. Follow package directions.

3. Caution: Larger doses may cause nausea, diarrhea, stomach upset, and vomiting.

Ginseng

1. What it is good for:

- Use to increase energy and to relieve stress

- May stimulate special enzymes that promote elimination of toxic foreign substances, and may increase the immune response by stimulating the number of antibodies in the body

- Use to stimulate memory, to counteract fatigue, and to soothe damage caused by stress.

2. How it is used: Available as tea, a powder, capsules, tablets, and an extract. Follow package directions.

3. Caution: Can cause headaches, insomnia, anxiety, breast soreness, or skin rash. More serious side effects include asthma attacks, heart palpitations, increased blood pressure, or uterine bleeding.

Goldenseal

1. What it is good for:

- Soothes inflammation of the respiratory, digestive, and genitourinary tracts caused by allergy or infection

- Enhances mucous membrane function

Bright Idea
If stress and tension have you tied in knots, try some eleuthero tea. This aromatic herb, also known as Siberian ginseng, can reduce blood pressure and can increase concentration. It's available in health food stores in liquid or capsule form.

2. How it is used: Available as dried roots, capsules, or a tincture. Follow package directions.

3. Caution: Pregnant women, people with hypoglycemia, children, and the elderly should not take goldenseal. It also is not recommended for long-term use.

Goto kola

1. What it is good for:
   - Use as brain food to promote memory, to alleviate mental fatigue, and to normalize blood pressure
   - Considered to be a nerve tonic

2. How it is used: Available as dry bulk, a tincture, or capsules. Follow package directions.

3. Caution: May have a narcotic effect and should not be used by young children or pregnant women.

Hawthorn berries

1. What it is good for:
   - Use to strengthen the muscles and nerves to the heart
   - May help regulate high or low blood pressure and battle arteriosclerosis, hypoglycemia, and heart disease

2. How it is used: Available as dried berries, leaves, or capsules. Follow package directions.

3. Caution: May cause a decrease in blood pressure and a feeling of faintness.

Hyssop

1. What it is good for:
   - Regulates blood pressure and promotes circulation

- Use to relieve hoarseness, lung congestion, and mucus buildup

2. How it is used: Available dried or as a tincture. Follow package directions.

3. Caution: May cause diarrhea or upset stomach.

Kava kava

1. What it is good for:

- Use to fend off anxiety and nervous tension

- Effective as a sedative, a diuretic, and a muscle relaxant

- Used as an anti-inflammatory pain reliever to replace aspirin, acetaminophen, or ibuprofen

2. How it is used: Available as tea, a tincture, or tablets. Follow package directions.

3. Caution: High doses of kava kava can lead to muscle weakness, visual impairment, dizziness, and drying of the skin. Long term use of the herb can contribute to hypertension, reduced protein levels, blood cell abnormalities, or liver damage. Alcohol consumption increases the toxicity of the herb. Do not use if pregnant, nursing, or being treated for depression.

Kelp

1. What it is good for:

- Provides energy and endurance, helps relieve nervous tension, and promotes circulation to the brain

- Heals goiter and hypothyroidism

2. How it is used: Available as capsules, a tincture, and dried bulk. Follow package directions.

3. Caution: Check with your doctor before using kelp if you have a history of high blood pressure or thyroid problems.

Lavender

1. What it is good for:

   - Has anti-inflammatory and antiseptic properties
   - Relieves insomnia, depression, and headache

2. How it is used: Available as capsules, an oil, a tincture, and dried bulk. Follow package directions.

3. Caution: Do not ingest lavender oil.

Licorice

1. What it is good for:

   - Use as an antiulcer drug, antibacterial, and decay-preventive.
   - Promotes healthy adrenal glands and acts as a sexual stimulant
   - Induces the adrenal cortex to produce more cortisone
   - Thins mucus and alleviates sore throats, coughs. and asthma

2. How it is used: Available as roots, syrups, and lozenges. Licorice is most effective when taken in lozenge form to soothe mucous membranes.

3. Caution: Can cause stomach distress, diarrhea, and fluid retention. Large amounts of licorice can lead to a sudden increase in blood pressure.

Meadowsweet

1. What it is good for:

   - Use to ease the pain of arthritis or rheumatism

Bright Idea
To make tea, steep one teaspoon dried flowers in one cup boiling water for 15 minutes. Drink one to three cups daily.

2. How it is used: Available as dried leaves and roots and as an extract.

3. Caution: Because of its aspirin-like qualities, be cautious taking it if you have a blood disorder or if you are on any nonsteroidal anti-inflammatory medications (NSAIDs).

Milk thistle

1. What it is good for:

   ▪ Increases levels of glutathione, the main vehicle of detoxification in the body

   ▪ Bolsters the immune system

   ▪ Supports the liver's ability to maintain normal liver function and stimulates production of new liver cells to replace old damaged ones

   ▪ Fights pollutants and prevents free-radical damage by acting as an antioxidant

2. How it is used: Available as capsules, a tincture, seeds, or dried bulk. Follow package directions.

3. Caution: There are no known toxic effects if used in small amounts as recommended.

Mullein

1. What it is good for:

   ▪ Use as a bone, flesh, and cartilage builder

   ▪ Works as an expectorant to relieve respiratory problems such as asthma, bronchitis, and sinus congestion

   ▪ Apply externally to heal ulcers, hemorrhoids, and benign tumors

2. How it is used: Available as dried leaves, stems, flowers, and an oil. Follow package directions.

3. Caution: You may get a mild stomach upset or diarrhea with mullein. Do not take mullein if you are pregnant or nursing or if you have a history of cancer.

Myrrh

1. What it is good for:

   - Has an antibacterial action that relieves sinusitis, respiratory congestion, asthma, coughs, and colds

   - Cleans the colon and soothes digestive system upset

   - Stimulates menstruation

   - Gargle with myrrh tea for irritated mouth or throat

   - Apply externally for wounds and cuts

2. How it is used: Available as resin, a tincture, an oil, and a powder. Follow package directions.

3. Caution: Large amounts may cause laxative action, sweating, vomiting, kidney problems, and rapid heart rate.

Nettle

1. What it is good for:

   - Use to relieve arthritis, gout, eczema, hemorrhoids, hay fever, and diarrhea

   - Has a diuretic effect

   - Helps stop excessive menstrual flow, premenstrual syndrome, vaginal yeast infections, and chronic cystitis

2. How it is used: Available as a tincture, dried leaves and stems, or capsules. Follow package directions.

3. Caution: Excessive amounts may cause stomach irritation, constipation, or burning skin.

Passionflower

1. What it is good for:
   - Use frequently as a mild tranquilizer and to ease insomnia, stress, and anxiety
   - Relieves shingles, hiccups, and asthma
2. How it is used: Available as a tincture, fruit, dried or fresh leaves, or capsules. Follow package directions.
3. Caution: Be careful not to combine passionflower with prescription sedatives. Do not take if you are pregnant, nursing, or a child under age 12.

Peppermint

1. What it is good for:
   - Aids in digestion, soothes the lining of the digestive tract, and stimulates the production of bile
   - Relieves nasal, sinus, and chest congestion
   - Stops cough by increasing saliva and freshens breath
2. How it is used: Available as dried peppermint leaves, crushed herb, an oil, tea, and an extract. Follow package directions.
3. Caution: Not recommended for children under age 5.

Psyllium

1. What it is good for:
   - Helps restore tone to the intestines and lubricates and heals irritated tissues

- Use as a natural laxative to clean accumulated toxic debris out of the colon

2. How it is used: Available as whole seeds, ground, powdered, and in laxative remedies. Follow package directions.

3. Caution: Can cause an allergic reaction if you have an allergy to dust or grasses. Do not take if you are pregnant, nursing, or a child under age 12.

Pycnogenol

1. What it is good for:

- As an antioxidant that boosts the action of serotonin in the body

- Contains a special blend of water-soluble bioflavonoids to boost immune function and to reduce the formation of histamine and inflammation

- Use to help alleviate symptoms of hay fever and many allergies

2. How it is used: Available as supplements, dried roots, and a tincture. Follow package directions.

3. Caution: In some chronic conditions (such as lupus), it has been found to worsen the illness.

Rosemary

1. What it is good for:

- Relieves respiratory-tract infections with a decongestant action

- Reduces indigestion and muscle pain

- Use externally to stimulate circulation, to soothe itchy skin, and to add shine to dull hair

Bright Idea
Add one tablespoon dried rosemary and two tablespoons dried chamomile to one cup of boiling water; steep 15 minutes and then strain the herbs. Apply this healing liquid toner to your face to remove makeup without alcohol or preservatives.

2. How it is used: Available as an oil, a tincture, and dried bulk. Follow package directions.

3. Caution: Rosemary oil may cause stomach distress, even in small doses. It can be poisonous in larger amounts.

Saw palmetto

1. What it is good for:

   - Use as a treatment for benign prostatic hypertrophy or enlarged prostate; relieves the main symptom of frequent urination

   - Relieves nasal congestion, asthma, bronchitis, and cough

2. How it is used: Available as capsules, a tincture, and fresh or dried berries. Follow package directions.

3. Caution: Appears to have no dangerous side effects when used in recommended amounts.

Slippery elm

1. What it is good for:

   - Relieves sore throats and soothes mucous membranes

   - Helps heal ulcers and relieves heartburn and common digestive complaints

2. How it is used: Available as a powder, dried roots, supplements, and lozenges. Follow package directions.

3. Caution: Some people are allergic to slippery elm, so use cautiously.

Spirulina

1. What it is good for:

   - Aids in weight control, allergies, and anemia

- Is a nutritious food that is an excellent blood and colon cleanser
- Boosts the immune system, reduces cholesterol, and aids mineral absorption

2. How it is used: Available as a whole plant, a tonic, and supplements. Follow package directions.

3. Caution: Appears to be safe.

St. John's wort

1. What it is good for:

- Use internally to relieve depression without the serious side effects of prescription antidepressants
- Use externally to aid in wound healing

2. How it is used: Available as capsules, a tincture, an extract, an oil, and dried leaves and flowers. Follow package directions.

3. Caution: Can cause sensitive skin in sunlight. Check with your doctor for correct dosage if using for depression.

Thyme

1. What it is good for:

- Use to remove mucus from head, lungs, and respiratory passages
- Helps fight infections
- Use externally to control fungal infections such as athlete's foot or to reduce pain and swelling of boils or abscesses

2. How it is used: Available as an oil or an entire plant and is found in toothpastes, gargles, and mouthwash products such as Listerine. Follow package directions.

3. Caution: Appears to be nontoxic.

> **"**
> "I was feeling sad after my mother died a few months ago, so a friend suggested I try St. John's wort. I took 300-milligram tablets each day and within 10 days, I was laughing again. I wasn't obsessing on the death of my mother and began to see joy in life."
> —Juanita, 58, teacher
> **"**

Turmeric

1. What it is good for:

   - Stimulates the flow of bile and helps digest fats

   - Aids digestion, treats dysentery, wards off ulcers, and protects the liver

   - May combat certain cancers

   - Helps prevent heart disease by lowering cholesterol

   - May prevent the formation of blood clots that trigger heart attacks and strokes

2. How it is used: Available as dried herbs, crushed herbs, and a powder.

3. Caution: Too much turmeric may cause stomach distress. Medicinal turmeric preparations should not be given to children under 2 years old. For older children and people over 65, start with low-strength preparations and increase strength if necessary.

Valerian

1. What it is good for:

   - Use to relieve stress and nervousness

   - Has a sedative effect and has been shown to help in treating insomnia

2. How it is used: Available as capsules, a tincture, and dried. Follow package directions.

3. Caution: If you are already taking antidepressants, you should stay away from valerian.

Wild Yam

1. What it is good for:

   - Take internally to ease morning sickness and menstrual cramps

- ▪ May help urinary tract disorders and gastro-intestinal problems

- ▪ Use to soothe nerves

2. How it is used: Available as capsules, a tincture, or dried roots. Follow package directions.

3. Caution: If using wild yam cream for a progesterone-like effect, check with your doctor for possible side effects.

Homeopathy

Homeopathy is a naturopathic form of medicine. The term comes from two Greek words: *homio* meaning "same" and *pathos* meaning "suffering." It based on the principle of "like cures like symptom." This means remedies that cause a potential problem in large doses actually will encourage the body to heal more rapidly if given in small doses. Homeopathetic remedies are made from plant, animal, or mineral substances and are regulated by the Food and Drug Administration (FDA).

Founded in the late 1700s by Dr. Hahnemann, a German physician, homeopathy did not gain popularity until the mid to late 1800s in the United States. At that time, 15 percent of U.S. doctors were homeopaths. With the advent of modern medicine and pharmaceuticals, homeopathy's popularity took a nosedive. With the resurgence of interest in alternative therapies in the late twentieth century, however, homeopathy has experienced a great revival.

How it works

Although there are several scientific theories on why homeopathy works, many believe the principle of "like cures like" works on a subtle yet powerful elec-tromagnetic level, gently acting to strengthen the body's healing and immune response. A homeo-pathic solution must be activated—a process called *succussion*—to make sure the original substance is diluted.

What it does

Homeopathic medicines affect allergic rhinitis, hay fever, migraine headaches, trauma, gastritis, allergic asthma, acute childhood diarrhea, fibromyalgia, and influenza. Some common homeopathic reme-dies are provided in Table 7.7.

Lack of convincing scientific proof is an obstacle preventing homeopathy's acceptance by conven-tional medical doctors. Critics believe that, because the medications are so diluted, the only benefit received is by placebo effect. Nonetheless, a survey of 107 clinical trials published in the *British Medical Journal* (February, 1991) showed that 80 percent were in favor of homeopathy. Other studies in British journals provided evidence that homeo-pathic remedies are beneficial in treating allergies, asthma, migraine, flu, and hay fever. One landmark review published in *The Lancet* said that homeopathy was shown to be nearly two and a half times more effective than placebos in the treatment of prob-lems such as arthritis, allergies, varicose veins, and gastrointestinal pain.

The basics

1. *How often should it be done?* You will need an ini-tial consultation with a homeopathic practi-tioner. You then check in with this person as necessary. Dosing is individualized, and usually two to three days of treatment is sufficient for most conditions. If you do not find relief within 24 hours, try another remedy. Because some

homeopathic remedies are derived from plants, they can be toxic if taken whole.

2. *How much does it cost?* The cost will vary depending on the practitioner you choose and the cost of the herbal remedy. Initial visits can run from $150 to $300 with $50 to $75 for follow-ups. Most insurance companies reimburse homeopathic treatment prescribed by a medical doctor or a doctor of osteopathy (see page 73).

3. *How long until it works?* This depends on the illness and whether it is chronic (longstanding, constant, or recurring) or acute (with a sudden onset and of short duration).

Table 7.7 lists the most common homeopathic remedies and what they treat. Though homeopathic remedy sales are growing at a rapid 25 percent each year, according to the National Center for Homeopathy, this type of alternative medical treatment always has received great criticism from the traditional medical community. If you seek advice from a homeopathic practitioner, make sure this person is a medical doctor. Ask where he or she studied homeopathy and whether a certification exam was passed. Licensing only is required in three states at this time (Arizona, Connecticut, and Nevada), and there are no formal guidelines or schools for homeopathy. Although true homeopathic remedies are diluted, allergic reactions are possible. It also is imperative that you check with your physician before taking any unknown substance or supplement that promises great cures.

TABLE 7.7   COMMON HOMEOPATHIC REMEDIES

Remedy	Ailment
Aconitum	PMS
Allium cepa	Allergies, colds
Apis	Bee stings
Arnica	Sore muscles, bruises, sprains
Belladonna	PMS, hot flashes
Bryonia	Constipation, vaginal dryness
Calendula	Cuts, scrapes
Chamomilla	Earache, PMS
Cimicifuga	PMS, anxiety, depression
Cocculus	Depression, sleep deprivation
Colocynthis	Menstrual cramps, irritability
Conium maculatum	Breast tenderness, swelling
Ferrum	Nausea, morning sickness
Gelsemium	Headache
Hepar sulph	Chronic itching, discharge
Ignatia amara	Depression, sadness
Ipecacuanha	Nausea
Lachesis	PMS, headaches, pain, hot flashes
Ledum	Sprains
Mag phosphorica	Menstrual cramps, bloating
Natrum muriatcum	Menopausal symptoms, vaginal dryness
Nux vomica	Diarrhea, hemorrhoids, constipation
Pulsatilla	Nausea, morning sickness, infections
Rhus tox	Sprains, flu, bruises
Ruta	Sprains
Sepia	PMS, menopausal symptoms, depression
Silica	Itching, discharge
Sulphur	Tender tissues, itching

Just the facts

- Aromatherapy is not a cure for cancer, but it can help your mind, body, and spirit rejuvenate.

- Bach Flowers are a soothing form of flower power that remind you to stop, to appreciate the moment, and to relax.

- Herbal therapies, particularly the use of St. John's wort to treat depression, are being studied by the National Institutes of Health.

- Homeopathy is based on the theory that remedies that cause a harmful problem in large doses actually will encourage the body to heal more rapidly if given in small doses.

GET THE SCOOP ON...
Mind/body therapies that ease symptoms of stress and
boost immune function ▪ How you can use autogenic
therapy to lower your heart rate and blood pressure ▪
How the creative arts are used in institutional and hospital settings for therapeutic purposes ▪ Biofeedback helps
alter the way you respond to life's stressors ▪ How light
boxes help people lessen depression

Mind/Body Therapy

Chapter 8

P opeye describes mind/body medicine per-
fectly when he says, "I yam what I yam." This
area of study centers on the idea that "we are
what we think." Many mind/body therapies are several thousand years old, but it was in the late 1970s
that researchers began to move toward a new way of
thinking about health and illness. Researcher
George Engel of the University of Rochester defined
the biopsychosocial model, in which health is the
outcome of many factors interacting together. In
this view, health is determined by an interaction
between our genetic vulnerabilities; environmental
inputs such as germs, viruses, or pollutants; psychological factors such as stress, lifestyle, attitudes, and
behavior; and social factors such as supportive relationships, economic well-being, access to health care,
and family and community patterns of behavior.

Although modern science confirms the funda-
mental truth that the mind and the body are related
in an intricate manner, many people do not realize
that we can actually empower this connection to
work in our benefit. In other words, we can make

the choice to focus on the negative, stressful aspects of life and to live with the resulting tear-down of our immune systems, or we can think positive, healing thoughts that work to keep us well.

Mind/body therapy

Psychoneuroimmunology (PNI) is the field that delves into the interplay between the mind and the body. *Mind/body medicine* (also known as *behavioral medicine*) is the influence of the mind in healing. It is addressed in virtually every medical tradition, from the ancient teachings of Chinese herbal medicine to modern allopathy.

How it works

Scientists know that our thoughts and feelings influence our body through the nervous system and the circulatory system. These are the pathways of communication between the brain and the rest of the body. When the body is exposed to a threatening situation, we prepare for confrontation. This physical response, called *fight or flight*, is controlled by our hormones and nervous system. Even though most of us don't live in the wild, the fight or flight response still occurs as it prepares our body to flee the situation we perceive as dangerous. The physiological changes that occur with the fight or flight response include increases in the following:

- Blood pressure
- Respiratory rate
- Heart rate
- Oxygen consumption
- Blood flow to muscles
- Perspiration
- Muscle tension

This adrenaline rush can be experienced whether the stressor is positive (eustress) or negative (distress). *Distress* is the term for the negative side of stressors; it can lead to loss of productivity, health problems, exhaustion, and burnout. *Eustress* is positive stress; it can increase productivity, happiness, and longevity (see Table 8.1).

Although we have no control over life's stressors, a number of mind/body therapies can be used to lessen the impact of these stressors on our bodies. Research has shown that a healthy mind can greatly improve the functioning of our immune system, and mind/body therapies can help switch your body into a calmer mode. Studies show that these therapies can put you back in control of your circumstances with positive thoughts, attitudes, beliefs, and emotions. When used with a nutritional diet, regular exercise, and social support, mind/body therapies can greatly increase your quality of life and your ability to fight illness.

> 66
> One week after I was promoted to Vice President at work, my wife had twins, and we had to purchase a larger home. It was all exciting, but even good stress can cause great anxiety.
> —Alan, 39, real estate broker
> 99

TABLE 8.1   TWO KINDS OF STRESS

Distress—Negative	Eustress—Positive
A test	A promotion
Losing your job	Buying a home
Divorce	Having a baby
Meeting with your boss	Graduation
Out-of-control kids	A pay raise
A medical test	A cruise
Health problems	Winning the lottery
Conflict with neighbors	Getting married

What it does
Mind/body treatments have been used successfully in treating both stress-related ailments such as

hypertension, chronic pain, and insomnia, and difficult illnesses such as cancer, AIDS, chronic fatigue,
immune dysfunction syndrome, and other immune-
related diseases. They also are used to reduce pain
before dental treatment and to lessen anxiety before
surgery.

Some mind/body approaches have been confirmed in scientific studies. When used prior to
surgery, research has shown that such preparation
can speed healing, can reduce complications and
bleeding, and can even result in an earlier discharge
from the hospital. These therapies can lower blood
pressure and heart rate, can boost immune
response, and can act as a protector against stress-
related illness.

The basics

1. *How often should it be done?* Because there are
   many different mind/body therapies, you could
   easily incorporate them frequently throughout
   the day to keep stress levels low.

2. *How much does it cost?* The cost of mind/body
   therapies is virtually nothing. Some people
   learn these tools quicker if they spend time with
   a counselor or a therapist, which could range
   from $40 to $100 for individual sessions or $25
   to $60 for group sessions. Once you understand
   how these therapies work, you can do them anywhere and anytime for free.

3. *How long until it works?* You might see benefits
   from mind/body tools within minutes of using
   them. For example, deep abdominal breathing
   actually alters your psychological state, making a
   painful moment diminish in intensity. Think
   about how your respiration quickens when you

Moneysaver
Many mind/body
therapies can be
learned by read-
ing how-to books
or by watching
an instructional
video. Before you
spend a great
deal of money,
try to teach
yourself methods
of relaxation and
stress reduction.

are fearful or in great pain. Then consider how taking a deep, slow breath can produce an immediate calming effect, reducing both stress and levels of pain. Likewise, music therapy can reduce your heart rate during the first experience if you fully believe in this response and mindfully focus on the music, the rhythm, and the resulting inner peace.

Mind/body therapies are for everyone. Although some people may want to lean on these tools for a miraculous disease cure, it probably is wiser to let the therapies complement your conventional medical treatment; thus, you get the best of both worlds. The main way these methods can help you stay well is by reducing your daily stress to keep your immune system functioning at an optimum level.

Mind/body therapies you can learn at home

Some mind/body therapies don't require you to see a specialist—you can learn them in the comfort of your own home. The following sections discuss some of the therapies you can get started on right now.

Autogenics

This method of cueing yourself to calm down and relax is easy to perform and can be done anywhere. Because the brain only needs a few reminders to calm down, autogenics teaches you to concentrate on raising the temperature of your hands and feet. Proponents claim that autogenics gives your heart a break from pumping so hard, opens blood vessels, reduces breathing rate and pulse, and lowers blood pressure. With autogenics:

- Sit quietly and put your left hand in your lap, palm up.

- Lay your right palm on top of it and clasp your fingers together.

- Concentrating on the feeling in your hands, mindfully work to raise the temperature of your hands for 10 minutes (then do the same with your feet). Counselors claim that, if this is done correctly, you will feel the heat rise in your hands and your feet.

Deep abdominal breathing

Many people breathe from their chest, taking shallow, rapid breaths. This type of breathing only hinders relaxation. Taking slow, deep, abdominal breaths not only oxygenates the brain, it helps end the stress cycle and enables your heart rate and blood pressure to return to normal. The brain makes its own morphine-like pain relievers, called *endorphins* and *enkephalins,* that are associated with a happy, positive feeling. These hormones can help relay "stop-pain" messages. During deep abdominal breathing, you add oxygen to the blood, cause your body to release endorphins, and decrease the release of stress hormones (see Table 8.2).

Faith factor

Even many scientists agree that the human body has a powerful sacramental dimension to it. People who acknowledge this with a strong sense of higher purpose—a body-soul connectedness—are more likely to stay with programs that lead to optimum health. This does not mean you should substitute faith in a higher power for medicine. However, faith in something greater than yourself offers a type of curative power; it can help you disconnect

Unofficially . . .
Believing that your mind and spirit can have a dramatic effect on the physical body is not a new revelation. The 2,000-year-old Hippocratic writings contain observations that "there is a measure of conscious thought throughout the body." More recently, a 30-year study conducted by the California Public Health Foundation found that frequent churchgoers were nearly twice as likely as nonchurchgoers to quit smoking and were one-third more likely to start an exercise program.

TABLE 8.2 USE DEEP ABDOMINAL BREATHING FOR IMMEDIATE STRESS REDUCTION

- Lie on your back in a quiet room with no distractions.

- Place your hands on your abdomen and take a slow, deliberate, deep breath in through your nostrils. If your hands are rising and your abdomen is expanding, you are breathing correctly. If your hands do not rise but your chest does, you are breathing incorrectly.

- Inhale to a count of five, pause for three seconds, and then exhale to a count of five. Start with 10 repetitions of this exercise and then increase to 25, twice daily.

unhealthy worries and replace them with soothing belief. Many recent studies have found that people who are active in religious organizations and who attend group functions regularly also are healthier and report lower blood pressure, less depression, and greater longevity.

At the National Institute for Healthcare Research, experts such as research psychiatrist David Larson, M.D., have compiled scientific studies supporting the positive link between faith and good health. One study concludes that people who attend church regularly have fewer stress-related health problems than those who do not attend church. The National Institute for Healthcare Research and the John Templeton Foundation awarded eight medical schools $25,000 each to offer courses about faith and healing. These grants bring the number of U.S. medical schools offering courses in spirituality to 19, including Georgetown University School of

Unofficially . . .
Norman Cousins was the first person to promote laughter as an antidote to disease. While editor of the *Saturday Review,* Cousins was diagnosed with a serious connective tissue disease. After his doctors said it was incurable, he was determined to get well. Cousins discovered that laughter affected his body chemistry in a positive, healing way. He filled his life with movies that made him laugh—a real belly laugh. He then documented his account of the "miraculous recovery from laughter" in the book *Anatomy of an Illness as Perceived by the Patient.* As he recovered from his so-called incurable illness, Cousins went on to tell others about the miracle power of laughter and the positive chemical changes in the body.

Medicine and the University of Chicago Pritzker School of Medicine.

Guided imagery

See *Visualization.*

Laughter therapy

Can a laugh a day keep the doctor away? Maybe, according to many researchers. Although the statistics are disheartening, it may come as no surprise that the average adult only laughs about 17 times a day, while a 6-year-old laughs as many as 300 times. Laughter increases the activity of body cells that attack tumor cells and viruses. It helps relieve anxiety, decreases stress-producing hormones, and increases immune system activity. In fact, many doctors are now prescribing humor therapy for chronically ill patients. Laughter may even have an aerobic benefit. Dr. William F. Fry, a psychiatrist at the Stanford University School of Medicine, has studied the aerobic, physical, and emotional benefits that laughter can provide. He found that 100 laughs is equivalent to 10 minutes spent rowing.

Meditation

Remember when transcendental meditation (page 49) was thought to be a cult? Today, meditation is recognized as a viable way to lower blood pressure, to alleviate insomnia, and to reduce chronic pain. This stress releaser seeks to integrate the mind, the body, and the spirit through intentionally focusing on the silent repetition of a focus word ("love"), sound ("om"), phrase ("peace heals"), or prayer ("thank you, God"). As thoughts intrude, you will continue to mindfully chant while facilitating the relaxation response.

This technique can guide you beyond the negative thoughts and agitations of the busy mind and can help you become unstuck from your fear and other disturbing emotions.

Mindfulness is a traditional Buddhist approach to meditation. It allows your mind to be full of whatever you are doing at that moment, whether you are dancing, gardening, writing, or listening to music. Intense focus is a key part of mindfulness, as is the ability to keep negative thoughts from intruding on the moment.

Music therapy

You can thank Pythagoras, the 6th-century B.C. philosopher and mathematician, for discovering this mind/body treatment. Music therapy uses music as an adjunctive therapy for treating neurological, mental, or behavioral disorders such as developmental and learning disabilities, Alzheimer's disease, and other aging-related problems, brain injuries, and acute and chronic pain. Today, more than 5,000 music therapists in our nation use music to soothe and heal physiological and psychological problems.

Music also may have therapeutic value in working with patients coping with autism, chronic pain, head injuries, poor motor control, and learning difficulties because it can help facilitate a change in behavior. In addition, studies are revealing that Mozart boosts intelligence. Groundbreaking research done at the University of California found that Mozart's *Sonata for Two Pianos in D Major* temporarily boosted students' abilities to distinguish shapes and objects—a higher-brain activity. Even surgeons report performing better when they can select the music played in the operating room.

Watch Out!
Some people who meditate occasionally have an opposite reaction, such as increased anxiety or fear, during a session. Researchers believe that these feelings may be responses to the sensation of being totally relaxed and uninhibited.

Moneysaver
Before you spend money on painkillers or anti-anxiety medications, first try music. At Saint Agnes Hospital in Baltimore, patients in critical care units listen to classical music. Researchers claim that listening to half an hour of classical music produces the same effect as 10 milligrams of Valium.

Composer and researcher Steven Halpern says that certain musical forms can transport the listener's brain into the alpha wave, a state of relaxation much like meditation.

Prayer

Prayer allows your thoughts to take a break from daily analytical routines and to give support to the spiritual dimension of life. When you pray or meditate, your body switches from the pumping fight or flight response to a calmer, more peaceful mood. Studies show that both prayer and meditation produce alpha and theta waves consistent with serenity and happiness. Prayer and meditation provide nourishment for your soul, satiate your inner spiritual hunger, and help you develop your ability to pay attention to all areas of life without distraction.

Can prayer help control the symptoms of stress-related illnesses? Again, there is no proof that this mind/body modality causes healing. More and more studies, however, show that people who find strength and comfort in their religion have greater survival rates from serious disease. An interesting study found that heart patients who were prayed for were less likely to die than those who were not prayed for.

Progressive muscle relaxation

Also known as deep muscle relaxation, this mind/body exercise involves concentrating on different muscle groups as you contract then relax all the major muscle groups in the body. You begin with the head and then move on to the neck, arms, chest, back, stomach, pelvis, legs, and feet. To do this exercise, you focus on each set of muscles, tense the muscles to the count of 10, and then release to the count of 10. Along with progressive muscle relaxation, it is

TABLE 8.3   LEARN THE RELAXATION RESPONSE

■ Set aside about 20 minutes that you can devote to relaxation practice.

■ Remove outside distractions that can disrupt your concentration. Turn off the radio, the television, and even the ringer on the telephone, if necessary.

■ Lie flat on a bed or floor. Recline comfortably so your whole body is supported, relieving as much tension or tightness in your muscles as you can. You can use a pillow or cushion under your head if it helps.

■ During the 20-minute period, remain as still as possible. Try to focus your thoughts as much as possible on the immediate moment; eliminate any outside thoughts that may compete for your attention.

■ As you go through these steps, try to imagine that every muscle in your body is now becoming loose, relaxed, and free of any excess tension. Picture all the muscles in your body beginning to unwind; imagine them beginning to go loose and limp.

■ Concentrate on making your breathing even. As you exhale, picture your muscles becoming even more relaxed, as if you somehow breathe the tension away. At the end of 20 minutes, take a few moments to study and focus on the feelings and sensations you achieved. Notice whether areas that felt tight and tense at first now feel more loose and relaxed, and whether any areas of tension or tightness remain.

important to perform deep abdominal breathing—breathing in while tensing the muscles and breathing out, or exhaling, while relaxing them.

Relaxation response

The relaxation response was first described by Dr. Herbert Benson more than 20 years ago. Benson realized that inducing the relaxation response at will can offer the potential to reduce physical strain and emotional, negative thoughts—and to increase your ability to self-manage stress.

Achieving relaxation through the relaxation response is an important part of reducing the emotional stress of daily living. It is done by developing an inner quiet and peacefulness, a calming of negative thoughts and worries, and a mental focus away from the pain itself (see Table 8.3). Each of these has a positive effect on your heart.

Visualization

Visualization (or guided imagery) is a stress-release activity that you can do wherever you are, any time of the day or night. Imagery is a flow of thoughts you can see, hear, feel, smell, or taste, an inner representation of your experience or fantasies. This is one way your mind codes, stores, and expresses information. Imagery also is the language of the emotions and the deeper self. Using visualization or imagery, you can allow your imagination to take over as you focus on your senses to create a desired state of relaxation in your mind (see Table 8.4).

Mind/body therapies that involve others

Some mind/body therapies require interaction. If you're a social creature, the following therapies may be for you.

66
After living with insomnia for years, I was finally able to sleep through the night—and feel rested the next day—using a combination of the relaxation response, meditation, and progressive muscle relaxation.
—Pat, 49, accountant
99

TABLE 8.4 TAKE THE FOLLOWING STEPS TO VISUALIZATION

- Find a place where you can be comfortable and set aside about 15 minutes for this exercise. Take several deep breaths while sitting or lying down and close your eyes.

- Imagine a relaxing place—preferably somewhere you have been so it can easily be pictured in your mind. This might be sitting on the seashore at sunset or sunrise, relaxing at a mountain cabin next to a babbling brook, or floating on a raft in a lake on a sunny day—whatever relaxes you.

- Continue to breathe slowly and keep this image in your mind. As you explore your mental picture of your relaxing spot, imagine all the stress, worries, and tension leaving your body. Feel the temperature of your special place. See the colors surrounding you. What sounds do you hear? Smell the freshness of the air. Touch the gentleness of the moment. Take in all the sensory details of your relaxing place and continue to destress.

- After about 15 minutes, slowly open your eyes and acclimate yourself to the surroundings in the room. Stretch your arms and legs; gently move your head from side to side and feel the tension release. Carry the calm feeling you now have with you through the day.

Art therapy

Art therapy is based on human developmental and psychological theories. Using a broad spectrum of creative and artistic methods, the art therapist will help you identify and then change inner emotional conflicts and behavioral problems. You also will increase self-awareness and will develop self-esteem. This mind/body therapy is especially effective for the educationally, socially, developmentally, medically, or psychologically challenged.

Counseling

Psychological counseling can help most people develop appropriate coping skills so life's stressors are not as overwhelming. This psychological intervention is an accepted component for everyone—not just people who have psychological problems. Some viable options include:

- **Individual counseling.** A one-on-one session takes place with a therapist and individual problem areas are addressed. These sessions may include specific help with alleviating depression, anxiety, or stress, or with other personal problem areas.

- **Family counseling.** Family members can gather to understand and accept your problems and the possible impact they may have on your family's lifestyle.

- **Group counseling.** The sessions, led by trained therapists, allow for sharing of feelings and the development of effective coping strategies. The exchange of ideas at group sessions often is the most productive way to revamp your thought processes.

Dance therapy

Dance or movement therapy came from the modern dance era in the 1940s. Using movement, positions, and various postures, the dance therapist helps you to get in touch with your innermost feelings. Once these feelings are brought out and identified, you can move forward in a healthy manner. This form of mind/body treatment often is used with developmentally or emotionally challenged children who cannot verbalize their feelings, adults who have buried painful memories, and the elderly, especially those who are confused or too depressed to talk about inner conflicts and the resulting emotions. Dance therapy is used in nursing homes, psychiatric hospitals, and schools for children with special needs, as well as in private psychotherapy practices.

Drama therapy

Drama therapy uses drama or theater methods to help you reduce symptoms of stress and anxiety, to integrate the mind and the body, or to move toward personal growth. It uses techniques such as role-play, theater games, mime, puppetry, and improvisation, among others.

Psychotherapy

Psychotherapy is an effective behavioral treatment that allows you to change your own biology (lower your heart rate, reduce your blood pressure) without invasive treatment or medications. Used especially for people who obsess on negative thoughts, are highly anxious, or are depressed about their situation in life, psychotherapy will let you identify and then verbalize inner conflicts as you learn positive coping skills.

Support groups

This form of mind/body therapy is geared toward the unique needs of its members. It provides both emotional support and education in dealing with illness or life's stressors. Support groups are not psychotherapy groups, but they can give you a safe and

Bright Idea
If you would like
to join a support
group but are
short on time,
you might find
support in the
privacy of your
home or office
on the Internet
via e-mail or
chat rooms.
When going
online, check the
World Wide Web
for the latest
information
about alternative
medicine or spe-
cific illnesses.

accepting place to vent frustrations, to share personal problems, and to receive encouragement from others. As people share their personal struggles, the assurance is given that "someone else knows what I am going through." Having a close bond with others is necessary to revamp your thought processes.

Biofeedback

This relaxation technique teaches you to read and control body functions such as skin temperature, heart rate, and brain waves. The main concept of biofeedback is centered around the idea that you may not be able to control what goes on around you, but you can learn to alter the way you respond to it. Biofeedback is *bio* because of biological monitoring; it is *feedback* when information from your body is returned to the source observer. Eastern mystics used biofeedback techniques thousands of years ago when they controlled their skin temperature, blood pressure, heart rate, and other involuntary functions through intense concentration.

How it works

With biofeedback, you are connected to a machine that informs you and your therapist when you are physically relaxing your body. Using sensors placed over specific muscle sites, the therapist will read the tension in your muscles, heart rate, breathing pattern, sweat, or body temperature. Any one or all of these readings can let the therapist know whether you are learning to relax. The ultimate goal of biofeedback is to use this skill outside the therapist's office when you are facing the real lions and tigers of life. If learned successfully, biofeedback can help you control your heart rate, blood pressure, breathing patterns, and muscle tension when you are *not* hooked up to the machine.

Some common types of biofeedback include:

- **Electromyographic (EMG) biofeedback.** This type of biofeedback provides feedback about muscle tension and works well for patients with anxiety disorders or chronic pain.

- **Electrodermal or Galvanic Skin Resistance (EDR).** This type of biofeedback measures subtle changes in amounts of perspiration.

- **Thermal biofeedback.** The temperature of the skin is measured and is used to teach hand warming. This helps relieve migraine headaches and can benefit people with Raynaud's disease.

- **Finger pulse biofeedback.** The finger pulse records heart rate and force and is useful for anxiety or cardiovascular symptoms.

- **Respiration feedback.** This type of biofeedback shows the rate, volume, rhythm, and location of each breath.

What it does
Any bodily process that can be measured can potentially be controlled through biofeedback. It is especially effective for relieving chronic pain, particularly tension headaches. It also can help relieve temporomandibular joint dysfunction (TMJ), neck and shoulder pain, anxiety, irritable bowel syndrome (IBS), epilepsy, asthma, Reynaud's syndrome, neuromuscular reeducation, attention deficit/hyperactivity disorder (ADHD), hypertension, and incontinence.

Although proponents some claim biofeedback can replace conventional medicine for chronic pain

Moneysaver
Most major med-
ical policies will
reimburse 80
percent of the
biofeedback fee;
counseling
usually is
reimbursed at 50
percent.

and anxiety-related problems, keep your analgesic close at hand. If you have trouble relaxing, this therapy may not be the best solution for you.

The basics

1. *How often should it be done?* Once a week is probably adequate.

2. *How much does it cost?* The fee should be discussed beforehand. Costs generally range from $50 to $125 a session, depending on the therapist's experience and the patient's ability to pay.

3. *How long until it works?* It takes time to learn biofeedback; it takes even longer to learn to use it outside the therapist's office. Some people can learn it in three or four sessions. A full treatment varies from 12 to 20 treatments.

For many people, biofeedback provides relatively fast, effective, long-lasting relief from the physical symptoms of stress. In some situations, however, biofeedback is inappropriate or only partially effective. For example, a person's individual cognitive ability, motivation, or psychological issues can prevent this treatment from working. Biofeedback is not always easy, but the skills acquired might be well worth the effort. Just be sure you don't forget them once you leave the therapist's office and face the real world!

Hypnotherapy

Hypnosis comes from the Greek word meaning "sleep." It is a temporary condition of altered attention, in which the brain shuts out external events. This intense state of concentration is used to control pain or stress or to alter negative behaviors.

Hypnosis has been used in therapy for centuries. You've probably read about ancient tribal leaders who induced trances in members during ritualistic ceremonies. In the past 50 years, the use of hypnotherapy by the medical community has greatly increased for a variety of medical and psychological purposes.

How it works

This mind/body technique allows you to concentrate deeply and fully on a single idea while including such factors as role-playing, imagination, motivation, and the power of suggestion. It also requires that you truly desire to change a type of behavior. In fact, success might be greater in people who are more desperate to change behaviors.

What it does

Hypnosis is effective in alleviating chronic pain associated with certain cancers and with tension headaches. It also is used for many illnesses that are difficult to manage by conventional treatment, including:

- Arthritis
- Asthma
- Depression
- Irritable bowel syndrome
- Migraine headache pain
- Psychosomatic illness
- Smoking cessation
- Surgical pain
- Weight loss

Not everyone can benefit from hypnosis when treating behavioral or habitual problems. Only about 15 percent of the population is thought to be highly hypnotizable, while 25 percent is thought to be not hypnotizable at all. According to the American Association of Professional Hypnotherapists, there is a 75 to 90 percent chance of changing behavior with hypnotherapy. In one controlled trial of chronic asthmatic patients who were inadequately controlled by drugs, after one year of hypnotherapy, the duration of hospitalization stays and the side effects of medications both were reduced. Although air flow measurements gave variable results, more than 62 percent of patients receiving hypnotherapy reported improvement in their symptoms.

The basics

1. *How often should it be done?* One session may be enough, or it might take as many as 5 to 10 sessions with semiannual or annual treatments to make sure you are doing it correctly.

2. *How much does it cost?* Hypnosis costs from $75.00 to $150.00 for a two hour initial session, depending on therapist's credentials and locale.

3. *How long until it works?* With most people, they can find help in just one to two sessions, although tougher cases may take longer.

Seek a qualified clinical psychologist or psychiatrist to help decide whether hypnosis would be helpful and safe for you. It has been highly endorsed by the American Psychiatric Association and the American Psychological Association.

Light therapy

Light therapy involves using natural or artificial light to cause physiological changes in the human body. It is well-documented that light entering the eyes influences the pituitary and pineal glands, which control the entire endocrine system.

Although people have used sunlight for healing for centuries, light therapy is a recent alternative treatment. Doctors use bright-light therapy to relieve the symptoms associated with seasonal affective disorder (SAD), a psychological problem that occurs with the change of seasons and less daytime exposure. People who have SAD feel depressed and fatigued and may crave carbohydrates, which boost levels of serotonin in the body.

How it works

In light therapy, a special kind of light called broad-spectrum light is used to give people the effect of having a few extra hours of daylight each day. Using specially made light boxes, people are exposed to bright light and, subsequently, produce serotonin. Because of this boost of serotonin, light therapy may ease depression. At night when it is dark, the brain produces less serotonin and more melatonin. *Serotonin* is a neurotransmitter in the brain that is associated with a calming, anxiety-reducing reaction. *Melatonin* is a hormone naturally produced in the brain that helps us sleep deeply.

What it does

Light therapy is thought to be helpful for many physical and emotional problems including:

■ Jaundice in newborns

■ PMS

■ Rashes and skin irritations

■ Seasonal affective disorder (SAD)

■ Migraines

■ High blood pressure

- Stress
- Insomnia
- Herpes simplex

Some new uses for light or photodynamic therapy include:

- Mesothelioma (a cancer of the lung lining usually caused by asbestos)
- Ovarian cancer
- Bladder cancer
- Macular degeneration
- Barrett's esophagus
- Early esophageal cancer
- Endometriosis

Some proponents claim that light therapy can replace antidepressants for people suffering from depression or other psychological problems. There is no scientific evidence to advocate throwing out your meds just yet, however, although some signs have been promising. Using broad-spectrum lights, women with PMS frequently report less depression, less moodiness, better sleep, and better concentration. Researchers have shown that serotonin levels drop just before ovulation in women; this drop correlates with the onset of PMS symptoms. Serotonin levels also rebound with the onset of menstruation or when PMS symptoms decrease. Recent research suggests that PMS occurs in women with low base levels of serotonin. When serotonin levels drop further at ovulation, these levels fall low enough in PMS sufferers for symptoms to appear. Using phototherapy, women with PMS can keep their serotonin levels high enough to prevent their PMS symptoms from appearing.

The basics

1. *How often should it be done?* The intensity of the light is a vital factor in determining your physiological response. Two standard intensities are suggested for use: 2,500 lux for an average of 2 hours per day or 10,000 lux for an average of 30 minutes per day.

2. *How much does it cost?* The cost of light fixtures can range from $50 to several hundred dollars. Many insurance companies have reimbursed the purchase price of light fixtures for the treatment of seasonal affective disorder (SAD), PMS, sleep disorders, and problems adapting to shift work.

3. *How long until it works?* This depends on what you are using light therapy to treat. Many mildly depressed individuals have seen improvement after just 30 minutes of bright-light exposure; others may need up to two hours daily.

Studies have shown that, with regular sessions, some individuals become happier and more energetic. More severe forms of seasonal depression may require a combination of phototherapy and antidepressant medications. This is consistent with the belief that light therapy helps people with winter depression because it makes up for light lost during shorter winter days.

Just the facts

- There are a host of effective mind/body treatments that are free and that can be done just about anywhere to relax and to reduce anxiety and tension.

- Biofeedback is an effective tool for destressing and for chronic health problems such as urinary incontinence.

- Hypnotherapy does not work in all people and should be used by people who find it easy to relax and daydream.

- Light therapy triggers physiological changes in the brain, causing a boost in serotonin and a sense of calmness.

Food as Medicine

Chapter 9

"You are what you eat." How many times did your mom say that when you were loading up on your favorite junk food? Simply stated, nutritional therapy is based on the premise that nutrients in food can help prevent disease and heal the body. As discussed in Chapter 2, being at the proper weight and eating healthful foods is important; it can minimize your chances of weight gain and can maximize energy and alertness. Nutritional therapy goes beyond counting fat grams and calories. It also focuses on how immune-boosting nutrients—vitamins, minerals, antioxidants, and phytochemicals, among others—work together to help optimize immune function.

Nutritional therapy

For centuries, civilizations have used food to heal the sick. It wasn't until the past decade, however, that nutritional therapy came into the limelight. Scientists who used to believe germs caused diseases now tell us that we have great control in our health and that lifestyle habits (such as the foods we eat) are an important key.

Nutritional therapy is based on eating the right foods to stay healthy, to feel productive, and to have energy. Just like a car needs the proper gasoline to make it run, our bodies need the right balance of protein, carbohydrates, and fat to stay well. They also need a host of vitamins, minerals, antioxidants, phytochemicals, and known and little-known nutrients to help balance it all.

How it works

> " Let food be thy medicine and thy medicine be thy food.
> —Hippocrates "

Because our bodies need specific nutrients to function properly, each vitamin or mineral regulates a bodily process. The mineral calcium, for example, keeps bones strong and helps prevent osteoporosis. Vitamin A is an important anti-aging nutrient that helps keep skin supple and smooth. When our bodies function well, we are given the bonus of delaying the onset of degenerative diseases. In fact, persuasive research shows that dietary habits play a key role in five of the nation's leading causes of death: cancer, stroke, heart disease, diabetes, and atherosclerosis. This is why nutritional therapy is crucial to help keep your body functioning at its best.

What it does

Nutritional therapy can keep you disease-free or can help you continue optimum health even with a chronic disease. The properties possessed by certain foods can help us feel alert, calm, or sleepy; can keep our bones strong, our blood pressure normal, and our heart healthy; and can help us stay at a normal weight and feel energetic.

Nutrient-dense foods can help heal your body and keep your immune system functioning at its highest level. Taking in fewer calories and exercising to burn more of them off will enable you to lose weight. A diet high in certain nutrients such as selenium can help your body stay cancer-free or can boost health if you have cancer. Although some people claim specific foods burn calories while you eat them or actually cure cancer, as of yet, there is no notable scientific research that singles out certain foods as miracle cures for cancer or obesity.

The basics

1. *How often should it be done?* Nutritional therapy should be ongoing. With every meal or snack you eat, the focus should be on feeding your body foods that will keep it healthy and running strong.

2. *How much does it cost?* Natural foods are an inexpensive form of healing therapy. Bottled vitamins, minerals, or other supplements can be quite costly depending on the type, your location, and how many you purchase.

3. *How long until it works?* Nutritional therapy begins to work as soon as the foods enter your body. If you are eating protein such as fish to increase alertness, you may notice a difference within the hour. But if you are adding more vegetables and fruits to your diet to ward off cancer or to prolong longevity, the benefits may not be noticed for years, even though chemical changes are occurring within the body each day.

There's not a magic food that carries the key to good health. The American Dietetic Association, the nation's largest organization of nutrition professionals, recommends obtaining adequate nutrients from a wide variety of foods to promote optimum health and to reduce the risk of chronic disease. Use the Food Guide Pyramid (page 31) as a basis for meal planning and lean heavily on fruits, vegetables, lentils, whole grains, and low-fat dairy products.

The new vita-mania

Recommended Dietary Allowances (RDAs) are issued by the Food and Nutrition Board of the National Academy of Sciences. These amounts are the levels of nutrients thought to be adequate to meet the known nutrient needs of most healthy individuals. This means the RDAs will help prevent deficiency-related diseases such as beriberi or scurvy. Overwhelming scientific evidence points to certain nutrients that should be ingested for disease prevention. Studies show, for example, that vitamin E is a protector against heart disease when taken in amounts greater than the recommended allowance. The RDAs, however, have not kept up with scientific breakthroughs.

So how do you know what is safe and what is not? Again, can easily be addressed by choosing a variety of healthful foods in your daily diet. If your eating habits are poor, you may need to take supplements. But which supplements do you choose? Although there are 50 known essential nutrients—almost all of which are vitamins and minerals—there are close to 1,000 dietary supplements. In fact, it is estimated that more than 100 million Americans spend $6.5 billion a year on vitamin and mineral pills, according to the Council for Responsible Nutrition in Washington, a trade group for the vitamin supplement industry. (See Table 9.1 to assess the type of supplement you take.)

TABLE 9.1   DIFFERENT TYPES OF SUPPLEMENTS

- **Time-released** supplements dissolve slowly in the intestine over a 6-to-12-hour period, increasing the absorption of a vitamin.

- **Chelated** minerals are designed to increase absorption in the body.

- **Superpotency or therapeutic** supplements contain at least one ingredient in a dose 10 or more times greater than the DV (daily value).

Healing nutrients repair the body

Nutrients are special compounds found in foods that support the body's repair, growth, and wellness.

They include vitamins, minerals, amino acids, essential fatty acids, water, and the calorie sources of carbohydrates, protein, and fat. Some nutrients can be made by the body (*nonessential nutrients*); others must come from the diet (*essential nutrients*). A deficiency of either nutrient type may lead to illness if left untreated. The essential nutrients fall into six categories:

- **Proteins** are found in meat, poultry, fish, eggs, cheese, milk and milk products, peas, and dried beans. They supply amino acids—the building blocks that build, repair, and maintain your body tissue.

- **Carbohydrates** are the body's main source of energy (or calories) and are classified as either complex carbohydrates (or starches) and sugars. **Fiber** is another carbohydrate that aids in digestion and that helps protect you from some diseases.

Moneysaver
Before you spend a fortune at a health food store, figure out what your body needs to stay well. Start with a supplement that has at least 20 vitamins and minerals known to be healthful. Add iron if you are a woman of child-bearing age. (Men and post-menopausal women do not need extra iron.) Then add at least 500 milligrams of vitamin C daily, calcium supplements of 500 to 1,500 milligrams daily (depending on your age and sex—women need more as they grow older), and 400 International Units (IUs) of vitamin D. If your fruit and vegetable intake is low, consider adding 15 milligrams (25,000 IUs) of beta-carotene. Talk to a certified nutritionist to determine whether you need to add other nutrients in the form of supplements.

TABLE 9.2   VITAMINS AND MINERALS

Water-Soluble Vitamins

- Vitamin C (ascorbic acid)
- Vitamin B_1 (thiamine)
- Vitamin B_2 (riboflavin)
- Vitamin B_3 (niacin)
- Vitamin B_5 (pantothenic acid)
- Vitamin B_6 (pyridoxine)
- Vitamin B_7 (biotin)
- Vitamin B_9 (folic acid)
- Vitamin B_{12} (cobalamin)

Fat-Soluble Vitamins

- Vitamin A
- Vitamin D
- Vitamin E
- Vitamin K

Minerals

- Boron
- Calcium
- Chloride
- Chromium
- Cobalt
- Copper
- Fluoride
- Iodine
- Iron
- Magnesium
- Manganese

- Molybdenum
- Phosphorus
- Potassium
- Selenium
- Sodium
- Sulfur
- Vanadium
- Zinc

- **Fats** supply energy and transport nutrients. Fats fall into three main categories: saturated (animal, dairy, coconut oil, and palm oil), monounsaturated (canola and olive oil), and polyunsaturated (sunflower, corn, soybean, and safflower oil).
- **Vitamins** regulate the body's processes, setting off chemical reactions in the cells. Each vitamin performs a specific function in the body, and no single food contains all vitamins (see Table 9.2).
- **Minerals** also help set off chemical reactions in cells. These substances are required for normal growth and development and for the maintenance of good health (see Table 9.2).
- **Water** helps regulate your body temperature and other body processes. It carries nutrients to cells and carries waste material away.

Antioxidants

Almost 9 out of 10 doctors endorse the role of antioxidants in fighting disease, according to an informal poll by *Medical Tribune,* a newspaper for physicians. These essential nutrients help protect your body against life's stressors. New studies have found that antioxidants can prevent or repair cell

Bright Idea
Even when you suffer from a mild illness such as a common cold, nutrition is vital. Researchers have found that sucking on zinc-gluconate lozenges at the start of a cold may lessen its severity. One study at Dartmouth College reported that students who took zinc lozenges at the onset of a cold had only five days of symptoms compared with nine days for students who received placebos. This may be because zinc has an antiviral effect in the mouth and the nose.

damage that initiates or promotes cancer and can actually block tumor growth. Antioxidant food sources are rich in beta-carotene and vitamins C and E. These nutrients are thought to play a role in protecting the body from free radicals, which destroy cell membranes, damage DNA, and may be a root cause of certain types of cancer, heart disease, and even the aging process itself. Eating to slow the aging process and to stay disease-free requires a diet rich in antioxidants.

The following are some antioxidant food sources you can add to your diet:

- **Beta-carotene.** Beta-carotene, found in apricots, carrots, cantaloupe, pumpkin, and spinach, is converted to vitamin A in the body. This antioxidant can protect against the damaging effects of the sun's ultraviolet rays; can protect the mucous membranes of the mouth, nose, throat, and lungs, thereby reducing susceptibility to infections; can counteract night-blindness and weak eyesight; can reduce the risk of lung cancer; and can aid in bone and teeth formation. Some preliminary studies indicate that beta-carotene may help stave off mental impairment. In a study of 5,100 people from age 55 to 95 at the Erasmus University Medical School in Rotterdam, the Netherlands, people who consumed less than 0.9 milligrams of beta-carotene were almost twice as likely to suffer memory impairment, disorientation, and difficulty solving problems than people who consumed 2.1 milligrams a day or more.

  Because of a great deal of media attention, most people think only beta-carotene has antioxidant properties. Many other carotenoid compounds also have antioxidant properties, however, including:

- **Alpha-carotene** (found in carrots, cantaloupe, and pumpkin)
- **Gamma-carotene** (found in apricots and tomatoes)
- **Beta-cryptoxanthin** (found in mangoes, nectarines, peaches, and tangerines)
- **Lycopene** (found in guava, pink grapefruit, tomatoes, and watermelon)
- **Lutein and zeaxanthin** (found in beets, corn, and collard and mustard greens)

  Current RDAs for vitamin A are 5,000 International Units (IUs) for men and 4,000 IUs for women. Although many people try to get vitamin A and beta-carotene from supplements, using natural foods is best (see Table 9.3). Because vitamin A can build up in your system, it is possible to take too much of the supplement, leading to toxicity. In addition, your supplement may not be fully absorbed into the body, and the potency can diminish over a period of time.

- **Vitamin C.** Vitamin C (ascorbic acid) protects against infection and aids in wound healing. It is especially important when you are under stress. Vitamin C also plays a vital role in boosting levels of *norepinephrine,* a brain chemical that produces a feeling of alertness and that increases concentration. A deficiency of vitamin C can influence your mood as well, leaving you less attentive. Although there is no direct research evaluating vitamin C in preventing colds, several studies have shown that taking

TABLE 9.3   FOOD SOURCES OF BETA-CAROTENE

Apricots	Mustard greens
Asparagus	Spinach
Beef liver	Squash, winter
Broccoli	Sweet potato
Cantaloupe	Watermelon
Carrots	Yellow corn
Kale	

1,000 milligrams daily may shorten the duration and the severity of a cold. Perhaps this is because vitamin C has an antihistamine effect. Recent studies also indicate that vitamin C can impede tumor growth, can protect blood vessels, and may even reduce blood pressure.

It is easy to get an ample supply of vitamin C through your diet if you choose from a variety of fresh fruits and vegetables (see Table 9.4).

▪ **Vitamin E.** Sophisticated research has found vitamin E to be a powerful antioxidant and to be important to the body for the maintenance of cell membranes. This vitamin, already praised for healthy hearts, has an antioxidant effect that can help prevent breast cancer and can delay Alzheimer's disease. In one study at the National Cancer Institute (1997), a derivative of vitamin E called VES blocked the growth of and even killed breast-cancer cells. Comprehensive research reported in *The New England Journal of Medicine* reported that large doses of vitamin E (2,000 IUs a day) dramatically delayed the progression of Alzheimer's disease. Some preliminary research shows possible prevention of

TABLE 9.4   FOOD SOURCES OF VITAMIN C

Broccoli	Papaya
Cantaloupe	Red, green, or yellow pepper
Cauliflower	Sweet potato
Kale	strawberries
Kiwi	Tomato juice
Orange juice	

gallstones and cataracts and treatment of asthma and male infertility with vitamin E.

Vitamin E supplements may help boost immune function in older adults, according to research done at Tufts University. In 88 healthy people 65 or older, taking 200 milligrams of vitamin E every day for eight months dramatically boosted immune functioning and cut infections by 30 percent. Vitamin E appears to stimulate the function of T-cells, which are important fighters in the immune system.

Vitamin E is taken in through vegetables and seed oils, but you would have to eat 930 almonds to get the benefit of 400 IUs of vitamin E—the amount necessary to benefit the heart. To get 400 IUs from food, you would have to eat about 20,000 calories a day of mostly fat! (See Table 9.5.) Some researchers feel the current Recommended Dietary Allowance (RDA) for vitamin E—15 International Units (IUs) for men and 12 IUs for women—may be too low for disease protection. Taking 400 IUs a day, 13 times the RDA amount, appears to lower heart disease risk.

TABLE 9.5   FOOD SOURCES OF VITAMIN E

Almonds	Lobster
Corn oil	Peanut butter
Cod-liver oil	Safflower oil
Corn oil margarine	Salmon steak
Hazelnuts	Sunflower seeds

Power-packed phytochemicals

These unique plant chemicals, found in certain fruits and vegetables, are essential in boosting immune function and in preventing diseases (see Table 9.6). *Crucifous vegetables* include bok choy, broccoli, Brussels sprouts, cabbage, and cauliflower, among others.

Flavonoids

Flavonoids (or bioflavonoids) include about 4,000 compounds responsible for the colors of fruits and flowers. Hosts of experiments on the bioflavonoids found in the soft white skin of citrus fruits have suggested that these key nutrients increase immune system activation and play numerous anticancer roles. These biochemically active substances accompany vitamin C in plants and act as an antioxidant. You can find bioflavonoids in citrus fruits, green peppers, lemons, limes, oranges, carrots, berries, parsley, squash, apples, grapes, cherries, eggplant, and tomatoes. Tea, red wine, and parsley also are good sources. Flavonoids may even help protect against heart disease, according to Finnish researchers in a study reported in The British Medical Journal (1996). In a recent study of 5,133 men and women who were followed for about 25 years, those whose diets were highest in flavonoids were less likely to die from heart disease than those whose diets contained fewer of these antioxidants.

TABLE 9.6

Phytochemical	Food Sources	Health Effect
Bioflavonoids	Most vegetables and fruits, licorice, flax seed, green tea	Cancer prevention
Capsaicin	Hot chili peppers, Thai peppers, jalapenos	Anti-inflammatory, cancer prevention
Carotenoids	Carrots, winter squash, sweet potatoes, apricots, spinach, kale, parsley, soybeans, cereal grains, cruciferous vegetables, citrus	Antioxidant, heart disease and cancer prevention, improved immune function
Ellagic acid	Grapes, raspberries, strawberries, apples	Heart disease and cancer prevention
Indoles	Cruciferous vegetables	Cancer prevention
Isoflavones	Soybeans, legumes	Cancer prevention, menopause symptom reduction
Isothiocyanates	Cruciferous vegetables, horseradish	Cancer prevention
Limonoids	Terpenes citrus fruits, cumin caraway seeds, ginger	Cancer prevention
Linolenic Acid	Leafy vegetables, seeds, flax seed	Heart disease and cancer prevention
Lycopene	Tomatoes, watermelon, pink grapefruit, guava, red peppers	Cancer prevention
Monoterpenes	Garlic, parsley, squash, basil, mint, eggplant, citrus, tomatoes, fennel, cruciferous vegetables	Antioxidant, heart disease and cancer prevention
Phenolic acids	Garlic, green tea, cereal grains, soybeans, fruits, vegetables, licorice root, flax seed	Antioxidant, heart disease and cancer prevention
Plant sterols	Broccoli, cabbage, soy products, peppers, whole grains	Cancer prevention
Sulfides (allyl)	Garlic, onions, cruciferous vegetables	Cancer prevention, suppression of tumor development
Sulforaphane	Cruciferous vegetables	Cancer prevention

Quercetin

This very highly concentrated form of bioflavonoid is found in citrus fruits, red and yellow onions, and broccoli. Quercetin can reduce inflammation associated with allergies, can inhibit the growth of head and neck cancers, and may reverse transcriptase, the method HIV uses to replicate itself. Other citrus flavonoids include *hesperidin,* which is said to raise blood levels of the "good" high-density lipoprotein and to lower the "bad" low-density lipoprotein and triglycerides, and *tangeritin,* which induces apoptosis (*programmed cell death*) in leukemia cells but does not harm normal cells.

Glutathione

Another nutrient found to strengthen the immune system so it can fight other infections is *glutathione.* This powerful antioxidant is most plentiful in the red, pulpy area of the watermelon near the rind. It also can be found in cruciferous vegetables.

Dietary fiber

Dietary fiber is another bonus we get from eating plenty of fruits and vegetables. Fiber moves foods and toxins quickly through the digestive tract, allowing less time for any possible cancer-causing agents to come in contact with the intestines, the colon, or the rectum. According to the National Cancer Institute, a diet high in fiber cuts the risk of colon cancer by up to 70 percent. It may also lower the risk of kidney and gallstones and may ease constipation. Fiber ferments in the colon and increases the amount of oxygen, which in turn diminishes the action of the harmful bacteria. The American Dietetic Association's recommendation for adults is 20 to 35 grams of fiber daily. About one-fourth of

TABLE 9.7   FOODS HIGH IN SOLUBLE FIBER

Acorn squash	Dates
Apples	Dried beans
Baked potatoes	Lentils
Blueberries	Peas
Broccoli	Prunes
Cabbage	Pumpkin
Carrots	Raspberries
Cauliflower	Strawberries
Citrus fruits	Sweet potatoes

your daily fiber intake should consist of the soluble type of fiber found in oats, beans, fruits, and vegetables (see Table 9.7). The rest of your fiber intake should be the insoluble type found in wheat bran and whole grains.

Essential building blocks: amino acids

Amino acids are supplied by protein and are the building blocks that build, repair, and maintain your body tissues. Nine of them are essential and must come from food because the body does not make them. Other amino acids are nonessential because the body makes them if you eat enough calories and amino acids each day. Besides building cells and repairing tissue, amino acids form antibodies to combat invading bacteria and viruses. (Check out Table 9.8 to understand the bodily functions of amino acids.)

Other healing foods

Dr. Judith Wurtman, a nutrition researcher at the Massachusetts Institute of Technology, has found that certain foods affect brain chemicals to influence our mood, our mental energy, our performance (see Table 9.9).

TABLE 9.8   AMINO ACIDS

Essential Amino Acids	Function in the Body
Leucine and Isoleucine	Keeps you alert, gives energy. Can be found in brown rice, beans, meats, nuts, soy flour, and whole wheat.
Lysine	Forms collagen, may be effective against herpes, aids in production of hormones. Can be found in cheese, fish, eggs, lima beans, milk, potatoes, red meat, soy.
Methionine	Prevents hair and skin problems, lowers cholesterol levels, protects kidneys. Can be found in beans, eggs, fish, garlic, lentils, meat, onions, yogurt.
Phenylalanine	Produces norepinephrine, keeps you alert, improves memory, reduces hunger. Can be found in meats and cheese.
Threonine	Aids digestive process, assists metabolism. Can be found in vegetables.
Tryptophan	Natural relaxant, alleviates insomnia, helps in treatment of migraines. Can be found in fish, beef, chicken, eggs, and soy.
Valine	Promotes mental alertness, calms emotions. Can be found in dairy products, grains, meat, mushrooms, peanuts, and soy.

Non-Essential Amino Acids	Function in the Body
Alanine	Energizes brain and central nervous system, strengthens immune function. Can be found in meats.
Arginine	Improves immune response, promotes wound healing, releases growth hormones. Can be found in carob, chocolate, coconut, dairy products, meat, oats, peanuts, and wheat germ.
Aspartic acid	Increases endurance, energizes. Can be found in plant protein, especially in sprouting seeds.

Cystine	Antioxidant, slows aging process, stimulates wound healing. Can be found in meat, poultry, fish, and soy.
Glutamic acid	Improves mental capabilities, controls cravings for sugar, energizes. Can be found in protein foods.
Glycine	Boosts immune function. Can be found in protein foods.
Histidine	Helps heal allergic diseases, arthritis, ulcers, and anemia. Can be found in rice, wheat, and rye.
Proline	Maintains and strengthens heart muscles. Can be found in meats.
Serine	Strengthens immune system. Can be found in meat, dairy products, wheat gluten, peanuts, and soy.
Taurine	Reduces changes of aging, clears free radical wastes. Can be found in eggs, fish, meat, and milk.
Tyrosine	Overcomes depression, increases alertness, promotes healthy thyroid function. Can be found in almonds, avocados, bananas, dairy products, lima beans, pumpkin seeds.

Pump you up, calm you down

Some "persuasive" foods high in protein—such as turkey, tuna, or chicken—are rich in an amino acid called *tyrosine,* which boosts levels of the brain chemicals dopamine and norepinephrine. This, in turn, creates a feeling of alertness and improves your concentration. Studies also have shown that foods high in tyrosine help counter the effects of stress in the body.

Calming foods—such as breads, cereal, pasta, or sherbet—are high in carbohydrates and cause the amino acid tryptophan to enter the brain in great amounts. Tryptophan is then converted into a

TABLE 9.9   FOODS THAT ENERGIZE OR RELAX THE BODY

Pump You Up Foods

Beans	Peas
Beef	Poultry
Cheese	Soy products
Fish	Yogurt
Milk	

Calm You Down Foods

Bagels	Pasta
Bread	Potatoes
Cereal	Rice
Crackers	Sherbet
Muffins	

neurotransmitter called *serotonin,* a mood-elevating brain chemical. When serotonin levels rise, we experience a calming effect and feel upbeat for a period of time. Revealing studies have shown that, by including plenty of foods high in complex carbohydrates in your diet, you can boost the level of serotonin and can reap the reward of a calming feeling throughout the day, along with a deeper, healing sleep.

10 nutrition superstars

1. **Broccoli.** This green tree-like vegetable is full of indoles, isothiocyanates, and sulforaphane—phytochemicals shown to trigger enzyme systems that block or suppress cellular DNA damage, to reduce tumor size (in animal studies), and to decrease the effectiveness of estrogen-like hormones. In other words, it packs a power punch of healing nutrition! If you want the highest concentration of these cancer-fighting compounds, get broccoli sprouts at your local

health food store. The sprouts have 10 to 100 times more sulphoraphane than mature broccoli.

2. **Dairy products.** Low-fat dairy products—such as low-fat milk, buttermilk, cheese and cheese products, cottage cheese, ice milk, and yogurt—will help protect you from several serious problems associated with aging. Studies show that a diet high in low-fat dairy products, fruits, and vegetables significantly lowers blood pressure. The calcium and vitamin D in dairy products helps to keep bones strong and to prevent osteoporosis and fractures.

3. **Fish.** New studies show that eating fish at least once a week can cut the risk of sudden cardiac death. One 11-year study of 20,551 male physicians found that men who ate fish once a week had half the risk of sudden cardiac death compared to men who ate fish less than once a month. Although this study focused on men, it wouldn't hurt women to get in on the bandwagon! Substances in fish called omega-3 fatty acids may have a protective effect against sudden cardiac death, possibly by preventing potentially dangerous arrhythmias or irregular heart beats. Some heart-healthy fish include:

- Anchovies
- Bluefish
- Lobster
- Mackerel
- Salmon
- Sardines
- Scallops

- Tuna
- Whitefish

4. **Garlic.** According to scientific research, garlic contains chemicals that act like ACE (angiotensin-converting enzyme) inhibitors, prescription drugs commonly given to lower blood pressure and cholesterol and to protect the heart. Garlic supplements reduce blood pressure by dilating blood vessels. In fact, some studies have revealed that ingesting as much as one or two cloves of fresh garlic can lower mild blood pressure an average of 8 percent in one to three months.

Researchers have found that garlic and onions can block formation of *nitrosamines,* which are powerful carcinogens that target several sites in the body (usually the liver, colon, and breasts). The more pungent the garlic or onion, the more abundant the sulfur compounds. The only problem is . . . you have to eat them raw!

5. **Green tea.** Green tea is a powerful antioxidant that may help prevent liver, pancreatic, breast, lung, esophageal, and skin cancers. It also has been found to help reduce the risk of cardiovascular disease and stroke, and some new studies indicate it may help prevent osteoporosis. Researchers report that a nontoxic chemical found in green tea, *epigallocatechin-3 gallate,* acts against *urokinase* (an enzyme crucial for cancer growth.) One cup of green tea contains between 100 and 200 milligrams of the antitumor ingredient.

6. **Olive oil.** Olive oil, a monounsaturated fat, also has been promoted recently as a heart-healthy oil that is preferable to other vegetable oils and

margarine. In Mediterranean countries, olive oil is widely used both for cooking and as a salad oil. Breast cancer rates are 50 percent lower in Mediterranean countries than in the United States.

7. **Red grapes.** A new super antioxidant called *Activin* has been discovered inside the seeds of red grapes. Byproducts of red grapes—such as red wine, juice, or seeds—may offer significant protection against certain types of cancer, heart disease, rheumatoid arthritis, cataracts, and many other chronic and degenerative diseases. Some studies show that Activin is up to seven times more powerful as an antioxidant than vitamins C, E, and beta-carotene. This may explain why red wine is healthier than white wine in protecting you from heart disease. Earlier studies have touted the cancer-fighting properties of Resveratrol, a compound extracted from red grape skins. Recent studies conclude that a glass of wine a day may also reduce the risk of age-associated vision loss.

8. **Soy.** Soy protein is an easy, inexpensive, and healthy alternative to meat. Soy products are dairy-free and do not contain saturated fat. For years, soybeans have played an integral part in the Asian culture. In fact, heart disease, breast cancer, prostate cancer, and osteoporosis rates for Asian men and women are much lower than for Americans. In a recent study of 1,000 people reported in the *American Journal of Epidemiology* (1996), people who ate soybeans in some form at least once a week had half the risk of developing the polyps that are precursors to colon cancer compared to people who did not eat soybeans.

Isoflavones are phytonutrients found in soy that are converted into phytoestrogens (plant estrogens that are close in structure to the body's form of estrogen) in the body (see Table 9.10 for Soy Superstars—foods high in isoflavones). These plant ingredients mimic the hormone estrogen. They appear to have no harmful side effects and can relieve menopausal symptoms that frequently occur because of plummeting estrogen levels. Studies show that soy isolate also can effectively prevent the rise in serum cholesterol associated with ovarian-hormone deficiency.

If you want to increase the soy in your diet but aren't fond of tofu, try soy-based products (see Table 9.11). Over the past decade, more than 2,000 new soy products have been introduced to consumers, from meatless pepperoni, salami, hot dogs, and bacon to puddings and dairy alternatives. Some calcium-rich soy foods include tahini, calcium-set tofu, fortified soy milk, textured vegetable protein, and soy nuts.

9. **Spinach.** You've probably heard a lot about *homocysteine* lately on the news. This naturally occuring blood protein promotes artery clogging and is a by-product of meals high in protein. With the latest health concerns about *homocysteine,* nutritionists tell us the cure is simple: Add more folic acid. Folic acid dramatically lowers elevated levels of homocysteine in the blood. Age-related macular degeneration (AMD), the leading cause of blindness in older people, also is significantly decreased by eating this green vegetable. Spinach is high in folacin, a nutrient crucial during early pregnancy to

TABLE 9.10   SOY SUPERSTARS

Food	Serving	Isoflavones (milligrams)
Roasted soy nuts	1/4 cup	62
Tempeh	1/2 cup	35
Low-fat tofu	1/2 cup	35
Regular tofu	1/2 cup	35
Soy milk	1 cup	30
Low-fat soy milk	1 cup	20

prevent neural-tube defects in children. This power vegetable also is abundant in beta-carotene, vitamins A and C, and potassium.

10. **Tomatoes.** Preliminary research confirms that the potent antioxidant *lycopene*, which is prominent in tomatoes, may be more powerful than beta-carotene, alpha-carotene, and vitamin E. This antioxidant is associated with protection against heart disease and certain cancers such as prostate and lung cancer. Cooking tomatoes releases the lycopene and makes it available for absorption into your body.

Healing diets

If you feel the need to concentrate on a particular condition or area of wellness, certain diet regimens can help you do just that. (Do not start any new diet regimen without first consulting your physician.)

■ **DASH diet.** This "miracle" diet rich in fruits and vegetables has been found to lower blood pressure in just eight weeks. In the study known as DASH (Dietary Approaches to Stop Hypertension), participants ate a diet low in fat (less than 30 percent of daily calories from fat) and high in fruits and vegetables (eight to 10 servings a day) and grains (seven to eight servings).

TABLE 9.11   THE LATEST IN SOY PRODUCTS

The following are just a few of the soy products available at supermarkets, natural food stores, and Asian markets:

- **Isolated soy protein.** This powder form of soy protein has a myriad of uses. You add it to casseroles, pasta dishes, drinks, and more. One ounce contains approximately 23 grams of soy protein.

- **Miso.** This rich, salty paste made from soybeans and grains is aged for one to three years in wooden vats. Used to flavor soups, sauces, and marinades, miso can taste delicate and sweet or savory and salty. Miso contains isoflavones, but since the serving size is small (1 teaspoon), you get a minimal amount of benefit.

- **Soya flour.** This finely ground powder has more flavor than soy flour and is milder in taste. One-half cup provides 20 grams of soy protein.

- **Soybeans.** Dried soybeans have a delicious nutty flavor and can be used in recipes such as baked beans or chili. Just remember to soak them first as you would any dried bean. You can add them to soups or use them in any recipe that calls for lentils. One-half cup provides 14.3 grams of soy protein.

- **Soy flour.** Soy flour is made from roasted soybeans that are ground into a very fine powder. You can purchase this flour in defatted, low-fat, or full-fat versions. One-half cup of full-fat soy flour contains 15 grams of soy protein, while the defatted soy flour has 24 grams of soy protein. Use soy flour to replace up to one-fourth of the regular flour in recipes.

- **Soy granules.** These tasty, nutty-like granules shake directly out of the container. You can soak them and then use them for a filler in recipes, or you can sprinkle them directly on food such as ice cream or yogurt. Soy granules have 23 grams of soy protein per one-fourth cup.

- **Soy milk.** This liquid can be used in virtually any recipe that calls for milk. The benefit is that eight ounces contains approximately 10 grams of soy protein. Be sure to look for soy milk that is calcium-fortified.

- **Tempeh.** This thin cake is made from fermented soybeans. It has an interesting nutty or smokey taste and a chewy texture. Four ounces contain almost 17 grams of soy protein. Tempeh frequently is used as a substitute for beef and contains more whole soybeans and fiber than soy milk or tofu.

- **Textured soy protein** *or* **Textured Vegetable Product (TVP).** This is a quick-cooking meat substitute made from low-fat soy flour. It can be used as a beef substitute for burgers, chili, sloppy Joes, and more. It is available in many forms including strips, chunks, flakes, and granular. One-half cup serving has 11 grams of soy protein. Veggie burgers made with soy protein may or may not have isoflavones. Some processed soy foods have had the isoflavones removed.

- **Tofu.** This soy product also is called bean curd. It is a tasteless food, but by blending it with herbs, spices, and other foods, it becomes very appetizing. Tofu comes in a myriad of varieties including soft, firm, extra firm, and silken and also is available in regular and low-fat forms. Four ounces of firm tofu contain 9 to 13 grams of soy protein; the same amount of soft tofu contains 9 grams of soy protein. Watch out for the fat in tofu. A three-ounce portion of lite tofu contains about 1 gram of fat; the same portion of regular firm tofu contains up to 7 grams of fat.

At the end of the study, systolic blood pressure readings (the top number) dropped an average of 11 points. The diastolic pressure (the bottom number) dropped more than five points. Speculation was that the diet was high in calcium, potassium, and magnesium from the fresh produce and naturally low in sodium.

Bright Idea
You can easily get the minimum daily intake of folate (400 micrograms) by adding the following to your diet:

Dark green vegetables

Fruits, especially citrus fruits or juices

Whole grains

Enriched breakfast cereals

- **High-protein diet.** It seems like every seven years the same high-protein diet crops up again. Although it has failed miserably in the past, this high-protein, high-fat, low-carbohydrate diet is based on the assertion that carbohydrates, not fats, make us fat. The diet allows you to eat until you are full, but only from certain food groups. Although such a diet is not recommended for long-term weight management, a recent study at Ohio State University showed that a high-protein, low-calorie diet may help obese hospital patients control their blood sugar levels. The study, which appeared in a recent issue of the *American Journal of Clinical Nutrition*, showed that the new diet allows obese patients to burn body fat for energy without endangering their health and to maintain a stable blood sugar level, which helps them avoid diabetes and hyperglycemia.

- **Low-fat diet.** Dr. Dean Ornish's very low-fat diet appeared to work for people seriously ill with heart disease, as he described in his book *Eat More, Weigh Less* (HarperCollins, 1993). This heart-healthy diet includes mostly carbohydrates, some protein, and very little fat (less than 10 percent). Although it was formulated to heal ailing hearts, it also has been found helpful for cancer prevention and weight loss. Before you start piling on the fruits and vegetables, however, you must know that the only way you can cut fat to 10 percent of calories is to eliminate more sources of animal protein from your diet. See Figure 9.1 and Table 9.12 for easy ways to read labels and to keep your diet lower in saturated fat.

- **Macrobiotic diet.** Macrobiotic is a semi-vegetarian diet that is claimed to improve health and to prolong life. It is based on the need to keep the principles of yin (the force of expansion) and yang (the force of contraction) balanced in the body. In this light, cooking appears to "yangize" yin vegetables with fire, salt, or pressure to keep balance. Brown rice is the basic staple in the diet, which is said to balance yin and yang; a myriad of vegetables, whole grains, and some fish are added as complements to the meal. Proponents suggest the diet is effective in preventing and treating cancer, heart disease, AIDS, and other serious medical problems, but there is no scientific evidence to support these claims. Some versions of macrobiotic diets contain adequate amounts of nutrients, but others do not. Deficiencies of

Watch Out! Although the high-protein, high-fat, low-carbohydrate diet works well for some people for quick weight reduction, this is a ketogenic diet (causing ketosis—when a shortage of glucose forces your body to burn fat as a source of energy) and has serious risks. Excreting potassium and sodium along with the ketones can disrupt heart rhythms, an increase in uric acid can cause kidney stones and gout attacks, and a loss of calcium in urine raises the risk of osteoporosis. Look out for rapid weight loss—it can be associated with gall stones.

"Staying on a 10-percent fat diet is probably one of the most difficult challenges I've undertaken, yet the results of losing 40 pounds and reducing my blood pressure were astonishing.
—Miriam, 58, legal secretary"

vitamin B_{12}, iron, and vitamin D also have been reported in people on strict macrobiotic diets for prolonged periods of time.

To see if a food is high, moderate, or low in fat, it is important to read the label. Package labels include the ingredients, calories, fat content, nutrients, sodium and fiber contents, and much more information for the consumer (see sample label).

Finely Shredded Parmesan Cheese

Ingredients: Part-skim milk, cheese culture, salt, enzymes, aged over 10 months.

Nutrition Facts

Serving size 2 Tsp (5g)
Servings per container 17

Amount Per Serving	
Calories 20	
Calories from Fat 10	
	% Daily Value*
Total Fat 1.5 g	2%
Saturated Fat 1 g	5%
Cholesterol less than 5 mg	1%
Sodium 75 mg	3%
Total Carbohydrate 0g	0%
Dietary Fiber 0g	0%
Sugars 0g	
Protein 2g	
Vitamin A 0%*	**Vitamin C** 0%
Calcium 4%*	**Iron** 0%

* Percent Daily Values are based on a 2,000-calorie diet. Your daily values may be higher or lower depending on your calorie needs.

Figure 9.1: Sample Food Package Label.

TABLE 9.12   HIGH OR LOW FAT?

After reading the label, you can figure out the fat content using the following information:

1 gram of fat = 9 calories

If the serving has 2 grams of fat, then:

$2 \times 9 = 18$ calories from fat

If the total calories for a serving are 100, then:

$18/100 = 18\%$ of calories from fat

■ **Mediterranean diet.** Recent studies have found that the dietary habits of many Mediterranean countries may be beneficial to the heart. The people in these countries, whose chief dietary fat is olive oil, have low cholesterol levels and lower rates of coronary artery disease than people in Western nations. There are many factors to look at when considering the Mediterranean diet. These people use plenty of olive oil, which is full of cholesterol-cutting monounsaturated fats, but they also eat a diet high in fruits and vegetables and low in meat. Grains, potatoes, pasta, legumes, vegetables, garlic, and, of course, olive oil make up the staples of this diet. Before you take the bottle of olive oil and pour it on your food, however, keep the total picture in mind. A balanced diet containing a variety of nutritious foods is the best diet.

■ **Vegetarian diet.** Some people believe vegetarianism is the new wave of medicine for the future because plants have many benefits in the prevention of chronic diseases. A vegetarian diet centers around high-fiber and low-fat meals consisting of fruits, vegetables, nuts, and seeds. Although 14 million Americans claim to be

Watch Out!
Labels can be confusing:

■ *Low-fat* means a product has no more than 3 grams of fat per serving.

■ *Low saturated fat* means it has no more than 1 gram of saturated fat per serving.

■ *Reduced fat* means the product has at least 25 percent less fat per serving than the traditional item.

■ *Light* means the product has 1/2 the fat or 1/3 the calories of its regular counterpart.

■ *Fat-free* has 1/2 gram of fat or less per serving.

strict vegetarians, more than 46 percent, or 120 million Americans, are reducing meat consumption. Review the terms in Table 9.13 to see what type of vegetarian you are or want to be.

Natural remedies and supplements

As you've learned throughout this chapter, dietary supplements include a host of products that contain vitamins, minerals, herbs, and amino acids as well as natural enzymes, organ tissues, metabolites, extracts, or concentrates. Some alternative practitioners recommend the following natural remedies for prevention and treatment of disease. Most are available at drugstores, grocery stores, or natural health food stores.

- **Chromium picolate** is an important trace mineral that helps cells break down sugar into energy for the body. Supplements can help regulate blood sugar, fat, and carbohydrate metabolism. Uncontrolled blood sugar levels can contribute to weight gain, high cholesterol, and high blood pressure in many people. Interestingly, chromium seems to normalize low blood sugar. A recent USDA study of 180 Type II diabetics in China documented spectacular results from taking 1,000 micrograms of chromium picolinate daily. Nearly all the subjects no longer had the classic signs of diabetes.

- **Conjugated linoleic acid (CLA)** is a fatty acid said to reduce fat by inhibiting the body's ability to store fats. It also has antioxidant properties, increases muscle tone, and improves how efficiently food is utilized in the body.

- **Coenzyme Q10** is a natural substance the body produces in smaller amounts as we age. It has

TABLE 9.13   WHAT TYPE OF VEGETARIAN ARE YOU?

You are a:

- **Quasi-vegetarian** if you eat fish and poultry but not red meat
- **Pescatarian** if you eat plants and fish
- **Lacto vegetarian** if you eat plants and dairy
- **Lacto-ovo** vegetarian if you eat plants, dairy, and eggs
- **Ovo-vegetarian** if you eat plants and eggs
- **Vegan** if you eat a strict plant-based diet with no animal byproducts such as milk or honey

been synthesized and is sold as a supplement that improves heart and immune function. It also is an antioxidant that helps lower cholesterol levels and that reduces oxidative damage to blood vessels.

- **Creatine** is a supplement that helps the body retain water in muscle tissue, helping to heal the muscle without bloating the body. This should be used in low doses to avoid toxic effects.

- **DHEA** is an anti-aging hormone; it is sometimes called the mother hormone because the body converts it into estrogen and testosterone. DHEA raises sex hormones and is said to make you feel younger and more sexy. But, as researchers are quick to point out, it also might increase your chances of developing ovarian, prostate, or other types of cancer. High doses of DHEA have been found to increase facial hair and to stop menstruation in women.

- **Essential Fatty Acids (EFAs)** are not manufactured by the body, but they are essential to cardiovascular health and normal brain development. EFAs are available in oils containing omega-3 (fish oils) and omega-6 (linolenic and gamma-linolenic [GLA], which are found in plant oils such as evening primrose, black currant, and borage).

- **Glucosamine** and **chondroitin** are two substances the human body produces to make cartilage. In supplement form, glucosamine comes from crab shells, and chondroitin comes from cow cartilage. Scientific studies have yet to call these the cure for arthritis, but in some studies of people with arthritis, the supplements were found to ease aches just well as over-the-counter pain killers (although more slowly). Their long-term safety has never been established, but they appear to have no side effects. Researchers do not yet know whether you must take the two supplements together or whether one is effective when taken by itself.

- **Lecithin** is commercially isolated from soybeans, corn, and eggs, and it may help ease the memory glitches that occur with aging. Just two tablespoons of lecithin a day stimulates the body's output of choline, a brain chemical important for recall and memory.

- **Melatonin** is a natural hormone secreted from the pineal gland in the brain. It has a major influence on the human body's inner clock, which governs the sleep-wake cycle and other biological functions. This hormone peaks in early childhood and then falls at puberty. It now is sold in pill form as a drug-free method of curing insomnia; it decreases the time to the onset of sleep without disturbing the typical phases of sleep. The problem is that the possible side effects are not widely publicized—worsening depression, decreased fertility, and excessively low body temperature (hypothermia). As with all natural dietary supplements, there is no regulatory control by the FDA at this time.

Just the facts

- The Recommended Dietary Allowance of vitamins and minerals may not be enough to prevent certain diseases.

- A host of different phytochemicals are available through fruits and vegetables, and each one plays a different role in keeping you well.

- Soy products may be the medicine of the future; they can help prevent some cancers and heart disease, can keep cholesterol low, and may be used for their estrogen effects at menopause.

- Just because a supplement is natural does not mean it is safe, and DHEA is a prime example.

Watch Out!
Super Blue Green Algae is one dietary supplement you might want to avoid until scientific tests are done. This freeze-dried algae is touted as a miracle cure, but it is not nearly as healthful as a simple multi-vitamin. Some people have complained that Super Blue Green Algae causes symptoms such as diarrhea, headaches, numbness, heart palpitations, and skin rashes.

What Ails You . . .

GET THE SCOOP ON...
How stress can contribute to acne ▪ Why body
odor may be a sign of a serious disease ▪
The latest treatments for hair loss ▪ How herbal
therapy, homeopathy, and aromatherapy
may hold the key to many stress-related
skin disorders

PART III

Skin Disorders

Chapter 10

Scientists are now finding that most skin disorders have a psychological or lifestyle basis, and alternative therapies can help bring balance to anxiety, stress, and unsettled emotions. Check out the following skin disorders and choose from the many alternative and conventional treatments to keep your skin supple, clear, and healthy.

Acne

These bumps, often called pimples, can appear anywhere on the body. Although acne is commonly associated with teenagers, it also can occur in children and adults. The symptoms are red, tiny bumps on the skin that sometimes have yellowish or white heads on top. The source of acne is Androgen, a hormone that, when abundant, causes the glands under the skin to make more oil. The oil ducts can get clogged and infected, resulting in tiny bumps called pimples. Adults can get an acne-like condition called *rosacea* (pages 222–24), and babies get acne from their mother's hormones. Stress, fluctuating hormones, greasy creams, or foods containing iodine—such as fish, beef, liver, broccoli and asparagus—all can contribute to acne.

How is it prevented?

Cleanliness is crucial to prevent acne. Wash the skin several times a day with soap and water. It also is important to use clean towels to dry the skin. Facial scrubs and astringents also can keep excess oil away. Acne products with benzoyl peroxide have a drying, healing effect and can help reduce inflammation. Avoid greasy face creams and make-up, and destress your body. Increased anxiety can cause fidgeting and picking at the skin, which increases break-outs.

What is the conventional treatment?

A host of over-the-counter creams, gels, and ointments containing benzoyl peroxide are designed to treat acne. (An *ointment* usually is made with a petroleum derivative that adds moisture to the skin, so use with caution if skin is oily. A *gel* is less greasy and does not clog pores as readily.) Prescription ointments containing retinoic acid, such as Retin-A or Renova, can be used if the acne worsens. In some cases, *antibiotics*—drugs that kill bacteria or that slow down its reproduction—can help control infection. For severe cases of cystic acne, isotretinoin (Accutane) is recommended. The possible side effects of cracked lips, conjunctivitis, gastrointestinal problems, and joint pain, however, can be debilitating. New reports about Accutane reveal that this medication can cause severe depression and possibly birth defects.

What are some alternative treatments?

- **Aromatherapy**—topical oils such as tea tree, lemon, peppermint, lavender, geranium, and sage

Watch Out!
If you use Retin-A, be sure to cover up before you go out in the sun. Prescription skin creams can cause skin sensitivity and can make you susceptible to sunburn.

- **Ayurvedic medicine**—foods that aid digestion such as fresh ginger, cilantro, cumin, and yogurt

- **Herbal therapy**—anise, cardamom, basil, cilantro, lavender, red clover

- **Nutritional therapy**—a low-fat diet high in beta-carotene; avoid white flour and sugar

- **Nutritional supplements**—zinc, copper, vitamin E, selenium, vitamin A, lactobacillus, folic acid, and B-complex vitamins

- **Mind/body therapy**—destress with art, music, or dance therapy

The basics

1. *What's been proven to work?* For guaranteed results, stick with products containing benzoyl peroxide for mild cases and use antibiotic and topical prescription creams containing tretinoin (Retin-A) for more persistent cases. Tretinoin removes dead skin, regenerates collagen, and allows the top layer of skin cells to mature normally. The herbal therapy tea tree oil (oil of melaleuca) is a powerful antiseptic and may help prevent a broad range of bacteria. Don't forget that you are what you eat, so fill your diet with foods rich in beta-carotene.

2. *How much does treatment cost?* Conventional treatments such as Retin-A and antibiotic therapy can cost as much as $30 to $50 a month, depending on the medication used. Tea tree oil costs about $8 a month.

3. *How long until it works?* A cream such as Renova can take from two weeks to one month before you will notice a significant difference.

66
Retin-A saved my life when I was in my early 20s. After graduating from college and taking my first teaching job, I had a massive acne attack. Just two weeks of applying Retin-A to my face got the problem under control.
—Mark, 26, economics teacher
99

Antibiotics may work as soon as three days to two weeks.

If you have already tried a healthy diet, vitamin supplements, stress reduction, and healing sleep, conventional medical therapy definitely is necessary to avoid pitted skin. Retin-A can cause stinging and burning, but newer acne medications such as Adapalen gel (Differin) and azelaic acid cream (Azelex) are available by prescription and may have fewer side effects.

Athlete's foot

This itchy foot problem is caused by a fungus. General symptoms include moist, scaly, cracked, and itchy skin between the toes. If that isn't enough misery, wait until it begins to blister, peel, and ooze.

How is it prevented?

Don't walk barefoot on the wet floors of a gym, public shower, or locker room. These areas are contaminated with fungus that grows from the constant moisture. Keep your feet clean and dry, especially between your toes. Wear open-toe sandals when you can to allow your skin to breathe or wear all-cotton socks to keep your feet dry. Use an antifungal spray or powder between your toes for prevention.

What is the conventional treatment?

Over-the-counter antifungal sprays or creams, such as Lotrimin AF Antifungal Cream, are available to help you keep the area dry and to kill the bacteria.

What are some alternative treatments?

- **Aromatherapy**—fungicide essential oils such as myrrh or tea tree (melaleuca), lavender (an anti-inflammatory or for cracked skin), calendula oil

Bright Idea
If you suffer from dry, cracked heels, keep a jar of petroleum jelly and a pair of white socks by your bed. Cover your entire foot with the petroleum jelly before bedtime and put on the white socks to protect your sheets. Do this for one week, and your heels will be noticeably smoother.

- **Herbal therapy**—chamomile and garlic
- **Nutritional therapy**—carrots, sweet potatoes, cantaloupe, and winter squash (foods high in vitamin A and beta-carotene)
- **Nutritional supplements**—fish oil; gamma-linolenic acid (GLA) found in evening primrose oil, borage, and black currant oils; and antioxidants (vitamins A, C, and E)

The basics

1. *What's been proven to work?* Unless you don't mind waiting for relief, better stick with the proven cures—over-the-counter antifungal sprays or creams along with the preventive measures of keeping the area clean and dry.

2. *How much does treatment cost?* Antifungal sprays or creams cost about $5 to $7.

3. *How long until it works?* You should feel great relief within 24 hours to two days.

To stop the fungus, use the proven conventional treatment and continue to use it for one to two weeks after symptoms have subsided. You can use lavender or other alternative therapies once the fungus is controlled to keep skin soft and supple.

Blisters

A blister is a raised area of skin, usually oval or circular in shape, that is filled with fluid. Although a blister can be sensitive or painful to touch, it provides protection to damaged tissue.

Blisters are caused by fluid collecting beneath the outer layer of skin. This fluid is leaked from blood vessels in underlying skin layers after minor damage such as a burn, a skin disease, friction, or other diseases such as chicken pox or shingles.

How is it prevented?

Avoid burns, sunburns, and any friction on the skin.
Apply petroleum jelly to your feet and then wear
acrylic socks to minimize friction.

What is the conventional treatment?

A blister protects damaged skin, so it is best to leave
it alone and allow it to heal on its own. Some physicians suggest taping the blister so the blister roof
sticks to the damaged skin. If the tissue becomes
infected, your doctor will need to see it for medical
treatment.

What are some alternative treatments?

- **Herbal therapy**—chamomile or calendula compresses; aloe vera juice from plant

- **Homeopathy**—calendula, cantharis, phosphorus, or urtica urens

- **Nutritional supplements**—vitamin E oil on the
  blister (break open a capsule, dab the oil on the
  blister, and then tape)

The basics

1. *What's been proven to work?* Soak and dry the
   affected area and apply triple antibiotic ointment to the blister. Cover with a loose gauze pad
   or Band-Aid so the blister stays intact. Aloe vera
   can be extremely healing for inflamed or blistered skin.

2. *How much does treatment cost?* Triple antibiotic
   ointment costs about $5. An aloe vera plant
   costs about $2 to $4 and can be grown in a small
   pot in your kitchen window.

3. *How long until it works?* It may take three days to
   a week or even longer for a blister to heal,

depending on the size of the injury. As the underlying, inflamed skin begins to heal, the blister will flatten, shrink in size, and then peel off. Aloe vera can help soothe the injury and its surrounding skin during this natural healing process.

A blister is a natural part of your body's healing process and protects damaged skin. Never pop a blister because bacteria can enter the broken skin.

Body odor

Body odor is exactly what the name suggests: a lingering, unpleasant odor that may stem from different underlying problems in the body.

There are a myriad of reasons for poor personal hygiene, from improper bathing or weak deodorants to dirty clothes or shoes. Body odor also can be caused by skin bacteria activity on dried sweat and hormonal or nutritional imbalances such as a deficiency in zinc. Gastrointestinal problems, liver dysfunction, diabetes, and yeast infections can cause some types of body odor, as can eating strong foods such as garlic, curry, and onions.

How is it prevented?

Check your hygiene and invest in a deodorant that contains an *antiperspirant*. If it stems from an internal problem, see your doctor for a diagnosis and proper treatment.

What is the conventional treatment?

Bathe thoroughly at least once daily and use an antiperspirant deodorant. If this does not work, your doctor may want to do diagnostic tests to see whether there is an underlying illness.

Timesaver
If you are low on deodorant, a thick paste of baking soda and water can act as a deodorant. Add your favorite essential oil; lavender, rose, or mint is particularly nice. Brush off the excess before putting your clothes on.

What are some alternative treatments?

- **Aromatherapy**—anise soap, thyme, yarrow

- **Detoxification**—fast for one or two days a month using juice, water, and fruit

- **Nutritional therapy**—parsley; avoid pungent foods such as garlic and onions

- **Nutritional supplements**—Lactobacillus acidophilus and bifidobacteria to boost intestinal flora quality

Bright Idea
To help with foot odor, fill a basin with warm water and mix in one-half cup of baking soda and 15 drops of peppermint essential oil. Soak your feet for 10 to 15 minutes and then dry.

The basics

1. *What's been proven to work?* Before getting a complete internal work-up to see what type of gastrointestinal problem you may have, try to bathe more frequently, avoid strongly flavored foods, and use an antiperspirant twice a day.

2. *How much does treatment cost?* A good antiperspirant deodorant costs around $5. An evaluation with an internist can cost $125 or more, depending on the diagnostic tests. A detoxification fast costs about $5 per day.

3. *How long until it works?* If bacteria on the skin is the problem, you should notice a difference within days.

A strong or unpleasant odor can be your body's warning sign of a serious or chronic illness. If the odor continues, see your doctor for further investigation.

Boils

Boils are inflamed, pus-filled nodules or *carbuncles* (clusters of boils) on the skin that generally are caused by a staph infection. Starting in the hair follicles, boils are itchy and then painful red lumps. As they fill with pus, they become round and form a yellowish tip. The shoulders, face, scalp, buttocks, and armpits are common sites.

How is it prevented?

Take showers instead of baths to avoid spreading the staph infection. Keep your immune system strong.

What is the conventional treatment?

Moist heat compresses applied every hour or two can help relieve pain. If the boil is large, antibiotics help the body get rid of the infection. You may need your physician to open (or lance) the boil to drain the pus using a sterile needle.

What are some alternative treatments?

- **Homeopathy**—a homeopathic remedy: echinacea spp. 3 parts, galium aparine 2 parts, iris versicolor 1 part, rumex crispus 1 part, phytolacca decandra 1 part to 5ml of tincture three times a day

- **Herbal therapy**—aloe vera, chickweed, black walnut, or garlic

- **Hydrotherapy**—warm, wet compresses bring it to a head and reduce inflammation

- **Nutritional supplements**—vitamins A, C, and E (antioxidants)

The basics

1. *What's been proven to work?* Although some alternative treatments might work, an antibiotic from your doctor is probably a better choice because you are dealing with a potentially dangerous staph infection.

2. *How much does treatment cost?* Antibiotics to treat this cost about $15 to $20.

> **"**
> Never use the same razor to shave with when you have boils. I suffered with underarm boils for several months until the doctor figured out that I was infecting myself each time I shaved under my arms.
> —Patricia, 35, artist
> **"**

3. *How long until it works?* Used in conjunction with moist heat applications, you will notice relief in one to two weeks. If a boil is painful, your lymph glands are swollen, or a fever occurs, call your doctor.

Boils are contagious and can spread to other parts of the body, so take precautions when treating this on your own.

Calluses

An area of flat, thickened skin on the body, usually on the ball or heel of the feet, on the hands, or on the knees. The main symptom of a callus is thickened skin that is hard and painless. A *corn* is a callus on a toe. Calluses are caused by repeated rubbing, squeezing, pressure, or friction on any part of the body.

How is it prevented?

Avoid ill-fitting shoes or activities that cause pressure or friction on the skin. Sometimes lamb's wool, pads, or orthotic devices are necessary to keep friction off sensitive areas.

What is the conventional treatment?

Watch Out!
Be careful not to remove healthy skin when using a pumice stone or an emery board on your callus. You can cause irritation or even bleeding.

The best way to treat a callus is to use a pumice stone or an emery board to remove dead skin and to smooth the callus. A podiatrist (foot specialist) will scrape away the hardened tissue using a scalpel. Chemical solutions often are used to peel away corns.

What are some alternative treatments?

- **Aromatherapy**—topical oils such as tea tree, lemon, peppermint, lavender, geranium, and sage (to soothe irritated skin)

- **Detoxification**—rub callus with a loofah
- **Hydrotherapy**—soften skin in warm water and then rub the area with a pumice stone

The basics

1. *What's been proven to work?* Because both conventional and alternative methods soften skin and remove dead, dry cells, you can try any of these methods to see which is best in your case.

2. *How much does treatment cost?* A loofah costs about $5. A pumice stone costs about $4, and topical oils cost from $8 to $12.

3. *How long until it works?* It can take from one to three weeks to completely rid your skin of the callus.

Again, prevention is important with problems like calluses. Make sure your shoes fit properly and keep your skin soft and supple using moisturizing lotion.

Dandruff

Dandruff is a common condition in which dead skin is shed from the scalp, leaving white flakes in the hair and on the clothes. It usually is caused by seborrheic dermatitis, an itchy, scaly rash on the scalp.

How is it prevented?

Dermatitis can be controlled with antidandruff shampoo.

What is the conventional treatment?

Use a shampoo that contains tar, zinc, selenium, sulfur, or salicylic acid. If the problem continues, consult your doctor; conditions such as psoriasis and eczema can resemble dandruff.

What are some alternative treatments?

- **Aromatherapy**—jojoba oil (a carrier oil), chamomile oil, rosemary oil, and vetiver oil
- **Herbal therapy**—chamomile
- **Nutritional supplements**—evening primrose oil, olive oil

The basics

1. *What's been proven to work?* If an over-the-counter antidandruff shampoo fails to control the flaking skin, a prescription corticosteroid cream or lotion or an antifungal cream applied to the scalp may help stop this condition.

2. *How much does treatment cost?* An antidandruff shampoo costs about $6 to $8.

3. *How long until it works?* If the shampoo works, you should see a difference within three days to one week.

The best way to control dandruff is to treat it before it gets out of hand. If antidandruff shampoos don't solve your problem, get an accurate diagnosis from a dermatologist.

Eczema

A chronic skin condition, eczema usually appears on the scalp, face, neck, or the creases of the elbows, wrists, hands, or knees. It can be caused by an allergy, but it also can occur for no known reason. Symptoms include an inflammation of the skin accompanied by small blisters and crusty scales. These may itch, turn red, and even bleed.

How is it prevented?

Avoid triggers of this skin disease such as wool fabric, sweating, too much sun, chapped or dry skin due to wind or cold, cosmetics, perfumes, lotions,

Bright Idea
If you get itchy, scaly hands after washing dishes, put an emollient such as petroleum jelly on your hands and cover them with plastic gloves. Your hands will stay dry, and the heat from the dish water will help the emollient penetrate into your skin, leaving your hands smooth and soft.

stress, and offending foods (frequently cow's milk, wheat, eggs, chocolate, peas, beans, tomatoes, nuts, some spices, fresh fruit, and seafood).

What is the conventional treatment?

Emollients such as petroleum jelly will keep skin soft and protected. Antihistamine drugs may help reduce itching. In severe cases, corticosteroid ointments and antibiotics are necessary to stop infection.

What are some alternative treatments?

- **Aromatherapy**—topical oils of rose, aloe, jasmine, and ylang-ylang.

- **Nutritional supplements**—gamma-linolenic acid (GLA) found in evening primrose oil, borage, and black currant oils

- **Nutritional therapy**—foods high in omega-3s, vitamin A, and vitamin E (or use supplements); avoid foods to which you are allergic

- **Mind/body treatments**—relaxation response, visualization, art or music therapy, and other stress-reduction tools

The basics

1. *What's been proven to work?* Avoid certain types of food and other triggers and use antihistamines and corticosteroid ointments.

2. *How much does treatment cost?* Avoiding foods that trigger eczema and destressing the body are free. Antihistamines cost about $4 for a two-week supply, and corticosteroid ointments cost from $5 to $20, depending on the brand.

3. *How long until it works?* You will notice a difference within four days to one week using corticosteroid ointments.

Once the eczema is under control with conventional treatments, use alternative methods such as mind/body treatments to reduce stress and nutritional therapy to keep the immune system strong.

Hair loss

As the name suggests, hair loss is an abnormal loss of hair from the face or scalp. Symptoms include thinning hair or patchy loss of hair over the scalp and other hair-bearing areas such as the beard or eyebrows. Inherited variables, stress, and hair injury caused by twisting, tugging, braiding, or tight rollers all can cause loss of hair. Sometimes hair loss also can be the result of a poor diet, infections of the scalp, an internal organ disease, hormonal changes such as pregnancy or menopause, or aging.

How is it prevented?

Use a wide-tooth comb and avoid brushes. Forget brushing your hair 100 times a night; it may actually pull your hair out. Avoid hair products such as gels, mousses, sprays, perms, and dyes that can damage or break your hair. Keep your hormones in check; they can influence hair loss. (If you are postmenopausal, for instance, ask your doctor whether estrogen may help your situation.) Make sure your diet is healthy with ample protein.

What is the conventional treatment?

Several products are now available to treat hair loss. One over-the-counter product, minoxidil (Rogaine), may help make thinning hair look fuller. There also is some evidence that finasteride (Proscar), a treatment for prostate problems, may stimulate hair growth. Another new prescription drug, Propecia, also has been used with good results.

Watch Out!
While it is normal to lose as many as 50 hairs a day, hair loss becomes abnormal if you lose more than 100 hairs a day. There are three types of hair loss:

■ *Androgenetic Alopecia,* or male pattern baldness (can affect both men and women)

■ *Alopecia Areata,* or patchy loss of hair with no known cause

■ *Telogen Effluvium,* or loss of hair occuring a few months following childbirth or from an acute illness, fever, physical or emotional stress, or improper diet

What are some alternative treatments?

- **Bach Flowers**—gentian and sweet chestnut (to reduce stress and worry)

- **Bodywork**—scalp massage

- **Nutritional supplements**—zinc, vitamin A, B-complex vitamins, gamma-linolenic acid (GLA) found in evening primrose oil, borage, and black currant oils

- **Nutritional therapy**—a healthful, balanced diet

The basics

1. *What's been proven to work?* Short of actually transplanting small plugs of hair—one hair at a time—there are not many options for growing a full head of hair.

2. *How much does treatment cost?* Hair transplantation costs about $15,000 for a complete scalp.

3. *How long until it works?* If new growth is going to appear, it usually occurs within a month to three months.

Many people depend on Rogaine for hair growth. Remember, though, that this new hair is lost if the treatment is stopped. At $40 for one month's supply, this is a costly investment for only temporary results.

Hives

Hives are an itchy, pinkish rash that usually occur on the limbs or the trunk. They consist of localized swellings of the skin that typically last a few hours before fading away.

Hives generally are caused by an allergic reaction when the chemical histamine is released from skin cells. An allergen is more likely to cause histamine release when stress hormones dilate

Watch Out!
Hives often are the first sign of anaphylaxis (see pages 343–46), a life-threatening allergic reaction. If hives are accompanied by shortness of breath, swelling of the lips, mouth, and ears, or difficulty swallowing, go to an emergency room immediately.

blood vessels, so stress is a factor in this allergic skin problem.

How is it prevented?

Avoid known allergens (foods, food additives, fabrics, mold or pollen, or drugs). Try to stay relaxed; stress can sometimes trigger hives within minutes of an upsetting event.

What is the conventional treatment?

First, identify and avoid the cause. Antihistamines, when taken orally, can relieve an already formed hive. In severe cases, corticosteroid drugs may be given to reduce inflammation. Epinephrine may be necessary if the swelling is life-threatening.

What are some alternative treatments?

- **Chinese medicine**—tai chi
- **Bodywork**—any form of massage (be careful if pressure on the skin causes inflammation or redness)
- **Herbal therapy**—chamomile, kava kava, and St. John's wort
- **Homeopathy**—allium cepa, sulphur, or silica
- **Mind/Body therapy**—relaxation response, biofeedback, self-hypnosis, visualization, art or music therapy, psychotherapy (to help destress the body and to resolve anxiety)

The basics

1. *What's been proven to work?* Therapies to destress, along with antihistamines taken orally.
2. *How much does treatment cost?* An over-the-counter antihistamine costs about $5 for 20 doses. Destressing your body is free.

3. *How long until it works?* It takes one to two hours for an antihistamine to fully affect the body, and most flare-ups subside within 24 hours.

Many skin conditions have psychological roots. Figure out what is causing anxiety in your life and try to resolve it. If you have allergies, stay away from triggers that cause hives and always keep an antihistamine with you—just in case.

Insect bites and stings

Insect bites and stings are tiny wounds in the skin caused by a variety of biting or stinging insects such as mosquitoes, wasps, gnats, horseflies, fleas, or chiggers.

How is it prevented?

Wear clothing that protects the body, apply insect repellent, burn citronella candles, avoid heavy perfumes or fragrances, and keep doors and windows closed.

What is the conventional treatment?

Wash carefully with non-perfumed soap and water, then apply a soothing anti-itch lotion such as calamine. If the itch is not resolved, you may try an antihistamine cream or take an antihistamine orally. In some cases, over-the-counter cortisone creams, such as Cortaid Maximum Strength, can stop the inflammation.

What are some alternative treatments?

- **Aromatherapy**—tea tree essential oil
- **Herbal therapy**—echinacea
- **Homeopathy**—apis, ledum, natrum mur (make into a paste), or urtica urens

Bright Idea
Ask your doctor about an Epi-Pen. This small, injectible shot of ephinephrine is only six inches in length and easily fits in your purse or briefcase. Having this can provide peace of mind if you suffer from life-threatening reactions to insect bites that require emergency attention.

- **Nutritional therapy**—avoid sweets and alcohol; for insect bites, use fresh, mashed papaya to cover the affected area; for bee stings, hold a slice of green, unripe plantain to the bite; for spider bites, mash half a white onion and spread on skin as a poultice

The basics

1. *What's been proven to work?* An antihistamine probably is your best bet after an insect sting, especially if there is a chance for an allergic reaction. Take an antihistamine orally (such as Benadryl) and then put an antihistamine or cortisone cream on the bite to stop external itching.

2. *How much does treatment cost?* Antihistamines cost about $5. Antihistamine cream costs about $4 for one ounce.

3. *How long until it works?* You should feel relief within 30 minutes to two hours.

If you have nausea, dizziness, diarrhea, or trouble breathing or swallowing after an insect bite, call your doctor or go to your local emergency room immediately.

Psoriasis

Psoriasis is a noncontagious, chronic skin disorder. Symptoms include raised, reddened, or silvery patches covered with scales and rashes. The rashes commonly affect the scalp, the back of the elbows, and the front of the knees. Fingernails may get crater-like pits and may thicken or separate from the nail's bed. Some patients develop pain and swelling in their joints, usually the hands and feet. This is known as *psoriatic arthritis,* and it is caused by a combination of an inherited tendency and environmental factors such as infection, injury, emotional stress, climate, and certain drugs. Some studies link psoriasis with a rapid growth of cells in the skin's outer later.

How is it prevented?

Eat your veggies. An Italian study reported in the *British Journal of Dermatology* (1996) revealed that people without psoriasis were more likely than people with psoriasis to eat fresh fruit two times a day, tomatoes every day, and carrots three times a week. Interestingly, psoriasis is rare in countries where people eat low-fat diets.

What is the conventional treatment?

For mild cases, creams and ointments containing steroids, anthralin, or tar usually can clear up the scaly patches. For severe cases, medications such as methotrexate and etretinate or ultraviolet light treatment may be used in addition to creams. Anti-inflammatory medications are used to treat joint pain and swelling.

What are some alternative treatments?

- **Chinese medicine**—acupuncture, acupressure, or shiatsu (helps remove the block in your body's pathways so energy can flow throughout the entire body)

- **Detoxification**—fast on fruits and clear liquids two days a month

- **Herbal therapy**—burdock root or yellow dock (helps detoxify the body)

- **Light therapy**—ultraviolet light (UVL) therapy (helps retard the production of new skin cells)

- **Nutritional supplements**—fish oil (or flaxseed oil), selenium, and antioxidants (vitamins A, C, and E)
- **Nutritional therapy**—fresh fruits and vegetables, especially those high in beta-carotene
- **Mind/body therapy**—relaxation response, visualization, music therapy

The basics

1. *What's been proven to work?* Try various therapies to find the one that removes your symptoms without causing serious side effects. Drugs such as methotrexate may work effectively for severe psoriasis, but it also can cause liver damage. Ultraviolet light therapy (UVL) can help, but you must use it cautiously to avoid skin damage or cancer. Tar sometimes is used to remove the scales.

2. *How long until it works?* The time varies depending on the persistence of the psoriasis and the treatment used.

3. *How much does treatment cost?* The cost can vary from $20 for a prescription cortisone cream to $50 for a treatment of UVL therapy.

Treat your psoriasis cautiously. Most remedies have side effects that are unwanted or even downright dangerous. You should generally try to keep your immune system boosted with nutritional supplements and healthful foods, and you should decrease stress.

Rosacea

Rosacea is a chronic inflammatory skin disorder that usually begins mid-life or later. Symptoms include redness of the skin, small pimples, flushing, and broken blood vessels in the middle areas of the face. It also sometimes occurs on the trunk and extremities. The cause is unknown, but the disease is most common in people with a fair complexion. Some studies have shown that astringents and skin toners can cause flare-ups of rosacea.

How is it prevented?
Avoid products that contain alcohol or witch hazel.

What is the conventional treatment?
Topical metronidazole gel or broad-spectrum oral antibiotics usually are effective. Tetracycline is the preferred antibiotic because it is the most effective and has few side effects with long-term use. Surgical correction may be required for rhinophyma (a bulbous red nose resulting from neglected rosacea).

What are some alternative treatments?

- **Ayurveda**—acupuncture, shiatsu, and spiritual awareness
- **Bodywork**—any massage technique
- **Herbal therapy**—chamomile, valerian, St. John's wort, or kava kava
- **Mind/body therapy**—autogenic therapy, biofeedback, music therapy, or the relaxation response

The basics

1. *What's been proven to work?* Use a combination of alternative treatments to reduce stress and anxiety, avoid foods and alcohol that trigger rosacea, and take oral antibiotics.

2. *How much does treatment cost?* Stress reduction and avoidance of triggers are free; oral antibiotics cost about $25 for one month's supply.

Unofficially . . .
It is suspected that W.C. Fields suffered from rosacea, which can result in an enlarged, red nose.

3. *How long until it works?* Give yourself two to three weeks of using a combination of treatments before you see results.

As with all skin problems, try to find the psychological root creating tension in the body. Strong emotions affect the blood vessels underneath the skin's surface, making you blush and turn red. In rosacea, these vessels remain dilated, causing the skin to look inflamed.

Scarring

A scar is a slightly raised mark that remains on the skin after damaged tissue has healed. Scars usually are narrow and are pale in color. When a wound is healing, the body increases the production of a fibrous protein called *collagen* at the wound site. The collagen helps make new tissue, which covers the area of the wound. The edges of the wound grow together, and the scar is left in the center. If the wound's edges are not completely drawn together, the scar may be larger.

How is it prevented?

Keep the wound clean so it does not get infected.

What is the conventional treatment?

If a scar is unsightly, you may consider having plastic surgery. Sometimes skin grafts can be taken from other healthy tissue and transplanted onto the healing wound and resulting scar.

What are some alternative treatments?

- **Aromatherapy**—topical oils of rose, aloe, jasmine, and ylang-ylang
- **Nutritional supplements**—evening primrose oil
- **Nutritional therapy**—foods containing omega-3s, vitamin A, and vitamin E

The basics

1. *What's been proven to work?* A new surgical technique called Z-plasty realigns a scar to lie with the natural creases in the skin—rather than across the crease—making it less noticeable.

2. *How much does treatment cost?* Z-plasty costs around $3,000 and up, depending on the problem and your location.

3. *How long until it works?* You should notice improvement within three weeks to two months after the redness dissipates.

Plastic surgery is effective for many people who have skin blemishes, birthmarks, deep wrinkles or freckles, and other discolorations on the skin. Be sure to research thoroughly before you have surgery and make sure your doctor has experience.

Skin changes

Spots, growths, color changes, or changes in skin texture can be caused by exposure to the sun and the wind, cigarette smoking or constant exposure to cigarette smoke, and aging. Symptoms include age spots, small growths, dryness, a breakdown in the collagen in the layers of the skin, enlarged blood vessels, skin thickness, spider or enlarged veins, and skin flaps or tags.

How is it prevented?

Use a sunscreen with a sun protective factor (SPF) of 15 or higher, wear protective clothing when outdoors, eat nutritious foods, and stop smoking cigarettes.

What is the conventional treatment?

Treatments include surface freezing, electrosurgery, chemical cauterization of small benign

Moneysaver
Before having any type of plastic surgery, have your doctor discuss the procedure and the diagnosis with your insurance agent. Many times insurance companies will not cover cosmetic surgery.

Watch Out!
See your doctor if you notice the following warning signs that a mole may be malignant:

■ A sudden change in the size of the mole

■ A sudden change of color

■ A persistent irritation such as itching, bleeding, or crumbling growths or spots, laser surgery, and sclerosis (a substance injected into a vein) to reduce unwanted purple veins. Moisturizers, bleaching creams, liquid nitrogen, and Retin-A or Renova can reduce pigment spots, dry skin, and wrinkling.

What are some alternative treatments?

- **Ayurveda**—yoga (keeps blood flowing)
- **Homeopathy**—over-the-counter calendula cream; rhus toxicodendron (take three times a day)
- **Nutritional supplements**—vitamins A and E, zinc, vitamin B-complex (particularly vitamin B_1 and vitamin B_5)

The basics

1. *What's been proven to work?* Prevention is the only method proven to avoid skin changes. Wear clothing to protect your skin when outdoors and always put on sunscreen before starting your day.

2. *How much does treatment cost?* Treatment for skin changes costs about $60 for a two- to three-month supply of a prescription facial cream. Procedures and surgery, of course, cost more.

3. *How long until it works?* It takes four to six weeks to notice a dramatic reduction in fine lines from sun damage. Age spots may take longer to fade.

Stay out of the sun and protect your skin from further damage. Talk to your dermatologist about any skin changes you may have to see whether further treatment, such as dermabrasion, is necessary.

Sunburn

Most people have experienced sunburn at some point in their lives. Sunburn is red, swollen, and often blistered skin caused by overexposure to ultra-violet (UV) light. The symptoms include painfully red and sensitive skin. If the sunburn is severe, you may feel nausea, chills, and fever.

How is it prevented?
Wear sunscreen with a UV factor of at least 15 (higher if you have sensitive skin), protective clothing, and a wide-brimmed hat. You should avoid the sun between 10 a.m. and 2 p.m. In addition, be careful of any medicine you may be taking. Some medications can make you more sensitive to the sun's harmful rays.

What is the conventional treatment?
Take a cool bath or shower, relieve pain with acetaminophen or ibuprofen, and use a soothing moisturizing cream to keep skin from drying out. Be sure to drink plenty of liquids to keep from dehydrating.

What are some alternative treatments?

- **Bach Flower Remedy**—Rescue Remedy (cream)
- **Herbal therapy**—aloe vera juice, chamomile
- **Homeopathy**—calendula (marigolds) spray or gel, urtica dioica, sulphur, and cantharis
- **Hydrotherapy**—cool water baths or sprays (helps ease the sting associated with sunburn)
- **Nutritional therapy**—milk bath

The basics
1. *What's been proven to work?* Anesthetic creams or sprays containing benzocaine or lidocaine can provide some pain relief. Some people prefer to gently sponge the body with a milk bath and then apply the juice from an aloe vera plant.

2. *How much does treatment cost?* Anesthetic sprays cost about $6. An aloe vera plant costs between $2 to $4.

3. *How long until it works?* You should feel some relief within 30 minutes to one hour. Sunburn pain can linger for two to four days, however, depending on the severity.

Why have pain at all? Stay out of the sun from 10 a.m. to 2 p.m., wear a wide-brimmed hat and long-sleeved clothes to protect your skin, and keep sunscreen on at all times when outdoors.

Warts

Watch Out!
If not treated in women, venereal or genital warts may cause pre-cancerous cells or even uterine cancer to form. If you or your partner suspect you have contracted genital warts, see your doctor immediately.

Warts generally are harmless skin growths caused by a virus. Growths can appear on any part of the body such as the face, the forearms, or a finger. Warts have a rough surface on which tiny, dark dots often can be seen. On pressure areas, such as the palms or the soles, they appear flat. Warts on the sole (called plantar warts) grow inward from the pressure of standing and walking and often are painful. Genital warts usually are white with a cauliflower-like appearance.

Warts may bleed if injured, but common warts never turn cancerous. (The exception is genital warts, which usually are acquired sexually.) Even though warts are contagious and may spread from one part of the body to another or to other people, researchers still do not know why some people get warts and others don't.

How is it prevented?
There is no way to prevent warts.

What is the conventional treatment?
Warts often disappear by themselves, especially in young children. This spontaneous disappearance is

less common in older children and adults. Treatment consists of destroying the outer layer of skin on which the wart grows. This can be done with surgery, laser ablation, electrocautery (destroying it with a weak electric current), by freezing it (with liquid nitrogen), or with chemicals such as salicylic acid. The treatment used depends on the location and the size of the warts and on the dermatologist. Sometimes new warts form while existing warts are being destroyed. All you can do is treat the new warts when they are large enough to be visible.

What are some alternative treatments?

- **Chinese medicine**—indirect moxibustion (a slice of ginger root covered with smoldering mugwort leaf is placed on the wart; the burning mugwort leaf is said to release antiviral constituents)

- **Herbal therapy**—aloe vera and dandelion

- **Homeopathy**—antimonium crudum, causticum, and nitric acid

The basics

1. *What's been proven to work?* You might try an over-the-counter product such as DuoFilm Wart Remover, but liquid nitrogen treatment (cryotherapy) is the most common treatment. This usually is done by a dermatologist or the family doctor. When applied to the skin, the liquid nitrogen usually results in a blister similar to a burn. The wart is lifted, and it will fall off when the blister dries. You may experience some pain, but it can easily be controlled with simple pain killers.

2. *How much does treatment cost?* Liquid nitrogen treatment costs about $50 to $100 and is covered by most insurance plans.

3. *How long until it works?* One week to 10 days.

No matter what treatment is used, warts occasionally fail to disappear.

Wrinkles

Wrinkles are an unavoidable sign of aging, dry, or damaged skin. Symptoms include sagging or folded skin, which usually occurs first on the forehead, lips (smile lines), and eyes (crow's feet). Because skin becomes looser over the face with age, wrinkles may sag on the eyelids. The skin under the chin and on the front of the neck also becomes looser and draped in appearance. This is caused by age, sun damage, and loose or sagging skin. Less fat tissue under the skin also can result in draping or sagging of the skin.

How is it prevented?

Stay out of the sun. If you must go in the sun, wear sunscreen and a large wide-brimmed hat. Keep hydrated and use moisturizing lotions to prevent dryness.

What is the conventional treatment?

Prescription skin creams containing retinoic acid (Retin-A or Renova) and plastic surgery.

What are some alternative treatments?

- **Ayurveda**— yoga (for improved blood flow)
- **Aromatherapy**—essential oils of chamomile and myrrh
- **Herbal therapy**—calendula, comfrey, ginger, parsley, and ginkgo biloba

- **Hydrotherapy**—drink two quarts of water a day to keep body hydrated; splash water on delicate tissues

- **Nutritional supplements**—evening primrose oil or black currant seed oil, vitamins A, C, and E

The basics

1. *What's been proven to work?* Ninety percent of skin changes associated with aging actually are caused by sun damage. Stay out of the sun and wear sunscreen with a sun protection factor (SPF) of at least 15 on all exposed skin during daylight hours. Retin-A and Renova are excellent prescription creams that can change the appearance of aging or sun-damaged skin. If your skin has deep wrinkles, newer chemical peels or laser techniques might help.

2. *How much does treatment cost?* A good sunscreen costs about $12 to $15 for one month. Prescription creams containing retinoic acid cost about $30 to $50 a month, depending on usage.

3. *How long until it works?* Prescription creams take two weeks to one month before you will see a noticeable difference in texture and tone of skin.

   It's hard to rejuvenate damaged, wrinkled skin because the effects of the sun are cumulative. It may take years before you notice any problems. Use preventive measures to avoid increased wrinkles and rely on prescription creams to change the texture of your skin.

Timesaver
Need a referral to a qualified plastic surgeon? Call the American Society of Plastic and Reconstructive Surgeons at 800-635-0635.

Just the facts

- Although Accutane has been proven to clear up severe cases of acne, recent studies claim this popular medication sometimes can cause depression.

- An oral antihistamine tablet, along with mind/body techniques to destress, is your best bet for preventing hives.

- Ultraviolet light therapy (UVL), a low-fat diet, and tomatoes all are new alternative ways to treat psoriasis.

- Z-plasty is a groundbreaking plastic surgery technique that can correct scarring.

- The best treatment for wrinkled skin is prevention—stay out of the sun, keep skin protected, wear a wide-brimmed hat, and stop cigarette smoking.

- Nutritional therapy, including a diet high in beta-carotene (carrots, sweet potatoes, winter squash, and cantaloupe), helps maintain proper immune function and healthy skin.

Why stress is a key in many gastrointestinal disorders ▪ The one herbal treatment that can keep constipation at bay ▪ Why hydrotherapy is a key treatment in many bowel problems ▪ Why antibiotics seem to be the treatment of choice for ulcers

Gastrointestinal Disorders

Colitis

Colitis is an inflammation of the large intestine that causes chronic diarrhea. This diarrhea is bloody, has mucus in it, and is accompanied by abdominal pain and possibly fever. It can be caused by an infection, a bacteria, a virus, or antibiotics, although sometimes the cause is unknown.

How is it prevented?

Avoiding raw fruits and vegetables to limit further trauma may reduce symptoms. A milk-free diet decreases symptoms in some people.

What is the conventional treatment?

A clear liquid diet is recommended until the diarrhea stops. See your doctor if the diarrhea lasts more than a few days. Some infections are treated with antibiotics such as metronidazole. In cases of Crohn's disease, an enema of hydrocortisone is given to settle the colitis.

Timesaver
If you are searching for an osteopath, an acupuncturist, a hypnotherapist or another practitioner, try the International Association of Healthcare Practitioners (IAHP) Directory, which lists more than 32,000 complementary-therapy professionals and their phone numbers. Call 800-311-9204, ext. 9359.

What are some alternative treatments?

- **Aromatherapy**—catnip, cayenne, cinnamon

- **Detoxification**—stick with clear liquids until diarrhea is over

- **Herbal therapy**—chamomile, feverfew, garlic, psyllium seed husks, or yarrow

- **Nutritional therapy**—the B.R.A.T. diet (bananas, rice, applesauce, dry toast) to stop the diarrhea, steamed vegetables

- **Nutritional supplements**—essential fatty acids (EFAs), flaxseed, or primrose oil

- **Mind/body therapy**—progressive muscle relaxation, relaxation response, or deep abdominal breathing

The basics

1. *What's been proven to work?* Colitis usually resolves itself without any medication. Decrease stress and increase healthful nutrients using any of the alternative treatments.

2. *How much does treatment cost?* Alternative methods that involve destressing or dietary changes are virtually free.

3. *How long until it works?* It may take several weeks to get your system regulated.

Preventing colitis is a lot easier than treating it. Stay on a well-balanced diet, avoid foods that aggravate the condition, and keep stressors controlled.

Constipation

Constipation is a condition in which you experience difficulty passing hard, dried feces. It can be caused by not drinking enough fluids, not eating enough dietary fiber (both soluble and insoluble), inactivity, overuse of stimulant laxatives, medications, ignoring the urge to use the bathroom, or medical problems such as hypothyroidism, irritable bowel syndrome, or hemorrhoids. Symptoms include bloating; abdominal pain; infrequent bowel movements; hard, formed feces; and difficulty in passing stool.

Watch Out!
Overuse of senna or cascara can, over time, damage the nerve cells of the colon and worsen constipation.

How is it prevented?

Add more fiber to your diet, especially bran, whole-grain bread, fresh fruit, and raw vegetables. Also, establish a regular bowel habit each day, exercise regularly, and drink at least eight glasses of water every day.

What is the conventional treatment?

For occasional constipation, you can use an over-the-counter stool softener, stimulant laxative, suppository, or enema. Using bulk-forming laxatives that contain psyllium and drinking plenty of liquids can keep you regular once you are relieved.

What are some alternative treatments?

- **Aromatherapy**—calendula, cascara, goldenseal
- **Ayurvedic medicine**—yoga, rose petal, triphala (herbal powder made from fruits of three trees: amalaki, haritaki, and bibhitaki)
- **Bodywork**—massage
- **Detoxification**—a cleansing fast or colonic irrigation
- **Herbal therapy**—psyllium seed husks, artichoke, senna, or turmeric
- **Nutritional therapy**—rhubarb root, foods high in beta-carotene, vitamin C, vitamin E, and selenium, as well as foods high in soluble and insoluble fiber, flaxseed

The basics

1. *What's been proven to work?* Psyllium seed husks are an excellent natural remedy for constipation and can be used all the time to prevent it from occurring.

2. *How much does it cost?* Psyllium cost about $6 for one week's supply.

3. *How long until it works?* It will take 24 hours to three days to reap the full colon-cleansing benefit of psyllium.

Alternative therapies are the answer for constipation, but the best treatment is to avoid constipation altogether with a fiber-rich diet.

Diarrhea

Diarrhea is an increase in the fluid, frequency, or volume of a bowel movement. It can be indicative of a variety of diseases that can be caused by an infection (dysentery), an inflammatory process (colitis), stress, or dietary indiscretion. One of the most common causes is food poisoning. Symptoms include frequent, loose stools in bowel movements that are different from a normal movement.

How is it prevented?

If possible, avoid situations that may aggravate diarrhea, such as eating spicy foods, drinking milk (if allergic), and stress.

What is the conventional treatment?

Replace the water and electrolytes (salts) lost during the attack of diarrhea. Use the B.R.A.T. diet (banana, rice, applesauce, toast). Antidiarrhea products—such as Imodium A-D or Pepto-Bismol—may be used, or your doctor may suggest a prescription drug.

> 66
>
> I found out that stress caused me to have stomach cramping and diarrhea when I was in bed for several days after a turnover in staff at my job. I couldn't eat anything without going to the bathroom. I knew I had to get in control, and learning to deal with my stress by using deep abdominal breathing and the relaxation response (page 154) gave me my life back.
> —Jacob, 44, CPA
>
> 99

What are some alternative treatments?

- **Chinese medicine**—acupuncture
- **Detoxification**—liquid diet
- **Herbal therapy**—chamomile tea
- **Nutritional therapy**—a tablespoon of carob powder mixed with applesauce and honey, the B.R.A.T. diet (banana, rice, applesauce, toast)

The basics

1. *What's been proven to work?* Drink clear liquids or use the B.R.A.T. diet.

2. *How much does treatment cost?* The B.R.A.T. diet costs under $5; the liquid diet is virtually free.

3. *How long until it works?* You should notice a difference in 6 to 12 hours on a liquid diet.

Don't let diarrhea go too long or it may cause dehydration. Call your doctor if it cannot be controlled using over-the-counter medications, clear liquids, or the B.R.A.T. diet.

Flatulence

Flatulence is the expulsion of intestinal gas through the anus. It can be caused by swallowed air, a diet high in fiber, legumes, a gastrointestinal virus, or fermentation. Symptoms include abdominal cramping or pain that is relieved when the intestinal gas is expelled.

How is it prevented?

Avoid chewing gum, eat a balanced diet, and keep anxiety and stress levels low. Sprinkle legumes with alpha-galactosidase (Beano) to neutralize the gas.

Bright Idea
Keep a product containing alpha-galactosidase (Beano) with you during the week in case you want to order legumes for lunch. Sprinkle this on the legumes to neutralize gas, preventing the problem of flatulence altogether.

What is the conventional treatment?

Flatulence usually passes without medical attention. You may try over-the-counter products containing simethicone to alleviate any abdominal discomfort. You also can monitor the foods you eat to see which are causing gas.

What are some alternative treatments?

- **Ayurvedic medicine**—ginger
- **Aromatherapy**—allspice, catnip, celery seed
- **Detoxification**—increasing liquids
- **Mind/body treatments**—relaxation response, progressive muscle relaxation
- **Nutritional therapy**—eat a balanced diet, eliminate foods that increase gas and then gradually reintroduce them into the diet

The basics

1. *What's been proven to work?* Watch what you eat! If you increase fiber in your diet, do so slowly. When you do get gas, try over-the-counter products that contain simethicone.

2. *How much does treatment cost?* Over-the-counter products that contain simethicone cost about $7 to $12 for one week's supply.

3. *How long until it works?* You will notice a difference within one to three hours.

Watch what you feed your mind and body to avoid flatulence. Stress can increase the incidence of excessive gas, as can lentils and a high fiber diet.

Gallstones

Gallstones are round lumps of solid matter found in the gallbladder. They're caused by an upset in the chemical composition of bile. When bile contains an abundance of cholesterol, a tiny particle forms and grows into a stone. There may be no symptoms at all, or you may feel intense pain in the right side of the abdomen between the shoulder blades. Vomiting and indigestion also may occur.

How is it prevented?
Stay at a normal weight, reduce sugar and fat intake, and increase fiber.

What is the conventional treatment?
Some stones can be dissolved with drugs or can be pulverized with sonic shock waves. Others require surgery to remove the gallbladder.

What are some alternative treatments?
- **Chinese medicine**—acupuncture and herbs
- **Nutritional therapy**—low-fat diet, elimination diet (avoid sugar), increased fiber

The basics
1. *What's been proven to work?* Dietary changes that result in weight loss can help you avoid problems with gallstones.
2. *How much does treatment cost?* Changing your diet to include more fiber and less sugar and fat will not alter your grocery bill.
3. *How long until it works?* You will notice a difference within two weeks to one month.

If you are overweight, get down to your normal weight. Change your diet to include extra fiber and choose foods low in saturated and trans-fats.

Heartburn
Heartburn is a burning pain in the center of the chest or in the middle of the torso under the ribs. It can be caused by overeating, spicy food, caffeine,

Watch Out!
If you are "female, fat, and forty," you had better eat a low-fat diet. You are a prime candidate for gallstones. Fill up on fresh fruits and vegetables; push high-fat meats and desserts away.

Watch Out!
Rapid weight loss also has been associated with gallstone formation. If you must pursue major weight loss, do so under a doctor's care to avoid this and other complications.

alcohol, peppermint, onions, garlic, chocolate, excessive stomach-acid production, and foods high in fat. Symptoms include a burning or stinging feeling in the chest and throat. Sometimes it can be associated with a chronic cough, a chronic sore throat, or asthma.

How is it prevented?

Destress your life, avoid your specific trigger foods, stay upright for a couple of hours after eating (don't lie down on the couch), and consider elevating the head of your bed a few inches.

What is the conventional treatment?

Over-the-counter heartburn-relief medications called H2 blockers (Pepcid AC, Axid AR, Tagament HB, and Zantac 75) are commonly used. Mylanta, an over-the-counter antacid containing magnesium hydroxide and calcium, is also sometimes helpful. Prescriptions such as Prilosec and Prevacid provide 24-hour acid control and are recommended for more complicated heartburn and acid reflux disease (gastroesophageal reflux disease, or GERD).

What are some alternative treatments?

- **Ayurvedic medicine**—ginger tea
- **Chinese medicine**—acupuncture, acupressure points on legs, hands, and feet
- **Herbal therapy**—aloe, chamomile, ginger, dandelion root, peppermint
- **Homeopathy**—arsenicum album (arsenic)
- **Mind/body therapy**— visualization and relaxation response (to manage stress)
- **Nutritional therapy**—avoid caffeine, alcohol, peppermint, tomatoes, and chocolate

Watch Out!
Last year, more than $3.7 billion was spent on heartburn medications in the U.S. Lifestyle changes—such as destressing, losing weight, avoiding trigger foods, quitting smoking, and eating small amounts of food at a time—can help prevent heartburn altogether.

The basics

1. *What's been proven to work?* If over-the-counter heartburn medications do not relieve your problem, Prilosec is extremely effective and easy to take.

2. *How much does treatment cost?* About $1 a day. Some, however, cost as much as $4 to $5 a day.

3. *How long until it works?* It usually takes at least 45 minutes to two hours for over-the-counter pills to work, although liquids may help sooner. Prilosec usually works within one to two days.

Not only is heartburn uncomfortable and irritating, it can be serious and can lead to problems such as GERD with asthma symptoms. Take care of heartburn in the early stages with the proper diet and medications. If you have risk factors for heart attack—obesity, family history, hypertension, or diabetes—call your doctor if you feel any unusual pain around the heart.

Hemorrhoids

Hemorrhoids are swollen veins in the lower rectum and in and around the anus. Excess pressure (such as straining to expell stool), inadequate diet, pregnancy, heredity, aging, and chronic constipation all increase the chances of developing this condition. An internal hemorrhoid (inside the anus) often is noticed when blood appears on the toilet paper. If the distended vein protrudes outside the body and becomes irritated and painful, it is called a *protruding* or *prolapsed hemorrhoid*. The other type, an external hemorrhoid, is the result of a blood clot forming under the skin around the anus. An external hemorrhoid can be extremely painful, especially when it becomes ulcerated. Excessive rubbing or cleaning can cause irritation, bleeding, or itching and can lead to an escalating cycle of pain.

How is it prevented?

Increase fiber and fluid in the diet; avoid straining during bowel movements.

What is the conventional treatment?

Most cases can be treated with over-the-counter suppositories or prescription corticosteroid suppositories and creams. Sitz baths or Epsom salts dissolved in warm bath water can help to reduce inflammation. In severe cases, surgery (hemorrhoidectomy) is necessary.

What are some alternative treatments?

- **Aromatherapy**—essential oils of chamomile or lavender (gently massage into irritated tissue)
- **Hydrotherapy**—warm sitz baths or moist heat applications to reduce inflammation
- **Nutritional therapy**—fiber rich foods (20 to 35 grams a day)

You can choose a high-fiber diet instead of medications to ease gastrointestinal problems (see Table 11.1).

The basics

1. *What's been proven to work?* High-fiber diets and shrinking the hemorrhoid with sitz baths or over-the-counter hemorrhoid suppositories.

2. *How much does it cost?* Over-the-counter hemorrhoid suppositories cost about $10 for a seven-day treatment.

3. *How long until it works?* You will notice a difference in three days to one week.

TABLE 11.1

Food	Serving Size	Total Fiber (grams)
Apple	1 medium	4
Banana	1 medium	3
Broccoli	1 cup, cooked	4
Cereal, high fiber	½ cup	10
Corn, kernel	½ cup, cooked	3.2
Kale	1 cup, cooked	4
Kidney beans	¾ cup, cooked	10
Oatmeal	¾ cup, dry	6
Orange	1 medium	4
Peach	1 medium	2
Prunes, dried	3	4
Raspberries	½ cup	4
Squash, summer	1 cup, cooked	4.4
Strawberries, raw	1¼ cup	6.5
Whole wheat bread	1 slice	2

If you notice blood after a bowel movement, do not assume it is caused by a hemorrhoid. Call your doctor and get it checked out. Sometimes bloody stools are caused by more serious gastrointestinal problems.

Irritable bowel syndrome (IBS)

Irritable bowel syndrome consists of intermittent abdominal cramps and constipation with alternating periods of diarrhea. Factors such as stress and lack of fiber in the diet have been implicated as the cause of this condition. The symptoms will get worse if you eat poorly, as people frequently do while on vacation or out of town. Periods of stress seem to worsen the symptoms. The cramps can be located in any part of the stomach. Sometimes the cramps are severe enough to cause a visit to the emergency

room. Degrees of severity can range from an occasional mild episode to a debilitating illness that
causes frequent absenteeism from work. It is important to realize that this illness will not shorten your
life. It is more of a nuisance like a headache.

How is it prevented?

Reduce stress, eat a diet high in soluble and insoluble fiber, and exercise regularly.

What is the conventional treatment?

Add fiber to your diet—high-fiber cereals, fruits,
and vegetables, as well as commercial brands of
fiber. Occasionally, antispasmodic medication must
be added to the treatment. Drinking plenty of liquids and getting daily exercise are very helpful in
reducing symptoms.

What are some alternative treatments?

- **Aromatherapy**—chickweed
- **Ayurvedic medicine**—yoga, allspice
- **Detoxification**—increased fiber and water
- **Herbal therapy**—psyllium seed husks
- **Mind/body treatments**—hypnotherapy or any
  relaxation technique
- **Nutritional supplements**—essential fatty acids
  (omega-3s, flaxseed, and evening primrose oils)
- **Nutritional therapy**—elimination diet (avoid
  sugar and fat), eat more fruits and vegetables

The basics

1. *What's been proven to work?* According to research
   published in *Medical Tribune*, patients with irritable bowel syndrome felt less anxiety, abdominal pain, and bloating after hypnotherapy.

2. *How much does it cost?* Costs vary from $50 to $75 per session, depending on location.

3. *How long until treatment works?* If you are able to be hypnotized, you may notice a difference in two days to one week.

Reducing stress and anxiety, avoiding dietary triggers, and eating a high-fiber diet seem to be the keys to coping with IBS.

Motion sickness

Motion sickness is an unpleasant, temporary disturbance that occurs while traveling. It is characterized by dizziness and stomach upset. It is the result of motion or movement that causes fluid changes in the semicircular canals of the inner ear, which transmit signals to the brain's nausea center. Symptoms include nausea, vomiting, weakness, and unsteadiness.

How is it prevented?
Avoid eating or drinking before and during travel, sit over the wings in an airplane, recline in your seat, avoid reading, avoid cigarette smoke, and breathe deeply.

What is the conventional treatment?
You can use over-the-counter medications such as Dramamine (meclizine hydrochloride) to prevent motion sickness before you travel, or you can wear scopolamine skin patches during the trip.

What are some alternative treatments?
■ **Chinese medicine**—acupuncture, dried tangerine peel (to prevent motion sickness), or acupressure (press the specific points on your wrist to ease feelings of nausea)

Bright Idea
Keep a diary of what you eat for a week or two when you have IBS symptoms. Try to correlate these symptoms with dietary triggers or foods that may not agree with your system.

Timesaver
The new prescription allergy medicine, Allegra, has been found to block motion sickness in many people. Keep some on hand when traveling.

- **Herbal therapy**—ginger or raspberry leaf (for motion sickness)
- **Homeopathy**—Nux vomica, Ferrum, and Pulsatilla

The basics

1. *What's been proven to work?* The National Institutes of Health has confirmed that acupuncture can help with nausea. Ginger has been found to help calm a weak stomach.

2. *How much does treatment cost?* Acupuncture costs $35 to $125 per session, but many insurance companies will foot the bill.

3. *How long until it works?* You should notice a difference within one treatment. Ginger may take several hours to provide the optimum effect.

Alternative methods are helpful with ailments such as nausea or motion sickness. If the nausea is associated with pregnancy, ask your doctor before using any treatment.

Nausea

Nausea is an unsettled feeling in the stomach that generally precedes vomiting. It can be caused by a host of physical disorders within the gastrointestinal tract such as peptic ulcer disease or gastroenteritis. Stress, heart disease, pregnancy, and psychological problems also can cause nausea. Symptoms include dizziness, churning in the stomach, feeling faint, and burning in the throat.

How is it prevented?

Avoid situations that make you feel nauseated, such as certain smells, fumes, foods, and traveling for long distances.

Bright Idea
Keep a supply of ginger ale on hand during cold and flu season to calm upset stomachs.

What is the conventional treatment?

Over-the-counter medications such as Emetrol can help stop feelings of nausea. If this doesn't work, your doctor may prescribe a drug such as Phenergan in either liquid, pill, or suppository form.

What are some alternative treatments?

- **Chinese medicine**—acupuncture, acupressure, shiatsu

- **Aromatherapy**—Add a drop of peppermint essential oil to a sugar cube and suck on it until the cube melts

- **Homeopathy**— Nux vomica and Ferrum (for nausea)

- **Herbal therapy**—Ginger, raspberry leaf, and horehound (to ease a queasy stomach and to squelch nausea).

The basics

1. *What's been proven to work?* You might try an acupressure wrist band, which is designed to apply pressure to the Neiguan point. This spot on the inside of the forearm just above the wrist is associated with nausea. Acupuncture also has been reported by the National Institutes of Health (NIH) to be safe and effective in ending nausea.

2. *How much does treatment cost?* Acupuncture costs from $35 to $125 per session and may be covered by your health insurance plan.

3. *How long until it works?* You may notice a decrease in nausea within minutes of trying acupuncture or acupressure.

If the nausea continues, it can be a sign of serious illness. Call your doctor.

Stomach ache

A stomach ache is abdominal pain associated with the stomach. It can be caused by a high-fiber diet, food poisoning, an ulcer, diverticulitis, gallstones, kidney stones, intestinal discomfort, stress, or a virus. It also may be caused by appendicitis, colic, an intestinal obstruction, endometriosis, ovarian cysts, ectopic pregnancy, or a very serious vascular accident. Symptoms may include bloating, burning or stinging pain, intestinal gas, vomiting, constipation, diarrhea, fever, heartburn, and mucus or blood in the stool.

How is it prevented?
Eat a balanced and nutritious diet, drink at least eight cups of water a day, exercise to avoid constipation, and reduce stress.

What is the conventional treatment?
Treatment varies depending on the cause of the stomach ache. For a stomach ache caused by a virus, treatment could include over-the-counter medications containing magnesium hydroxide.

What are some alternative treatments?

- **Aromatherapy**—chamomile
- **Mind/body treatments**—relaxation response or any mind/body therapy (to destress)
- **Nutritional therapy**—B.R.A.T. diet (bananas, rice, applesauce, dry toast), blueberries

The basics
1. *What's been proven to work?* Use a combination of stress-reduction techniques and a bland diet until the stomach calms down.

2. *How much does treatment cost?* Over-the-counter medications cost from $5 to $8 for one week's supply.

3. *How long until it works?* You should notice a difference within two to six hours.

If the stomach ache is caused by a virus, sometimes the best treatment is no treatment. Let the virus pass, introduce bland foods (B.R.A.T. diet) and flat cola, and the stomach gradually will feel less queasy.

Ulcer

An ulcer is a sore or an area of raw tissue in the stomach (gastric ulcers) or in the part of the intestine that drains food from the stomach (duodenal ulcers). Ninety percent of all ulcers are caused by a bacterium, Helicobacter pylori (H. pylori), that adheres to the cells in the lining of the stomach and causes tissue damage. Other causes include excessive acidity, arthritis medicine, inflammatory drugs, inflammation, and irritation. Symptoms include burning, belching, and bloating in the stomach. Sometimes gas and nausea are felt.

How is it prevented?

Avoid overuse of aspirin or anti-inflammatory drugs; they can cause damage to the lining of the stomach.

What is the conventional treatment?

You may find relief with H2 blockers, a class of drug traditionally prescribed for ulcers. Over-the-counter heartburn-relief medications (Pepcid AC, Zantac 75, Tagament HB, Axid AR) are low-dose versions of prescription H2 blockers. Temporary relief can be provided by antacid tablets (medicine that counteracts or neutralizes acids). The prescription drugs

Prilosec or Prevacid completely shut down the production of stomach acid and can be used with a combination of antibiotics that treat H. pylori bacteria.

What are some alternative treatments?

- **Aromatherapy**—chamomile
- **Mind/body treatments**—relaxation response, autogenic training, visualization

The basics

1. *What's been proven to work?* Antibiotic therapy works in most cases caused by a bacterium.

2. *How much does it cost?* Antibiotic therapy costs from $30 to $100. Prilosec costs about $3 to $5 a pill.

3. *How long until it works?* With an antibiotic, you will notice a difference in one to two weeks. Prilosec will bring relief in one to three days.

New findings on ulcers dramatically change the way they are treated. Doctors used to think ulcers were caused by diet and stress; now it is known that the H. pylori bacteria or arthritis and anti-inflammatory drugs are responsible in most cases. If you have an ulcer or think you might have one, see your doctor for a diagnosis and treatment.

Just the facts

- Nausea is one ailment that can easily be treated with acupuncture or acupressure, according to the National Institutes of Health.

- Irritable bowel syndrome (IBS) frequently ends when you use stress-reduction techniques to calm anxiety and tension.

- Doctors used to blame ulcers on stress, but now they know the H. pylori bacteria is responsible in most cases.

- Constipation can be easily avoided by introducing more fiber into the diet and by increasing liquids.

Musculoskeletal Disorders

Chapter 12

Arthritis

Arthritis is inflammation in or around the joints and muscles, and it affects more than 40 million people in the U.S. There are two main categories of arthritis:

Osteoarthritis	Inflammatory Arthritis
Fibromyalgia	Rheumatoid arthritis
Bursitis	Ankylosing Spondylitis
Tendinitis	Systemic Lupus Erythemetosus
	Gout (Gouty arthritis)
	Pseudogout
	Polymyalgia Rheumatica (PMR)

Arthritis is caused by inflammation, wear-and-tear, aging, and immune system dysfunction. Symptoms include joint and muscle pain, stiffness in the joints, and swelling. At times, the joints may be warm or red. In osteoarthritis, the pain is limited to the joints. In rheumatoid arthritis, a person may

Watch Out!
A startling 9 out of 10 cases of back pain are not caused by herniated discs—they are simply muscle strain, which goes away within a month with nonoperative treatment. In spite of this, more than 181,000 men underwent a discectomy (removal of disc) last year, a rate that is five times higher than in other Western countries. After the discectomy, the number of fusions done on the back has increased 100 percent over the past decade, yet 60 percent of fusions do not reduce the pain. Ten percent of people get new, unrelated back pain after fusions.

suffer from pain and deformities in the joints, fever, weight loss, and severe fatigue. There also may be inflammation around the heart, the lungs, and the eyes in rheumatoid arthritis.

How is it prevented?

Protect your joints with exercise and keep the muscles strong with strength training, which supports the joints and helps prevent injury. Stay at a normal weight because obesity can add unnecessary pressure to aging joints.

What is the conventional treatment?

Treatments include twice daily applications of moist heat or ice on the joints (20 minutes each time), exercises, nonsteroidal anti-inflammatory drugs (NSAIDS), cortisone-like medications, muscle relaxants, pain medications, and anti-depressants.

What are some alternative treatments?

- **Herbal therapy**——ginger, capsaicin (ointment or cream)
- **Homeopathy**—arnica
- **Hydrotherapy**—moist heat, spas, whirlpools
- **Nutritional supplements**—glucosamine and chondroitin, fish oil supplements, and flaxseed or evening primrose oil
- **Nutritional therapy**—pineapple (contains the enzyme bromelain, which helps reduce inflammation)

The basics

1. *What's been proven to work?* There is nothing like moist heat for tender, arthritic joints, especially when combined with nonsteroidal anti-inflammatory medications (NSAIDs) to reduce swelling, to increase mobility, and to reduce

pain. Applications of a topical cream, Capsaicin, also can help. Although some people believe glucosamine and chondroitin can cure arthritis, these medications have only been shown to give relief similar to that provided by over-the-counter pain medications such as ibuprofen.

2. *How much does treatment cost?* Moist heat can cost pennies a day if you use a warm bath or shower. Nonsteroidal anti-inflammatory drugs can cost from fifty cents to over a dollar a day. Capsaicin creams cost about $5 a week.

3. *How long until it works?* You will notice a difference in pain within three days to two weeks if you keep up the twice daily applications of moist heat (20 minutes each time) along with the recommended dose of NSAIDs.

It is important to remember that, in arthritis treatment, the benefits should outweigh the risks, and the chances for improvement should be greater than the risks of side effects from medications. Try to prevent pain by following an exercise plan that keeps joints and muscles strong, and lean on alternative therapies such as hydrotherapy (the use of moist heat on aching joints) before taking medications that could have deleterious effects such as nausea, abdominal pain, or a peptic ulcer.

Backache

A sharp or dull pain in the back usually is caused by strained muscles in the lower back. Other causes include back injuries such as a slipped or herniated disk, arthritis, osteoporosis, and urinary tract infections. Symptoms can include severe pain (sharp, shooting, or the electrical-shock type) in the back or pain felt in the low back that travels down the back

Unofficially . . .
In a study of 66 patients with rheumatoid arthritis (published in the *Journal of Arthritis and Rheumatism)*, of the participants who took fish-oil supplements, about half had less joint tenderness and morning stiffness and had less pain overall. The fish-oil patients also experienced a drop in blood levels of interleukin 1-beta, a growth factor that causes joint inflammation.

of one leg. Sometimes the pain worsens with movement or activity and is accompanied by numbness or tingling in the back, leg, or foot.

How is it prevented?

Use safe lifting techniques, keep the muscles of the back strong, and stay at a normal weight. Also, silly as it may sound, you should avoid falling, especially if you are older.

What is the conventional treatment?

Get a few days rest, apply moist heat or ice, and use anti-inflammatory medications (if necessary). Exercise as the pain lessens and use a moist heating pad, a hot-water bottle, hot compresses, a hot tub, hot baths, or hot showers. Use heat for 20 minutes and then take the heat off for 20 minutes. Do this up to three hours a day. Be careful not to burn the skin. Stretching, exercises, and avoiding too much bed rest also are important.

What are some alternative treatments?

- **Aromatherapy**—myrrh
- **Bodywork**—Swedish massage
- **Chinese medicine**—acupuncture, acupressure, shiatsu, or tai chi
- **Chiropractic**—spinal adjustment
- **Homeopathy**—rhus toxicodendron (poison ivy)
- **Hydrotherapy**—moist heat or ice
- **Nutritional therapy**—pineapple (contains the enzyme *bromelain*, which helps reduce inflammation)

The basics

1. *What's been proven to work?* In a study of 741 men and women with chronic back pain, London

researchers found that, after three years, people treated by chiropractors showed almost a 30 percent greater improvement than people treated by therapists in hospital-based outpatient clinics. Chiropractic patients paid more frequent visits, however, and underwent care for a longer period of time than the other patients. This may have accounted for at least part of the difference, as reported in the *British Medical Journal.*

2. *How much does it cost?* A visit to a chiropractor for spinal adjustment costs about $50 to $100 for an initial visit.

3. *How long until it works?* Chiropractic can ease tense muscles on the first visit, or it may take weeks to months to feel relief. Most people find relief within 10 to 12 days.

Most back pain resolves itself without any treatment at all. But moist heat, analgesics or anti-inflammatory medications, and exercise also are important to decrease pain and to increase mobility.

Bursitis

A bursa is a fibrous sac or tissue space that is lined with joint tissue and that contains a small amount of joint fluid. They are found between tendon and bones, skin and bones, and muscles. They work by helping fluid move. Bursitis is an acute or chronic inflammation of a bursa.

The cause of bursitis is unknown, although repetitive direct pressure, such as kneeling or leaning on your elbow, is a key factor. Symptoms include pain and difficulty moving the muscle or tendon around a joint (such as the shoulder, hip, elbow, or knee). You also might feel severe pain when lying down on one side, which can interfere with sleep.

"

Because I cannot take aspirin, I started taking fish oil capsules to help alleviate some of the inflammation of bursitis in my shoulder. Within two weeks of taking two capsules per day, I felt great relief. I now stay on one capsule each day to prevent a flare up.
—Sadie, 59, bank teller

"

How is it prevented?

Avoid constant or direct pressure on muscles or tendons.

What is the conventional treatment?

Treatment includes twice daily applications of moist heat (20 minutes each time) along with non-steroidal anti-inflammatory drugs (NSAIDs) to reduce inflammation and to alleviate pain and stiffness. A local injection of cortisone in the bursa may be necessary.

What are some alternative treatments?

- **Bodywork**—Swedish massage, reiki, Alexander technique

- **Chinese medicine**—acupuncture, Chinese herbs

- **Chiropractic**—spinal adjustment

- **Homeopathy**—arnica or lobelia inflata, viburnum opulus (anti-spasmotic rub)

- **Hydrotherapy**—warm whirlpool bath or spa

- **Nutritional therapy**—pineapple (contains the enzyme *bromelain*, which helps reduce inflammation)

The basics

1. *What's been proven to work?* Stick with the conventional treatment of moist heat and NSAIDs for optimum pain relief. If this does not work, ask your doctor about an injection in the bursa.

2. *How much does treatment cost?* NSAIDS cost about $5 to $10 for seven days.

3. *How long until it works?* You should notice a difference in three days to one week. If not, see your doctor.

Using a combination of NSAIDS, moist heat, and stretching exercises, most cases of bursitis will easily resolve in time.

Carpal tunnel syndrome

Carpal tunnel syndrome is a common cause of pain, numbness, and tingling in the thumb, index, and middle fingers. It's caused by pressure on the median nerve as it passes through the wrist's carpal tunnel. Any process that causes swelling in this small area will create pressure on the nerve. Arthritis, injury, diabetes mellitus, pregnancy, an underactive thyroid gland, and other medical problems all can cause carpal tunnel syndrome. Symptoms include pain and numbness that affect the thumb, index, and middle fingers and that may extend to the forearm or the entire hand. The pain or discomfort usually is worse at night. Sometimes, instead of pain, you may feel as if your hand went to sleep.

How is it prevented?

Avoid injury to the wrist. Wrist guards can be used with computer keyboards, splints can be worn at night, and exercises can be done to relax the wrists.

What is the conventional treatment?

A special splint can be worn to alleviate pressure on the median nerve. Twice daily applications of moist heat (20 minutes each time) and anti-inflammatory medications (NSAIDs) also are used to decrease swelling and pain. In severe cases, surgery or injection of steroids is necessary.

What are some alternative treatments?

- **Chinese medicine**—acupuncture, acupressure
- **Homeopathy**—arnica, rhus toxicodendron

Unofficially . . .
Carpal tunnel syndrome, which affects 2 million Americans and costs business a staggering $20 billion annually, is reported 1.7 times more often by working women than men. More women than men also experience musculoskeletal injuries to the hand, wrist, arm, and shoulder caused by child care responsibilities requiring lifting and bending.

Unofficially . . .
A recent National
Health Survey
reported that, of
the 697 million
visits to physi-
cians' offices
annually, a star-
tling 81.6 mil-
lion are injury
related. Of this
number, approxi-
mately 14 mil-
lion are home
accidents and
five million are
sports-related
injuries.

Bright Idea
If you have been
diagnosed with
fibromyalgia,
destressing your
life using
mind/body
therapies (see
Chapter 8) is an
excellent way to
reduce symp-
toms. Stress
heightens symp-
toms in some
people, but ther-
apies such as the
relaxation
response, music
therapy, and
deep abdominal
breathing can
help reduce
them.

■ **Hydrotherapy**—moist heating pad, warm paraffin wax

■ **Nutritional supplements**—vitamin B complex

The basics

1. *What's been proven to work?* Use a combination of protecting the wrist with special splints so it can heal, NSAIDS, moist heat, and exercise.

2. *How much does treatment cost?* NSAIDS cost about $5 to $10 for seven days. A wrist guard costs from $20 to $40 at a medical supply store.

3. *How long until it works?* You will notice a decrease in pain within one week after starting a regular treatment program of moist heat, NSAIDS, and protecting the wrist.

If possible, avoid repetitive motions that will cause this injury. If you already have this condition, wear the wrist guard day and night until you feel relief and try to avoid further injury.

Fibromyalgia

Fibromyalgia is an arthritis-like syndrome that affects more than 10 million people, mostly women in mid-life. The cause is unknown. It may happen after an injury, or a virus may cause it. Some researchers believe it is associated with a sleep disorder or chronic fatigue syndrome. Symptoms include widespread deep-muscle aches and pain, ongoing fatigue, difficulty in acquiring restful sleep, depression, and anxiety, among others.

How is it prevented?

No one knows how to prevent fibromyalgia.

What is the conventional treatment?

Use medications such as analgesics, nonsteroidal anti-inflammatories, muscle relaxers, local injections to reduce pain, and antidepressants; along with twice daily moist heat, stress reduction, and exercise.

What are some alternative treatments?

- **Aromatherapy**—lime, lemon, marjoram

- **Bodywork**—massage therapy

- **Chinese medicine**—acupuncture, acupressure, shiatsu, tai chi

- **Chiropractic**—spinal manipulation

- **Herbal therapy**—capsaicin ointment on painful trigger points

- **Hydrotherapy**—moist heat applications

- **Mind/body treatment**—relaxation response, guided imagery, biofeedback

- **Nutritional therapy**—a varied diet high in antioxidants and phytochemicals

The basics

1. *What's been proven to work?* A multidimensional treatment plan appears to work best for fibromyalgia symptoms. This includes moist heat, pain medications, antidepressants, and lifestyle changes to reduce stress.

2. *How much does treatment cost?* Anti-inflammatory medications cost about $10 a week; antidepressants cost about $20 to $35 a month.

3. *How long until it works?* You may notice a difference in three days to three weeks, although some fibromyalgia patients have difficulty finding any relief at all.

Using a combination of treatments, most people can feel relief from symptoms. Capsaicin ointment rubbed on painful muscles may help bring relief because capsaicin depletes the bodily reserves of Substance P (believed to be high in fibromyalgia patients), which prolongs inflammation and pain.

Gout

Gout is a form of arthritis that may cause a sudden onset of severe pain. It's caused by a buildup of uric acid in the body. Symptoms include pain and swelling, usually in the large toe. The joint usually is warm and tender to touch, and it can be difficult to walk. Sometimes more than one joint may be attacked at one time.

How is it prevented?

Avoid foods that are high in purine such as liver, organ meats, poultry, and legumes. Also avoid excessive alcohol consumption.

What is the conventional treatment?

Treatment of gout includes large doses of non-steroidal anti-inflammatory medications (NSAIDs) and colchicine. Sometimes injections into the painful joint with a corticosteroid drug may be necessary. Allopurinol tablets can prevent gout altogether if taken regularly.

What are some alternative treatments?

- **Homeopathy**—rhus toxicodendron (poison ivy)
- **Hydrotherapy**—moist heat or ice
- **Nutritional supplements**—flaxseed or evening primrose oil, omega-3s
- **Nutritional therapy**—elimination diet (avoid meat and alcohol)

The basics

1. *What's been proven to work?* Gout is so painful that conventional treatment should initially be used

to quickly treat the gout and to reduce the inflammation.

2. *How much does treatment cost?* Medications for gout cost from $15 to $35 for seven days. NSAIDs cost from $5 to $10 for seven days.

3. *How long until it works?* Using NSAIDs, you should feel relief within four days to two weeks. An injection of cortisone should bring relief within one day to one week.

Prevention is the key with gout. Avoid meat and alcohol to stay gout-free.

Heel spurs

A heel spur is a hard bony shelf as wide as the width of the heel bone. It is the result of a repeated pulling away of periosteum (tissue around the heel bone) from the heel bone.

A heel spur can be caused by obesity, constant pressure on the foot from prolonged standing, repeated injuries to the foot, running, or fast walking. Chronic inflammation of the connective tissues can lead to a heel spur. Symptoms include throbbing pain, warm to touch, and tenderness. Firm pressure applied directly to the center of the heel will elicit further pain.

How is it prevented?

Wear low-heeled shoes, avoid activities that put undue pressure on the heel, and wear well-cushioned athletic shoes for exercise.

What is the conventional treatment?

You can take ibuprofen, acetaminophen, or aspirin to alleviate pain. You also can ice the heel, elevate the heel to the level of the heart to prevent swelling, inject corticosteroids, strap the heel to ease tension,

Moneysaver
A simple and inexpensive heel cup can be purchased at drug stores or grocery stores. Studies have found that this device will, in many cases, protect the heel from further injury.

and use orthotic devices such as a heel cup to protect from further trauma or irritation to the tissues.

What are some alternative treatments?

- **Chinese medicine**—acupuncture, acupressure, or shiatsu

- **Chiropractic**—realign the pelvic bones and spine

- **Homeopathy**—rhus toxicodendron (poison ivy)

- **Hydrotherapy**—ice packs or moist heat

- **Reflexology**—massage to relax tissues

The basics

1. *What's been proven to work?* Chiropractic balancing of the pelvic bones and vertebra may help reduce the cause of the inflammation and allow the tissue to heal. A stretching program and reflexology to soften and relax the tissues also may be helpful. A simple heel cup purchased at a drug store can help take pressure off the injured foot and give it time to heal.

2. *What does treatment cost?* A chiropractic session can cost from $50 to $100 for an initial visit and from $25 to $65 for a follow up visit. A simple heel cup purchased at the drugstore costs about $8.

3. *How long until it works?* It may take several weeks or months for you to feel total relief from heel pain.

Make sure your shoes fit comfortably and try to keep pressure off the injured heel. Consult with a podiatrist as necessary.

Muscle strain

Muscle strain occurs when a muscle is damaged by excessive stretching. Symptoms include aching or sharp pain in the injured muscle.

How is it prevented?

Make sure to do a proper warm-up before exercise, including stretching muscles.

What is the conventional treatment?

Treatments include ice, nonsteroidal anti-inflammatory medications to reduce pain and swelling, elevation of the injured muscle, and strengthening exercises.

What are some alternative treatments?

- **Ayurvedic medicine**—vetivier root

- **Bodywork**—massage

- **Chinese medicine**—tai chi, acupuncture, acupressure, or shiatsu

- **Homeopathy**—rhus toxicodendron (poison ivy), arnica

- **Hydrotherapy**—R.I.C.E. (rest, ice, compression, elevation) followed by applications of moist heat

- **Nutritional supplements**—essential fatty acids (EFAs)

The basics

1. *What's been proven to work?* Stick to NSAIDS and R.I.C.E., a combination of conventional and alternative treatments.

2. *How much does treatment cost?* NSAIDS cost about $5 to $10 for seven days.

3. *How long until it works?* Using this combination, you will feel relief within two days to one week.

Prevention is the focus. Stretch carefully before exercise to warm up tight muscles. Don't work beyond your capabilities. Go slow if you are just starting to exercise to avoid muscle injury. You may want to consult a personal trainer or a professional at your health club or purchase a video tape if you're unsure about the proper method of stretching.

Neck pain

Neck pain occurs when you feel tension and pain in the upper back, shoulders, and neck. You may experience difficulty turning the neck, stiffness, muscle tightness, and burning pain. The many causes include stress, tightness of the muscles, osteoarthritis, osteoporosis, frozen shoulder, bone spurs, pinched nerves, broken collarbone, herniated disk, and sleeping in a bad position, among others.

How is it prevented?

Keep the shoulder, upper back, and neck muscles strong and flexible with frequent stretching and strengthening exercises. Avoid repetitive strain injuries or sudden movements of the neck.

Bright Idea
Place an old stool in your bathtub or shower, sit on it, and let warm water from the shower flow down the back of your neck. Try this for 20 minutes twice a day, and you will notice reduced pain and increased mobility within days to two weeks.

What is the conventional treatment?

You can use twice daily moist heat (20 minutes each time), nonsteroidal anti-inflammatory medications, exercises to strengthen the upper back and neck, and stress reduction.

What are some alternative treatments?

- **Aromatherapy**—lime, lemon, marjoram
- **Ayurvedic medicine**—yoga
- **Bodywork**—massage
- **Chiropractic**—spinal manipulation
- **Herbal therapy**—capsicum, cat's claw, or lavender for inflamation; valerian to relax muscles

- **Hydrotherapy**—moist heat or ice packs
- **Mind/Body treatment**—biofeedback, relaxation response, or hypnosis

The basics

1. *What's been proven to work?* The relaxation response, or any of the mind/body therapies, may reduce emotional stress by calming negative thoughts and keeping the mental focus away from the pain. Hydrotherapy using moist heat can help relax inflamed muscles resulting from injury or repetitive stress.

2. *How much does treatment cost?* The relaxation response is free and can be used along with moist heat, ibuprofen, and exercises. If you take the maximum dose of ibuprofen tablets each day for two weeks, you will pay approximately $12.

3. *How long until it works?* You should begin to feel relief within three days to one week.

If neck pain stems from stress—such as sitting at a computer, using the telephone frequently, or carrying a shoulder bag—try to take periodic time-outs throughout the day to stretch these neck muscles.

Osteoporosis

Osteoporosis is a debilitating disease that causes bones to thin and become easier to break.

Many risk factors contribute to osteoporosis. Some you can control or change; others are out of your control, as you can see from the following:

Risk Factors You *Can't* Control	Risk Factors You *Can* Control
Family history	Low calcium in the diet
Race	Having a bone density test

Watch Out!
Better get your calcium and exercise or osteoporosis may be in your near future. Studies show that 20 percent of American men will suffer at least one fracture because their bones have become too thin and weak to withstand the normal stresses of life. One-third of men who break their hips die within a year from complications of the fracture or its treatment.

Risk Factors You *Can't* Control	Risk Factors You *Can* Control
Sex	Lack of regular exercise
Age	Being underweight
Menopause	Heavy alcohol consumption
Certain diseases	Smoking cigarettes
	Diet high in sodium and protein
	Certain medications
	Excessive exercise in athletes
	Estrogen replacement after menopause

With osteoporosis, there are no symptoms until a fracture occurs. If osteoporosis progresses for years, you may see a bending of the spine called a Dowager's hump, which indicates that compression fractures have occurred. Your doctor can do a bone density test to see whether you have osteoporosis, and treatment can begin early in the disease to prevent fractures from happening.

How is it prevented?

Change the risk factors you can control—increase your calcium intake (through dairy products such as skim milk, foods or beverages fortified with extra calcium, or calcium supplements), avoid smoking or heavy alcohol use, and exercise regularly. Estrogen replacement can help postmenopausal women keep bones strong.

What is the conventional treatment?

Remove risk factors you can control, increase calcium and vitamin D, add daily weight-bearing exercise, use newer medications that help build bone mass, and add estrogen if you are a postmenopausal woman. The drugs Fosamax and Evista can restore bone mass in most cases of osteoporosis without the dangerous side effects of estrogen.

What are some alternative treatments?

- **Herbal therapy**—horsetail, licorice, sourdock

- **Nutritional supplements**— magnesium, vitamin D supplements, and at least 1,000 to 1,500 milligrams of calcium

- **Nutritional therapy**—calcium, vitamin D, magnesium, and soy; avoid alcohol, caffeine, and a diet high in sodium and animal protein

The basics

1. *What's been proven to work?* A diet high in calcium, magnesium, and vitamin D, along with regular weight-bearing exercise (biking, walking, running, skating, climbing stairs, or aerobics), can help prevent osteoporosis. Studies reveal that 80 percent of all women do not get adequate amounts of calcium each day. Calcium requirements vary from 800 mg (milligram) per day for a small child to 1,500 mg per day for older children, teenage girls, pregnant women, postmenopausal women not taking ERT, and men and women over age 65. The average adult between ages 25 to 65 needs at least 1,000 to 1,200 milligrams per day.

2. *How much does treatment cost?* You can get adequate calcium through food for less than $1 to $1.50 a day. Fosamax costs about $50 for one month's supply.

3. *How long until it works?* Studies of Fosamax show that 90 percent of people with osteoporosis who take this medication see an increase in bone mass within the first year, lowering the risk of hip and fracture by 50 percent.

If you can build strong bones during your childhood and teenage years, you can keep them strong

Moneysaver
If you are not lactose intolerant or opposed to consuming dairy products, you can avoid unnecessarily spending money on supplements by drinking two glasses of milk and eating one cup of yogurt and one ounce of cheese each day (or the equivalent of more than 1,000 milligrams of calcium) to guarantee strong bones.

TABLE 12.1 OSTEOPOROSIS TEST

Take the following quiz to assess your risk for osteoporosis.

1. What is your current age? _____ years

   Take this number, multiply by three, and enter the result in this space

   Start _____

2. What is your race or ethnic group? (Check one)

   African-American ____ (Enter 0)

   Caucasian ____   Hispanic ____   Asian ____ (Enter 5)

   Native American ____ Other ____ (Enter 5)

   _____

3. Have you ever been treated for or told you have rheumatoid arthritis?

   Yes____ No____

   If yes, enter 4. If no, enter 0._____

4. Since the age of 45, have you experienced a fracture (broken bone) at any of the following sites?

   *Hip   Yes ____ No ____ If yes, enter 4.

   _____

   *Rib   Yes ____ No ____ If yes, enter 4.

   _____

   *Wrist   Yes ____ No _____ If yes, enter 4.

   _____

5. Do you currently take or have you ever taken estrogen? (Examples include Premarin, Estrace, Estraderm, and Estratab)

   Yes____ No____

   If no, enter 1._____

Add your scores from questions one to five.
Subtotal _____

6. What is your current weight? _____ pounds

_____

Take your weight and subtract it from the subtotal to receive your score.
Score _____

If your final score is 6 or greater, it may be a good idea to have a bone density test. Talk to your doctor.

during adulthood. If you do so, osteoporosis is less likely to occur. People most at risk include post-menopausal, petite women with a family history. If you have two or more risk factors for osteoporosis, see your doctor for a bone density scan, which measures the amount of bone mass you currently have.

Shin splints
Medial tibial stress syndrome (MTSS), or shin splints, causes pain and tenderness in the lower leg. It's caused by overuse of muscles, soft tissue damage, and inflammation. Symptoms include pain in the shin when the heel strikes the ground during running and severe muscle tenderness.

How is it prevented?
Avoid overuse, run on a soft surface, wear cushioned shoes, and do proper warm-ups before exercising or running.

What is the conventional treatment?
Stop running, ice the injury, take nonsteroidal anti-inflammatory medications (NSAIDs), and do stretching exercises.

What are some alternative treatments?

- **Bodyworks**—massage
- **Homeopathy**—rhus toxicodendron (poison ivy)
- **Hydrotherapy**—R.I.C.E. (rest, ice, compression, elevation), then applications of moist heat
- **Reflexology**—deep foot massage

The basics

1. *What's been proven to work?* Stick to R.I.C.E. followed by moist heat. Take NSAIDS to alleviate inflammation.

2. *How long until it works?* You will notice a difference within a few days to one week.

3. *How much does treatment cost?* NSAIDS cost from $5 to $10 per week.

Again, prevention is crucial. Avoid overuse, warm up properly, and wear supportive shoes.

Tendinitis

Tendinitis is an inflammation of a tendon that attaches muscle to a bone. It most often is caused by overuse or wear-and-tear changes in the tissues that make up the tendon. If you are experiencing tendinitis, you may feel pain, swelling, warmth, and difficulty using the nearby joint. This usually occurs in the elbow, shoulder, and the Achilles tendon near the heel.

How is it prevented?

Build up strength, do proper warm-ups before exercise or sports, and understand the technique of the game or exercise before you engage in it.

What is the conventional treatment?

Use R.I.C.E. immediately. The pain could linger for weeks, but with proper and immediate treatment, it

66
If you suffer from tendonitis, don't be afraid to get a cortisone shot if needed. I pulled my tendon from swinging a golf club the wrong way and tried to heal it with moist heat and Advil. Finally, after two months, I conceded and let my doctor give me a shot of cortisone. Within 24 hours, I had no more pain.
—Josh, 26, computer analyst
99

usually disappears in a few days. Twice-daily applications of moist heat (20 minutes each time) and non-steroidal anti-inflammatory medications can help alleviate pain and promote healing. Injections of cortisone may be necessary in more severe cases.

What are some alternative treatments?

- **Aromatherapy**—lime, lemon, marjoram
- **Bodywork**—Swedish massage
- **Chinese medicine**—acupuncture, acupressure, or shiatsu
- **Chiropractic**—spinal adjustment
- **Homeopathy**—rhus toxicodendron (poison ivy)
- **Hydrotherapy**—moist heat or ice
- **Reflexology**—foot massage (if Achilles tendon is involved)

The basics

1. *What's been proven to work?* You can blend conventional and alternative treatments for tendinitis, using R.I.C.E. with acupuncture, acupressure, or Swedish massage.

2. *How much does treatment cost?* Acupuncture costs from $35 to $125 per session. R.I.C.E. is virtually free.

3. *How long until it works?* You will notice a reduction in pain within three days to one week. If pain lingers, ask your doctor about an injection of cortisone.

It's not difficult to prevent tendinitis by doing strengthening exercises and avoiding overuse.

Just the facts

- Glucosamine and chondroitin are two supplements that have been found to alleviate the pain of osteoarthritis (the wear-and-tear disease).

- Mind/body treatments such as the relaxation response may help fibromyalgia patients reduce stress and sleep more soundly.

- Soy foods help keep bones strong and prevent fractures associated with osteoporosis.

- Fosamax and Evista are new medications that help increase bone mass in most patients.

GET THE SCOOP ON...
Why a wait-and-see attitude probably is best
when treating benign fibroid tumors in the
uterus ▪ How, in Japan, no word exists for the
term *hot flash* because of the high soy content
in the diet ▪ A scientific study that proves cranberry juice can be helpful in preventing urinary
tract infections

Sex-Specific and Genitourinary Disorders

Women

Because the female anatomy is so intricate, attention must be paid to a host of potential problems. From menstrual pain to hot flashes, women need to consider all the options before making a wise, healthy decision about treatment. Many ailments are conducive to alternative therapies, while others depend entirely on conventional medical care.

Endometriosis

Endometriosis is the presence of uterine tissue outside its usual location on the inner lining of the uterus. Hormones, late pregnancy, and implants may contribute to it; however, the exact cause is still unknown. Most researchers believe that, when the uterine lining tissue peels off and is sloughed out in the menstrual flow, some material builds up and passes backwards out of the Fallopian tubes into the pelvic cavity. This material implants itself into other tissues and reacts monthly as if it were still in the uterus, thickening and peeling away. Newly peeled off tissues start new implants. The growing tissue between pelvic organs may cause them to stick together, causing pain and other symptoms. Symptoms include abdominal or rectal pain, severe menstrual cramps, abnormal menstrual bleeding, scar tissue, and infertility.

How is it prevented?
Having your first pregnancy at a young age can help prevent endometriosis.

What is the conventional treatment?
Surgery often is used to remove scar tissue.

What are some alternative treatments?

- **Chinese medicine**—acupuncture, acupressure, shiatsu

- **Herbal therapy**—astragalus, dong quai, echinacea

- **Nutritional supplements**—antioxidants, calcium, evening primrose or flaxseed oil, omega-3s

- **Nutritional therapy**—soy foods

The basics

1. *What's been proven to work?* Increased consumption of soy foods has been linked with a decreased risk of endometrial cancer, according to a report published in the *American Journal of Epidemiology*. The data suggests that plant-based diets that are low in fat, high in fiber, and rich in legumes (soybeans), whole grain foods, vegetables, and fruits reduce the risk of endometrial cancer.

2. *What does it cost?* A healthy diet including soy products costs from $5 to $15 a day.

3. *How long until it works?* It will take weeks before you notice a difference, if any is noticed at all.

Endometriosis is a complicated problem that some people now are associating with poor nutrition and a reduced immune response. Examine your lifestyle habits to determine whether increasing healthy nutrition, sleep, and exercise and decreasing stress may help.

Fibrocystic breast disease

Fibrocystic breast disease is a common nonmalignant breast disease. It is caused by fibrous tissue growth that most frequently appears when a woman is in her 30s or 40s but disappears with menopause. Symptoms include cysts that become larger and more painful just prior to the onset of menstrual bleeding.

How is it prevented?

Keep your hormones in balance by avoiding weight gain, having children early in life, and reducing stress.

What is the conventional treatment?

The key to successful treatment is normalizing hormonal fluctuations. This is especially important because the role of low levels of estrogen and/or high levels of progesterone is not clear.

What are some alternative treatments?

- **Ayurvedic medicine**—a combination of herbs, diet, exercise, and stress reduction
- **Chinese medicine**—acupuncture, herbs, tai chi
- **Homeopathy**—bryonia, conium maculatum
- **Mind/body treatment**—relaxation response or any stress-reduction therapy

- **Nutritional supplements**—vitamins A and E, evening primrose oil
- **Nutritional therapy**—soy foods, foods rich in vitamin A (carrots, spinach, cantaloupe), and avoidance of caffeine

The basics

1. *What's proven to work?* There is no easy answer to fibrocystic disease. A combination of eliminating caffeine, adding vitamins A and E to the diet, and reducing stress has helped many.

2. *How long until treatment works?* If alternative measures work, you will notice a difference in three to six weeks.

3. *How much does it cost?* These measures are not expensive. A vitamin supplement will cost about $8 for one month's supply.

If you have painful or lumpy breasts, make sure your physician is aware of this in case something else is going on. If you notice any lumps or changes in the shape of your breasts, or if you are experiencing unusual pain or discomfort in your breasts, make sure to have your doctor check this out immediately. If you haven't already, ask your physician teach you the proper way to do self-examination and do monthly check-ups yourself. Better to be safe than sorry!

Fibroids

Fibroid tumors are common benign tumors of the uterus that occur in premenopausal women.

The cause of fibroids is unknown. Estrogen and heredity both may play an important factor in their development. There may be no signs or symptoms of fibroid tumors, or you may have abdominal cramping, heavy periods, abnormal bleeding from the vagina, and possibly anemia.

How are they prevented?

Some researchers believe staying at a normal weight and avoiding hypertension may help prevent fibroids.

What is the conventional treatment?

Although fibroids are the most common reason for a hysterectomy, this only is warranted in extreme situations. Frequently, no treatment is necessary other than keeping an eye on the problem. In some situations—such as suspicion of cancer, rapidly enlarging tumors, uncontrolled bleeding, or problems with fertility—surgery may be required. Surgery called a *myomectomy* can remove the tumors but spare the uterus.

What are some alternative treatments?

- **Aromatherapy**—essential oils of chamomile, sage, lavender
- **Chinese medicine**—acupuncture treatments called *chong mo*
- **Herbal therapy**—black cohosh, crampbark, dong quai, ginger, raspberry leaf, licorice, and ginseng
- **Homeopathy**—medorrhinum, phosphorus, ustilago maydis, magnesia phosphorica, and folliculinum
- **Nutritional therapy**—soy foods, low-fat diet

The basics

1. *What's been proven to work?* Unless the fibroids are large and symptomatic, the best treatment is to manage the annoying symptoms of pain or

Unofficially . . .
Fibroids remain the leading reason for hysterectomies in this country, according to the American College of Obstetricians and Gynecologists. Of the 583,000 hysterectomies performed in 1995, more than one-third were due to fibroids, reports the National Center for Health Statistics. The NCHS claims that between 20 and 40 percent of women of reproductive age have fibroids, but some research indicates that this may be as high as 60 or 70 percent because many women do not realize they have them.

bleeding until the woman becomes meno-pausal. Fibroids tend to shrink at that time due to reduced estrogen levels. No alternative medicine shrinks fibroid tumors.

2. *How much does treatment cost?* The wait-and-see approach is free.

3. *How long until it works?* If you are in your 30s, you have around 10 to 15 years of dealing with the cramping and bleeding of fibroids. See your physician regularly to monitor the problem.

An herbal practitioner or naturopath may give you progesterone-like herbs such as chasteberry, trillium, cotton, cinnamon oil, or ergot, but because they are so potent, it might be best to stick with your conventional medical doctor for proven treatment. Some women report positive results from alternative therapies such as herbs, hydrotherapy, Ayurveda, and Chinese medicine.

Hot flashes

Hot flashes are sudden hot sensations that usually occur in the neck or upper body. They are caused by low levels of the female estrogen hormones during menopause (see page 281). If you are experiencing hot flashes, you will often feel sudden hot sensations in the neck, the upper body, or throughout the entire body. There often is flushing of the skin, a feeling of intense warmth, and sweating. There may be shivering, nausea, dizziness, fainting, and palpitations. The episodes usually last a few minutes, but because they frequently happen at night, they can disturb sleep and can increase daytime sleepiness.

How is it prevented?

Reduce stress, dress in layers so you don't become overheated, avoid hot and spicy foods, avoid caffeine, and keep room temperatures cool.

Bright Idea
If you are between the ages of 35 and 50 and are having menopausal symptoms of anxiety, insomnia, irritability, hot flashes, or night sweats, ask your doctor to check your estrogen level during the second, third, or fourth days of your menstrual cycle. Your doctor also might choose to test for FSH (follicle-stimulating hormone, produced by the pituitary gland). This test ideally should be done on blood drawn during the first six days of the menstrual cycle and should be repeated the next month.

What is the conventional treatment?

Estrogen-replacement therapy can help treat hot flashes.

What are some alternative treatments?

- **Chinese medicine**—acupressure points in the ankle and forearm
- **Herbal therapy**—black cohosh, Siberian or American ginseng
- **Homeopathy**—belladonna, lachesis, and sulphuric acid
- **Mind/Body treatment**—relaxation response, aromatherapy, deep abdominal breathing
- **Nutritional therapy**—soy foods with isoflavones

The basics

1. *What's been proven to work?* In Japan, there is no word for the term *hot flash*. This is due, in part, to the high soy concentration in the diet.

2. *How much does treatment cost?* Soy beans cost about $3 to $4 at a health food store. Tofu costs about $3 at a grocery store.

3. *How long until it works?* It may take four to six weeks to notice a difference, if any is noticed at all.

There is no need to suffer from hot flashes, especially with the options women have. If soy products do not agree with you, try hormone-replacement therapy. Ask your doctor what is best in your situation.

Menopause

Menopause refers to a woman's final menstrual period and the phase of life following a woman's reproductive stage—climacteric. *Climacteric* is a transitional phase lasting 15 to 20 years during which

Watch Out!
Heart disease is the leading killer of women 50 to 75 years old, claiming five times as many lives as breast cancer. To prevent this from happening to you, follow a low-fat, heart-healthy diet, get plenty of exercise, and take estrogen if recommended by your doctor.

hormone production declines. After age 35, a grad-
ual decrease occurs that lowers the levels of female
estrogen hormones. This is due to reduced production of estrogens by the ovaries.

Because of reduced estrogen, one symptom is
the loss of monthly menstrual periods. About 85
percent of women experience hot flashes around
the time of menopause, and sleep disturbances are
common. Other symptoms may include headaches,
anxiety, feelings of inadequacy, and decreased concentration. Dryness of skin and membranes can
result in dryness of the vagina with discharge, and
intercourse may become painful. There may be frequency of urination with a feeling of urgency to
empty the bladder. Osteoporosis (thinning of the
bone) and heart disease also may occur.

How is it prevented?
You cannot prevent menopause; it is a normal stage
in life.

What is the conventional treatment?
Estrogen treatment improves and often controls hot
flashes, dryness in the vagina, and urinary symptoms. It also can help control the risk of osteoporosis and heart disease. Alendronate (Fosamax) and
raloxifene (Evista) are newer medications that can
help with some of the problems associated with
menopause.

What are some alternative treatments?
- **Aromatherapy**—essential oils of cypress, fennel,
  and sage for vaginal dryness; lavender to induce
  healing sleep

- **Herbal therapy**—black cohosh, gota kola, kava
  kava, St. John's wort to balance moods; cinnamon to lift spirit

- **Homeopathy**—bryonia, natrum muriatcum
- **Nutritional supplements**—essential fatty acids (EFAs), calcium, magnesium, B-complex vitamins
- **Nutritional therapy**—soy foods, foods rich in calcium

The basics

1. *What is proven to work?* Estrogen is the most prescribed remedy for symptoms of menopause.
2. *How much does treatment cost?* Estrogen costs about $20 to $40 for one month's supply, depending on brand and your location.
3. *How long until it works?* You will notice a difference within several days to two weeks.

Talk with your doctor about the best possible solution for you. Even though estrogen has been proven to work, there are side effects that may not be beneficial for every woman.

Menstrual pain

During menstruation, it is common to experience severe pain in the abdomen, upper thighs, and/or lower back, uterine cramping, nausea, diarrhea, dizziness, and sometimes even vomiting. All this is caused by uterine contractions brought on by substances called prostaglandins, which are manufactured in the cells of the uterine lining. During menstruation, the uterus may contract more strongly and more frequently than normal, cutting off the blood supply—and therefore oxygen—to the uterus. Pelvic lesions or disease, post-surgical adhesions, and tumors also can cause pain.

Timesaver
Exercise provides many benefits such as keeping bones strong and dense, helping you maintain a normal weight, and preventing coronary artery disease. If you don't have time to exercise, take advantage of small opportunities to exercise during the day—they add up. You can park at the back of the parking lot at the mall or the grocery store, walk the stairs frequently at work, do your own housework and yard work, and run or skate with your children or grandchildren.

How is it prevented?

Exercising, eating a balanced diet, reducing stress, and getting plenty of rest all can help quell menstrual pain.

What is the conventional treatment?

Applications of heat—whether from a hot pad, a bath, or a cup of tea—can help soothe cramps by relaxing the uterus. Exercise also can reduce cramping because it improves circulation and promotes relaxation. Aspirin, naproxen, and ibuprofen can relieve pain and can slow the release of prostaglandins. Ibuprofen should be taken regularly for two days to be most effective and should be taken with food. Birth control pills can help prevent cramps because they block the production of prostaglandins.

What are some alternative treatments?

- **Aromatherapy**—essential oils of chamomile, sage, and lavender to relieve pain

- **Ayurvedic medicine**—yoga

- **Herbal therapy**—bearberry (uva ursi), blessed thistle, hyssop, dong quai, chamomile, valerian, yarrow (antispasmodic property)

- **Nutritional supplements**—vitamins C and E, B-complex vitamins (especially B_6), calcium, magnesium, and essential fatty acids (EFAs)

- **Nutritional therapy**—soy foods, broccoli, complex carbohydrates such as pasta, sherbet (calming effect)

The basics

1. *What's been proven to work?* Nonsteroidal anti-inflammatory drugs (NSAIDS) seem to work for

most women, combined with applications of moist heat and exercise.

2. *How much does treatment cost?* NSAIDs cost from $7 to $10 for one week's supply.

3. *How long until it works?* To feel optimum relief, it's important to take NSAIDS (Nonsteroid anti-inflammatory drugs) before cramping begins and to continue this therapy during the most painful days of your period. You should notice relief within one to two hours of taking the medication.

If your cramps are severe, ask your doctor about new prescription medications that may help.

Premenstrual syndrome

Premenstrual syndrome is a condition characterized by nervousness, irritability, emotional instability, depression, and possibly headaches that occurs around one week before menstruation. It's caused by hormonal and chemical changes within the body.

How is it prevented?

Keep hormones balanced by reducing stress, getting plenty of sleep, and avoiding salt, caffeine, fatty foods, sugar, and alcohol during this time of the month.

What is the conventional treatment?

You can use nonsteroidal anti-inflammatory medications (to reduce swelling), hormone therapy, and antidepressants such as sertraline (Zoloft).

What are some alternative treatments?

- **Aromatherapy**—ylang-ylang
- **Chinese medicine**—acupressure points on ankle and wrist

Watch Out!
Millions of American women between the ages of 35 and 50 are now in peri-menopause, a transition time that precedes menopause. Ask your doctor for an explanation of common symptoms and for ways to cope with them. Estrogen is sometimes given during this period to reduce symptoms such as insomnia, hot flashes, and irritability. A good book about this topic is *Perimenopause: Preparing for the Change* by Dr. Nancy Lee Teaff and Kim Wright Wiley (Prima, Rocklin, CA, 1996, $12).

- **Herbal therapy**—blessed thistle, caraway, hyssop
- **Homeopathy**—lachesis (for pain and tenderness)
- **Mind/body treatments**—relaxation response, visualization, music therapy, deep abdominal breathing
- **Nutritional supplements**—essential fatty acids (EFAs) such as evening primrose oil or flaxseed oil, calcium, manganese, magnesium, B_6, zinc, vitamin C, and chromium
- **Reflexology**—foot massage

The basics

1. *What's been proven to work?* According to researchers at The University of Texas Southwestern Medical Center at Dallas, 62 percent of women given sertraline showed marked improvement in PMS symptoms.

2. *How much does treatment cost?* It depends on the amount you take. Generally, it costs about $60 for 30 50-milligram tablets.

3. *How long until it works?* Some women notice a dramatic difference within one to two weeks.

If alternative therapies such as reducing sugar and caffeine, destressing, and taking vitamin and mineral supplements do not help, ask your doctor about sertraline, which seems to work in many severe cases.

Vaginitis

Vaginitis is an infection of the vagina most commonly caused by Candida organisms (yeast infection). Other causes include sexually transmitted infections such as trichomonas, genital herpes, gonorrhea, and syphilis. The symptoms of vaginitis may vary as follows:

- Candida (yeast) causes itching and a thick, white, curd-like discharge from the vagina.

- Trichomonas infection causes a foul-smelling yellow vaginal discharge.

- Genital herpes causes fever, chills, pain, and swelling around the opening of the vagina, as well as difficulty in urination.

- Gonorrhea causes fever, chills, and pain in the abdomen and pelvis, as well as a thick discharge from the vagina.

- Syphilis causes a painless sore outside the vagina. It can progress into a rash and even permanent damage to the heart, brain, and other organs if untreated.

How is it prevented?
Wear cotton underwear to keep the area dry and practice monogamous or safe sex.

What is the conventional treatment?
Treatment varies depending on the infection, but it can include over-the-counter creams and suppositories for yeast infections, pain medications, acyclovir (a medication for herpes), and antibiotics such as penicillin or tetracycline.

What are some alternative treatments?

- **Herbal therapy**—echinacea, garlic, goldenseal, and yarrow (to boost immune function)

- **Homeopathy**—hepar sulph, silica, pulsatilla (brand name Yeast Gard™, Lake Consumer Products)

- **Hydrotherapy**—cool, damp compresses

■ **Nutritional therapy**—eight ounces of yogurt daily (to replace "good" bacteria), elimination diet (avoid yeast products such as pasta, bread, cheese, and beer)

The basics

1. *What's been proven to work?* If vaginitis is caused by a yeast infection, over-the-counter creams and suppositories usually work. Prevention also is important so keep the area dry.

2. *How much does treatment cost?* Over-the-counter products cost about $14 to treat one infection.

3. *How long until it works?* You should feel relief within two to seven days.

Feminine burning and itching are facts of life for most women. If alternative preventive measures do not work to reduce the occurrence of yeast infections, get an accurate diagnosis, recognize symptoms early, and treat it with the proper medication.

Yeast infection

A yeast infection is a common infection in the vaginal area caused by an overgrowth of the Candida organisms. If you have a yeast infection, there may be a thick, white, curd-like discharge from the vagina, and there may be itching.

How is it prevented?

Wear cotton underwear and avoid wearing wet bathing suits for long periods of time.

What is the conventional treatment?

A host of vaginal creams and suppositories are available. In many cases, however, the male partner may also need treatment.

What are some alternative treatments?

- **Herbal therapy**—echinacea, garlic, goldenseal, yarrow

- **Homeopathy**—hepar sulph, silica, pulsatilla (brand name Yeast Gard(TM), Lake Consumer Products)

- **Hydrotherapy**—cool water applications to burning area

- **Nutritional therapy**—vinegar douches, or eat 8 ounces of yogurt daily

The basics

1. *What's been proven to work?* Stick with vaginal creams or suppositories for fast relief.

2. *How much does treatment cost?* One week's treatment usually costs about $12.

3. *How long until it works?* You will notice relief in one to three days.

Once the infection is healed, use preventative methods such as wearing cotton underwear, avoiding damp swimsuits, and eating yogurt daily to keep infections at bay.

Men

Years ago, men's health problems were not discussed in public. Today, numerous campaigns advise men about the warning signs of prostate cancer and make sure men understand how to do a monthly testicle exam. Good health and an increase in life-span are results of this new awareness of the male anatomy. Read through the following common ailments and then weigh the benefits of each treatment before making a decision.

Impotence

Impotence is a male's inability to have an erection when sexually stimulated. It can be caused by stress, psychological problems, chronic illness (such as diabetes), hardening and narrowing of the arteries (atherosclerosis), low levels of testosterone, age, adverse reaction to prescription medications (such as antihypertensives, antidepressants or antihistamines), or excessive alcohol consumption.

How is it prevented?

Avoid alcohol, reduce stress, and talk openly with your doctor if medications cause impotence. There may be another alternative.

What is the conventional treatment?

Treatments for impotence include medications, injections, a pump-like device to increase blood flow, and prosthetic surgery in which a prosthesis is inserted into the penis. Some of the new pharmaceutical treatments include a tiny capsule that is inserted into the urethra (Muse) and a new pill called Viagra (Pfizer).

What are some alternative treatments?

- **Aromatherapy**—rose, jasmine, ylang ylang, and cinnamon
- **Ayurveda**—spiritual awareness and Transcendental Meditation
- **Herbal therapy**—yohimbe (an herb that occurs naturally in the bark of evergreen trees and has been used as an aphrodisiac for centuries by Indians and Africans), ginseng, ginkgo biloba
- **Hydrotherapy**—a cold shower (to stimulate circulation)

- **Mind/body therapy**—deep abdominal breathing, relaxation response, music therapy, visualization, psychotherapy

The basics

1. *What's been proven to work?* In one German study, 20 impotent men took an 80-milligram capsule of the herb ginkgo biloba three times a day. After nine months, all were able to have spontaneous erections. Another herb called *yohimbe* heightens potency by increasing blood flow to the penis. It does not increase testosterone, but it does increase the body's production of the adrenal hormone norepinephrine. One study in California found that this herb was especially effective for treating impotence in men with diabetes and heart disease. A tiny capsule called Muse works for some men, and a much-awaited pill called Viagra is now available.

2. *How much does treatment cost?* Herbal treatment costs about 50 cents a day. Viagra costs about $7 to $10 per pill.

3. *How long until it works?* It may take three to nine months to see a difference in potency.

Before you take any alternative or conventional medication, get a good work-up with a board-certified urologist and talk with a qualified psychologist, marriage and family counselor, or social worker to fully evaluate the causes of impotence. Although there are some positive results with herbal therapy, there also are warnings of side effects such as low blood pressure, increased anxiety, abdominal distress, elevated heart rate, or kidney disease. This does not mean you will have these side effects, but

Bright Idea
Eating certain foods may have an amorous effect on the body. For example, chocolate contains phenylethylamine (PEA), a chemical the body produces when we are in love, which may give the libido a lift. Likewise, studies show that the smell of pumpkin pie and doughnuts can arouse sexual desires in men.

to be safe, check with your doctor about any alternative treatment.

Premature ejaculation

Male orgasm and ejaculation follows sexual stimulation. Premature ejaculation occurs before a sexual partner is stimulated. This common disorder affects men of all ages and usually is caused by psychological problems such as poor communication with a sexual partner, anxiety about sexual performance, or religious conflicts.

How is it prevented?

Couples can perform exercises in which each partner caresses the other's body without intercourse to learn pleasurable ways of touching. The stop-and-start technique, in which the man is stimulated through controlled intercourse or masturbation until he feels an impending ejaculation, also may be effective. Stimulation is stopped and then resumed in 20 to 30 seconds.

What is the conventional treatment?

If prevention measures are not effective in ending premature ejaculation, counseling from a qualified sex therapist may be necessary. No medication is needed.

What are some alternative treatments?

- **Ayurveda**—spiritual awareness, yoga
- **Chinese medicine**—acupuncture, shiatsu
- **Herbal therapy**—ginseng
- **Mind/Body treatment**—counseling, relaxation techniques
- **Naturopathy**—exercise, check level of testosterone

The basics

1. *What's been proven to work?* Counseling and the stop-and-start technique are most effective.

2. *How long until treatment works?* It may take several months for these measures work.

3. *How much does it cost?* Counseling costs around $50 to $75 per hour.

Many sexual problems that seem embarrassing to men are very common. Talking with a knowledgeable professional about the problem often can identify sources of tension and anxiety that can easily be remedied.

Prostate enlargement

The medical term for prostate enlargement is benign prostatic hypertrophy (BPH). Prostate enlargement is brought on by aging. The walnut-shaped gland is present in men at the base of the bladder around the urethra (the tube that conducts urine out of the bladder). Symptoms include decreased force in the urine stream, frequency of urination, difficulty starting and stopping urination, and arising several times each night to empty the bladder. Eventually, prostate enlargement may cause complete blockage of urine flow.

How is it prevented?

Stay sexually active, urinate frequently, drink eight cups of water a day (but not before bedtime), limit caffeine and alcohol, and reduce stress.

What is the conventional treatment?

Alpha blockers that help relax muscles in the prostate are given for BPH treatment. Finasteride (Proscar) is another medication that claims to cause the prostate to shrink. These medications, however,

Watch Out!
If you take medication such as Propecia to restore hair, make sure you know the side effects. Because Propecia causes birth defects, it is not approved for women. It must be taken every day for the rest of your life to be effective and possibly can cause impotence for as long as it's taken.

Watch Out!
Do you know the warning signs of testicular cancer? The most common symptom is a small, painless lump in a testicle or a slightly enlarged testicle. Other possible symptoms include a feeling of heaviness in the scrotum, a dull ache in the lower stomach or groin, a change in the way a testicle feels, or a sudden accumulation of blood or fluid in the scrotum. It is important for men to be familiar with the size and the feel of their normal testicles, so they can any detect changes that may occur.

may not reduce the rate of BPH complications or the need for future surgery. Another treatment is *balloon dilation*, a surgical procedure in which a balloon-tipped catheter is inserted into the penis through the urethra and into the bladder. The balloon is inflated to stretch the urethra; this should allowing urine to flow more easily. In some severe cases, surgery is necessary.

What are some alternative treatments?

- **Herbal therapy**—saw palmetto, ginkgo biloba
- **Nutritional therapy**—soy foods

The basics

1. *What's been proven to work?* In one study of 110 men with BPH symptoms, the herb saw palmetto decreased nighttime urination by 45 percent, increased the urinary flow rate over 50 percent, and reduced posturination residual volume (the amount of urine left in the bladder after urination) by 42 percent.

2. *How much does treatment cost?* Saw palmetto costs about 45 cents a day.

3. *How long until it works?* It make take up to three months before you notice an improvement in symptoms.

More than 80 percent of men over age 50 have enlarged prostates (benign prostatic hyperplasia, or BPH). Lifestyle changes such as limiting caffeine and alcohol, having regular bowel habits, and emptying the bladder before bedtime can sometimes lessen symptoms.

Genitourinary

Bladder infections are one of the milder genitourinary problems you can have. If the bladder infection goes untreated, however, it can result in a full-blown kidney infection complete with pain, fever, blood in the urine, and damage to this vital organ. This is why it's important to know the various signs and symptoms of common genitourinary ailments, as well as the safest and most effective treatments. Read on for information that can make your life healthier and more comfortable.

Bladder infection

Commonly called *cystitis*, a bladder infection is an inflammation of the wall and lining of the urinary bladder, usually caused by bacterial infections. There may be no warning signs, or you may feel abdominal pain, localized pain or burning upon urination, and frequency of urination. Blood may appear in the urine. Prostate disease in men may cause obstruction in the urine flow, leading to pain and infection.

How is it prevented?

Wear cotton underwear to keep the area dry, avoid wet bathing suits, drink at least 8 to 10 glasses of water daily, drink cranberry juice, and urinate frequently. Avoid wiping bacteria onto the urethral opening after a bowel movement and stay away from antibacterial soaps, sprays, douches, feminine deodorants, contraceptive jellies, and creams that may cause irritation.

What is the conventional treatment?

Antibiotics are effective for ending infection. In some cases, surgery may be necessary to remove an obstruction or a stone.

Unofficially . . .
Each year, urinary tract infections (UTIs) account for about a million doctor visits, according to the National Institute of Diabetes and Digestive and Kidney Diseases.

What are some alternative treatments?

- **Aromatherapy**—essential oils of bergamot, lavender, thyme, and ylang-ylang (add oils to bath water, all have disinfectant properties)

- **Detoxification**—drink at least 8 to 12 glasses of water daily at the first sign of a possible infection

- **Herbal therapy**—alfalfa, bearberry (uva ursi), burdock, bladderwrack

- **Nutritional therapy**—cranberry juice

The basics

1. *What's been proven to work?* The most common home remedy, cranberry juice, might help prevent a urinary tract infection. In one study reported in the *Journal of the American Medical Association*, cranberry juice drinkers were 58 percent less likely to develop a UTI than people who drank a placebo, and existing infections were 27 percent less likely to continue. If this does not help your symptoms, see your doctor for antibiotic treatment.

2. *How much does treatment cost?* Cranberry juice costs about $4 a week. Antibiotics cost $20 or more for seven days.

3. *How long until it works?* If you drink plenty of liquids and cranberry juice when you first notice the symptoms, it is possible to get rid the infection before it worsens. Antibiotic therapy takes two to three days before you will notice a difference.

66
I have lived on cranberry juice—as much as two glasses a day—after getting a horrible bladder infection in college. Interestingly, I have never had another infection since!
—Britt, 34, homemaker
99

You can prevent UTIs with alternative treatments if you catch it early, but if symptoms linger or worsen, see your doctor immediately. Urinary tract infections can lead to kidney infections and serious damage if not treated effectively.

Herpes

Herpes is a lifelong sexually transmitted disease that affects roughly one in five Americans over age 12. It is caused by a virus called *herpes simplex* that is spread by skin-to-skin contact during genital, oral, or anal sex.

Symptoms can include many painful sores on the penis of the male (or the vagina of the female), fever, enlarged lymph nodes in the groin area, burning upon urination, headache, and flu-like symptoms. A first outbreak can last several weeks. Subsequent outbreaks can occur as frequently as several times a year or never again. About 70 percent of the 40 million Americans with genital herpes have no symptoms at all.

How is it prevented?

Maintain a monogamous sexual relationship and/or practice safe sex using condoms.

What is the conventional treatment?

Use cool compresses to alleviate burning, take care of the infected skin, drink plenty of fluids, and take pain and antiviral medications directed against the herpes virus.

What are some alternative treatments?

- **Hydrotherapy**—cool compresses on infected skin, increased liquids

- **Mind/body treatments**—relaxation response, progressive muscle relaxation, or visualization (to destress)

The basics

1. *What's been proven to work?* Taking antiviral medication such as Valtrex (Glaxo Wellcome and Zovirax) or Famvir (SmithKline Beecham) at

Watch Out!
The common cold sore also is caused by a herpes virus. It invades the skin and can remain for months or even years before becoming active. This virus is transmitted by person-to-person contact or by contact with saliva, stools, urine, or discharge from an infected eye. The blisters and ulcers of herpes simplex are contagious until they heal, initially and in subsequent flare-ups.

the first sign of genital herpes may decrease the severity of the disease.

2. *How much does it cost?* Valtrex costs about $75 for a 10-day supply.

3 *How long until treatment works?* You may notice a difference in a few days, if it is caught early.

Early diagnosis and treatment of herpes within the first 72 hours of symptoms is the key to stopping it.

Incontinence

Incontinence is urinary leakage that occurs when a person coughs or strains with physical activity. The many causes include a blockage of the usual urine flow, a "dropped bladder" (cystocele), a weakness in the muscles that control urine flow from the bladder, irritability of the bladder with spasms or contractions that may force urine out of the bladder, an infection, or diseases that can damage the nerve supply to the bladder. Diuretic medicines also can aggravate an incontinence problem.

How is it prevented?

To prevent incontinence, avoid getting dehydrated; concentrated urine can irritate your bladder. Avoid taking diuretics because they will make you produce too much urine. Stay away from caffeine; it is irritating as well as being a diuretic. Treat urinary tract infections immediately to avoid injury. Another method of preventing incontinence is to keep your pelvic floor muscles strong.

What is the conventional treatment?

Kegel exercises, which strengthen the pelvic-floor muscles, are a mainstay for treating stress incontinence. Dietary modification also may help.

Irritating substances—such as acidic drinks like orange juice or drinks sweetened with aspartame—can affect urge incontinence. Tampons can be used with mild stress problems, as they help support the pelvic organs by pushing against the urethra and helping it close. Bladder training is good if you have mild urge or stress incontinence. Try to withhold urination for longer and longer periods to strengthen the bladder muscles. Ask your doctor about Kegal exercises or see a specialist in biofeedback.

What are some alternative treatments?
- **Mind/body treatment**—biofeedback

The basics

1. *What's been proven to work?* A combination of Kegel exercises and biofeedback may be your best bet to treat incontinence nonsurgically.

2. *How much does treatment cost?* Biofeedback costs $50 to $125 per session; Kegel exercises are free.

3. *How long until it works?* You should notice a difference in two weeks to two months.

The chances of regaining the same muscle strength you had in younger years are slim, but you can make a difference by continuing to practice the Kegel exercises.

Infertility

Infertility is the inability to conceive human life after one year of intercourse without the use of contraception. Causes include low sperm count, blocked sperm ducts, premature ejaculation, an inability to attain an erection, and trauma to the scrotum or testes of the male.

Unofficially . . .
More than five million people of childbearing age in the U.S. experience infertility, but did you know that infertility is not just a woman's problem? It is a female problem in 35 percent of the cases, a male problem in 35 percent of the cases, a combined problem in 20 percent of the cases, and is unexplained in 10 percent of the cases. It is essential that both the man and the woman be evaluated during an infertility work-up.

For females, infertility can be caused by endometriosis, pelvic inflammatory disease (PID), abnormalities in the size or the shape of the uterus, infectious disease, previous surgery, cervical mucus not conducive to sperm, or extended periods of strenuous exercise. Obesity, excessive alcohol consumption or drug abuse, and prolonged stress also are contributing factors.

What is the conventional treatment?

Treatments include fertility drugs, reconstructive surgery, artificial insemination, and therapeutic donor insemination (TDI), in which sperm from a donor is transferred to the woman's uterus. In-vitro fertilization (IVF)—in which the ova are retrieved from the ovary, the eggs are fertilized with sperm in a test tube, and the embryos then are transferred back into the woman's uterus—also can be effective.

What are some alternative treatments?

- **Nutritional supplements**—zinc, vitamins C and E, selenium

The basics

1. *What has been proven to work?* Moderate doses of vitamins C and E enhance the ability of sperm to fertilize an egg, according to animal research discussed in *Obstetrics and Gynecology* (1995). High levels of the vitamins can be toxic to sperm, however, rapidly decreasing their ability to move and eventually killing them. The studies also showed that the mineral selenium is essential for sperm development. In animal tests, when moderate doses of vitamins E and C were given, cellular damage was prevented, and sperm movement and function were enhanced. The suggested dose for humans is 250

milligrams of vitamin C and 400 international units (IU) of vitamin E—but no more. The recommended dietary allowances of vitamin C is 60 milligrams, and the RDA of vitamin E is 12 to 15 IUs. In addition, don't smoke; cigarette smoking is known to deplete the body's natural army of antioxidants.

2. *How much does treatment cost?* A week's supply of vitamins C and E costs about $2 dollars. Quitting smoking is free!

3. *How long until it works?* This treatment has no time frame; you just have to wait and see. If you are still having fertility problems in four to six months, you may want to pursue conventional infertility treatments.

No matter what method is used to conceive, all moms-to-be must make sure they get the full recommended 400 micrograms (mcg) of folic acid daily before conception. This B vitamin is crucial for preventing birth defects, low birth weight, and premature delivery. Eat beans (pink, pinto, and garbanzo), citrus fruits, and dark green vegetables or take supplements.

Kidney stones

Kidney stones are a hard material produced by the kidney. They can lodge in the kidney or can pass through the ureter, the bladder, and finally the urethra to exit the body. Kidney stones are caused by an excessive buildup of mineral crystals in the kidney. Symptoms include excruciating lower-back pain, abdominal pain, urinary tract infections, fever, a burning sensation while urinating, and blood in the urine.

Watch Out!
Men should avoid cigarette smoking and drugs. Destressing your life also is vital. Researchers have found that the stress of losing a loved one can be tied to male infertility.

66
I felt like such a failure when I could not conceive a baby and blamed myself entirely. Imagine my surprise when the doctor said my husband had a low sperm count and that was why I couldn't get pregnant. I think so many times everyone thinks it's the woman's problem. The good news is that most problems can be overcome with medical intervention.
—Rachel, 29, secretary

99

How is it prevented?

Drink 8 to 12 glasses of liquid a day, urinate frequently, and avoid foods that can lead to stones in some people. New studies show that a high intake of dietary calcium appears to decrease the risk of kidney stones; an intake of calcium supplements, however, may increase risk.

What is the conventional treatment?

Lithotripsy is the standard treatment—shock waves crumble the stones and then the fragments flow out with the urine.

What are some alternative treatments?

- **Hydrotherapy**—increased liquids to hydrate the body

- **Nutritional therapy**—cranberry juice, cranberries, elimination diet (avoid foods that cause stones such as grape juice, grapefruit juice, spinach, black tea, and asparagus)

The basics

1. *What's been proven to work?* Lithotripsy is an outpatient procedure that zaps stones so they can pass—without pain.

2. *How long until treatment works?* The stones usually will begin to pass within three hours of treatment.

3. *How much does it cost?* The cost varies depending you location, but it will cost in excess of $5,000 to $6,000 for the procedure, the physicians, and the facility.

If at all possible, prevent kidney stones altogether. Drink plenty of liquids (12 cups a day), increase calcium-rich foods in your diet, and avoid calcium supplements and offending foods that cause kidney stones.

Just the facts

- Eating just one cup of yogurt each day can help prevent many types of yeast infections.

- Saw palmetto is a common herb used by millions of men to treating benign prostate disease and to help increase urine flow.

- Folate is important for women of childbearing age. It helps prevent birth defects and premature delivery.

- Lithotripsy is a common outpatient procedure that blasts kidney stones.

How to distinguish the pain of angina from the pain of a heart attack ▪ Common fruits and vegetables that can dramatically reduce your risk of hypertension ▪ How to reduce your cholesterol level with diet and exercise ▪ The one herbal therapy that has been found effective in reducing headache pain

Cardiovascular and Whole-Body Disorders

Chapter 14

Each year millions of Americans are diagnosed with heart disease. In many cases, it can be prevented with a program of nutrition, exercise, and medication (if necessary). This chapter explains the most common types of cardiovascular problems. As you read, focus on the hands-on alternative therapies you can start today to keep your heart healthy.

Angina

Angina is chest pain or pressure, usually beneath the sternum (breastbone), and is frequently associated with exertion. It is caused by inadequate blood supply to the heart, which often is triggered by strong emotions, exercise, or heavy meals in someone who has heart disease.

Angina pain has been described as heaviness, tightness, burning, pressure, or squeezing behind the breast bone. A sharp chest pain that lasts a few seconds usually is not angina, but it could be related

to a muscle, a tendon, or heartburn. When in doubt,
see your doctor.

How is it prevented?

Keep stress levels low, avoid smoking, lose weight,
avoid overeating, take prescribed drugs to treat
hypertension, and practice healthy eating habits.

What is the conventional treatment?

Exercise helps some patients because it reduces the
heart rate and blood pressure. Nitroglycerin tablets
taken under the tongue can resolve the pain. Taking
aspirin each day can cut the rate of unstable angina.

What are some alternative treatments?

- **Aryurvedic medicine**—Transcendental Meditation

- **Chinese medicine**—tai chi, qigong

- **Nutritional supplements**—omega-3s (fish oil),
  Coenzyme Q10, magnesium, calcium, potassium, vitamin E

- **Nutritional therapy**—DASH diet, Mediterranean diet, vegetarian diet, low-fat diet

- **Mind/body treatments**—relaxation response,
  any destressing technique

The basics

1. *What's been proven to work?* You can use a combination of lifestyle techniques to reduce weight,
   to stop smoking, to increase exercise, and to
   eliminate contributing risk factors such as
   hypertension. Taking aspirin is important to
   reduce the risk of dying from a heart attack.

2. *How long until treatment works?* You should notice
   a difference within one to two months if you are
   committed to a holistic program to reduce risk
   factors.

3. *How much does it cost?* Making lifestyle changes costs virtually nothing, but the benefits you will gain—reduced chest pain and reduced chance of heart disease—are priceless.

If you have chest pain, don't guess whether it is angina or a heart attack. Call your doctor immediately. The only way to distinguish angina from a heart attack is to measure heart function with an electrocardiogram and other tests. You should get to the emergency room of the nearest hospital if you experience intense, unexpected, or prolonged chest pain.

Heart disease

The number one killer in the United States, heart disease, often has no symptoms. Angina (chest pain, see preceding section) at rest, however, usually indicates the presence of severe coronary artery disease (CAD) and a serious risk of a heart attack (see Table 14.2). A heart attack can be caused by smoking, high blood pressure, high cholesterol, genetics, obesity, diabetes, and age (see Table 14.1). Atherosclerosis, caused by the wear and tear of the inside lining of the arteries (especially the coronary arteries that supply the heart muscle), is the basic problem of most heart attacks. This buildup eventually decreases the diameter of the artery, and an angioplasty or surgery is performed to reduce the blockage in the coronary artery. Depression also is strongly associated with hypertension and heart disease. Nearly 50 percent of heart patients have suffered an episode of major depression.

Control any risk factors you can—stop smoking, lose weight, and reduce blood pressure and cholesterol to normal limits.

Watch Out!
Vitamins do not take the place of healing foods. Try to get the required vitamins and minerals through a healthy diet; use supplements to fill in what your diet lacks. Usually vitamin E is difficult to get through foods.

Watch Out!
Common symp-
toms of a heart
attack are:

■ A feeling in
the chest of
tightness, pres-
sure, dull pain,
squeezing, heavi-
ness, aching,
indigestion,
burning, or other
discomfort (or
any combination
of these)

■ Pain felt in the
shoulder, arm,
neck, jaw, or
back

■ Shortness of
breath

■ Nausea and
sweating

TABLE 14.1   RISK FACTORS FOR HEART ATTACK

| High blood pressure (hypertension) |
| High blood cholesterol (hypercholesterolemia) |
| Cigarette smoking |
| Poor diet |
| Lack of exercise |
| Obesity |
| Stress |
| Personality traits—hostility and anger |
| Gender |
| Menopause |
| Diabetes mellitus |
| Family history of heart disease |
| Increasing age |

What is the conventional treatment?

Following a diet in which only 10 percent of calories
are from fat has been shown to reduce plaque
buildup. This type of diet relies primarily on vegetables, beans, whole grains, fruits, fat-free dairy products, and no red meat. Medications such as nitrates
(nitroglycerin), beta blockers, calcium antagonists,
and aspirin frequently are prescribed for people
with heart disease. Women at menopause can take
hormone replacement therapy (HRT).

What are some alternative treatments?

- **Ayurvedic medicine**—yoga, Transcendental
  Meditation

- **Nutritional therapy**—soy foods; DASH diet;
  Mediterranean diet; vegetarian diet; low-fat diet
  with only 10 percent of calories coming from
  fat; red wine and grapes; carrots, spinach, and
  cantaloupe (rich in beta-carotene); potatoes,
  bananas, and orange juice (high in potassium);
  and foods high in folic acid

- **Nutritional supplements**—increase vitamins A, C, and E (antioxidants may help prevent clogged arteries by altering the process in which cholesterol becomes damaging to cell membranes), folic acid, omega-3s, calcium, potassium, magnesium

Bright Idea
Eat cooked carrots instead of raw ones—cooking them unleashes more healing beta-carotene. To take advantage of all nutrients, use the liquid in which vegetables are cooked as stock to make soups.

The basics

1. *What's been proven to work?* Nutrition is the best way to lower cholesterol. Resveratrol, found in grapes, is thought to lower levels of harmful cholesterol (LDL) and to decrease arterial plaque. In one study, Harvard Medical School doctors found that, when men with a history of cardiac disease were given the antioxidant beta-carotene as a 50-milligram supplement every other day, they suffered half as many heart attacks, strokes, and deaths as men taking a placebo pill. Folic acid also is important in preventing heart disease, according to a study in the *Journal of the American Medical Association.* Still another study from the Harvard School of Public Health (reported in *The New England Journal of Medicine*) found that trans-fatty acids greatly contribute to heart disease. In this report, women who ate diets high in saturated fat and trans-fatty acids were more likely to develop heart disease than women who consumed less of these fats. (Trans-fatty acids are found in foods such as potato chips, cookies, and pastry.)

2. *How long until treatment works?* You may notice a beneficial effect within weeks of changing your diet, adding exercise, stopping smoking, and losing weight.

3. *How much does it cost?* There should be no additional cost for making these lifestyle changes. In fact, stopping smoking will allow you to save money.

Risk factors play a key role in many serious diseases. Eliminating any risk factors you can while taking medications to treat high blood pressure, high cholesterol, or high triglycerides will help you greatly reduce the chance of heart disease and the resulting heart attack.

Hypertension (High blood pressure)

Hypertension is an increase in the force of blood against the arteries as blood circulates through them. Blood is forced through the arteries using systolic pressure; when the heart rests between beats, a diastolic pressure remains. Blood pressure is the measure of these two pressures. Normal pressure is considered to be 120/80. Blood pressure usually goes up as a result of stress or physical activity, but a person with hypertension has high blood pressure at rest.

Hypertension is caused by smoking, obesity, alcoholism, heredity, a diet high in saturated fat or sodium, and unhealthy lifestyle habits. Sometimes birth control pills, chronic diseases, or certain medications can increase blood pressure. Anxiety, restlessness, tension, tightness, and headaches all are associated with hypertension. This often is referred to as the silent disease because many times there are no symptoms.

How is it prevented?

Reduce all risk factors for the disease.

Bright Idea
If you are struggling with high blood pressure, try limiting your intake of processed foods with 480 mg or more of sodium per serving to only one serving per day. This includes foods such as canned soups, pizzas, hot dogs, and frozen dinners. Seventy-five percent of the sodium in American's diets comes from these types of foods.

TABLE 14.2 CATEGORIES OF HYPERTENSION

Systolic (upper number)		Diastolic (lower number)
Normal blood pressure less than 130	and	less than 85
High normal 130-139	or	85-89
Hypertension		
Stage 1 (Mild) 140-159	or	90-99
Stage 2 (Moderate) 160-179	or	100-109
Stage 3 (Severe) 180-209	or	110-119
Stage 4 (Very severe) 210 or higher	or	120 or higher

TABLE 14.3 COMMON MEDICATIONS FOR HYPERTENSION

Medication	Function in the Body
Diuretics	Reduce the fluid level in the body
Beta blockers	Alter the body's chemistry to ignore adrenaline
Calcium channel blockers	Prevent blood vessels from constricting
Vasodilators	Cause muscles in the walls of blood vessels to relax and dilate

What is the conventional treatment?

Reducing obesity and salt intake can lessen hypertension in some people, but many people with high blood pressure need antihypertensive drugs such as ACE inhibitors and calcium channel blockers (see Table 14.4).

What are some alternative treatments?

- **Ayurvedic medicine**—Transcendental Meditation
- **Chinese medicine**—tai chi, qigong
- **Herbal therapy**—garlic

- **Mind/body treatments**—relaxation response, autogenic therapy, deep abdominal breathing
- **Nutritional therapy**—DASH diet; a low-fat, low-salt diet (restricted to 2 grams of sodium per day, called a no-added-salt diet); eliminate animal and dairy products

The basics

1. *What's been proven to work?* Weight loss, regular exercise, reduced salt, and medications. If you have hypertension, try the new DASH diet (Dietary Approaches to Stop Hypertension), which has been found to reduce blood pressure in about two weeks. The daily diet includes seven to eight servings of grains or grain products, four to five servings of fruit, four to five servings of vegetables, two to three servings of nonfat or low-fat dairy products, ½ serving of nuts, and two or fewer servings of lean meat. Transcendental Meditation also has been found to reduce blood pressure.

2. *How long until treatment works?* In the DASH diet study, participants experienced drops in blood pressure within two weeks.

3. *How much does it cost?* Adding fruits and vegetables while reducing animal products should not increase your regular grocery expense.

Although diet is crucial for reducing hypertension, another goal is to adopt a lifelong, regular exercise program—at least 20 to 30 minutes a day. Stress can cause an increase in blood pressure, so it also is beneficial to reduce stressful situations and to learn mind/body treatments to control the fight or flight response.

TABLE 14.4   FOODS HIGH IN SODIUM

Type of food	Amount	Milligrams
Beef broth	1 cube	1,150 mg
Cheeseburger, fast food	¼ lb.	1,200 mg
Chicken noodle soup	1 cup	1,100 mg
Cottage cheese	4 ounces	450 mg
Frankfurter	1½ ounces	500 mg
Garlic salt	1 tsp.	1,850 mg
Ham	3 ounces	1,000 mg
Luncheon meat	1 slice	575 mg
Meat tenderizer	1 tsp.	1,750 mg
Olives, green	3	720 mg
Onion salt	1 tsp.	1,620 mg
Peas, green canned	1 cup	493 mg
Potato, instant	1 cup	475 mg
Salt	¼ tsp	500 mg
Sauerkraut	⅔ cup	740 mg
Soy sauce	1 tbsp.	1,030 mg

High cholesterol (hypercholesterolemia)

With high cholesterol, there are no warning signs until blockage of an artery occurs. Cholesterol is a main component of the plaque that builds up on arterial walls. A total blood cholesterol higher than the safe range is considered too high. Total blood cholesterol is made up of *low-density lipoprotein (LDL)*, *high-density lipoprotein (HDL)*, and *very low-density lipoprotein (VLDL)*. Increased levels of LDL are associated with the plaque deposits on artery walls that narrow them and restrict blood flow. HDL, or "good" cholesterol, helps prevent plaque. It comes from a diet high in saturated fat and from genetics.

How is it prevented?

Maintain a diet that is low in saturated fat and high in fruits, vegetables, and fiber. Exercise regularly, lose weight, quit smoking, reduce alcohol intake, and watch medications taken for diseases.

Watch Out!
Some medications taken for heart problems can elevate liver enzymes. Make sure your doctor checks your blood chemistry periodically.

What is the conventional treatment?

Change to a low-fat, high-fiber diet; reduce dietary cholesterol; increase exercise; stop smoking; and reduce stress. Sometimes medications are prescribed if lifestyle changes do not work. Common medications include Zocor (Simvastatin), Mevacor (Lovastatin), Provachol (Pravastatin) and Questran (Cholestyramine). Women can take hormone replacement therapy at menopause to reduce cholesterol.

What are some alternative treatments?

- **Herbal therapy**—psyllium seed husks
- **Nutritional supplements**—niacin, Coenzyme Q10
- **Nutritional therapy**—red wine, soy foods, oat bran, oatmeal, and other high-fiber foods

The basics

1. *What's been proven to work?* In many cases, changing your diet, losing weight, and adding exercise to your daily routine will result in reduced cholesterol. Garlic tablets and fish oil capsules also lower cholesterol. Millions of people, however, still may need medication. Coenzyme Q10 is an antioxidant that may help lower cholesterol levels and reduce oxidative damage to blood vessels. Hormone-replacement therapy decreases the risk of heart disease in women by 40 to 60 percent by reducing the "bad" LDL

TABLE 14.5   DIETARY STEPS TO LOWER CHOLESTEROL

- Avoid saturated fats and trans-fatty acids
- Use low-fat or fat-free milk
- Eat more fish and poultry
- Use only lean and fat-trimmed meat
- Eat more fresh fruits and vegetables
- Add more fiber to your diet
- Add garlic supplements to your diet
- Increase omega-3 fatty acids (fish oil)
- Use monounsaturated fats (olive oil)

cholesterol and increasing the "good" HDL cholesterol in the blood. One mind/body therapy that can help lower cholesterol is increasing social support. Researchers at Osijek University in Croatia found that, among 137 volunteers, those who felt loved by family and friends had lower cholesterol levels than those who lacked emotional support.

2. *How long until treatment works?* You should notice a difference within a few weeks to two months.

3. *How much does it cost?* Dietary changes are virtually free because you purchase fewer foods with saturated fats (including many processed and snack foods) and add more fresh fruits, vegetables, and foods low in cholesterol (see Table 14.6).

Exercise can lower LDL cholesterol and triglycerides, and it can raise HDL cholesterol, especially in men—even after heart attack. Dietary changes to control cholesterol seem to have a beneficial effect

TABLE 14.6   CHOLESTEROL CONTENT
OF SELECTED FOODS

Food	Amount	Milligrams
Dairy		
Butter	1 tsp	11
Margarine	1 tsp	0
Skim milk	1 cup	5
1%	1 cup	10
2%	1 cup	18
Whole milk	1 cup	34
Sherbet	½ cup	7
Ice cream	½ cup	30
Cream	1 Tbsp	20
Half and half	1 Tbsp	6
American cheese	1 ounce	16
Cheddar cheese	1 ounce	30
Mozzarella, part skim	1 ounce	15
Swiss cheese	1 ounce	26
Cottage cheese, 1% fat	1 cup	10
Poultry		
Chicken, dark (no skin)	3 ounces	81
Chicken, white (no skin)	3 ounces	72
Turkey, dark (no skin)	3 ounces	87
Turkey, white (no skin)	3 ounces	66
Red meat		
Bacon	1 slice	5
Beef, lean	3 ounces	78
Frankfurter	1.6 ounces	45
Ham (boiled)	3 ounces	75
Pork (lean)	3 ounces	75
Veal (lean)	3 ounces	84
Seafood/fish		
Crab	3 ounces	85
Flounder	3 ounces	70
Haddock	3 ounces	40
Lobster	3 ounces	70

Oysters	3 ounces	42
Shrimp	3 ounces	128
Tuna	3 ounces	55
Breads/Cereals/Grains		
Bread	1 slice	0
Bagel	1 whole	0
Doughnut, yeast	1	21
Oatmeal	½ cup	0
Rice, plain	½ cup	0
Cookie, plain	1	1
Fruits/Vegetables		
Potato, baked	1 small	0
Potato, fried	10 strips	0
Cabbage	½ cup	0
Apple	1 medium	0
Banana	1 medium	0
Miscellaneous		
Cereal		0
Egg noodles	1 cup	50
Egg whites		0
Egg yolk	1 large	272
Fruits		0
Nuts		0
Vegetables		0

in most people, but they may not help if the only abnormality is low HDL cholesterol. Stopping smoking results in an increase in HDL cholesterol. Adding estrogen treatment in women after menopause also increases HDL cholesterol.

Migraine

A migraine headache is an intense, incapacitating headache (often accompanied by other symptoms) that occurs repeatedly in some children and adults. Migraines usually are caused by an enlargement (dilation) of arteries in and around the head, causing the pain.

Watch Out!
If your headache worsens and cannot be relieved with over-the-counter medications, see your doctor. It could be a symptom of something more serious.

The pain may last a few hours or several days and can be dull, throbbing, constant, and severe. The pain is most often (but not always) on one side of the head and usually is felt in the front or on the side of the head. Nausea or vomiting can accompany the headache and, occasionally, the sufferer will have diarrhea. Lights and a bright room may make the headache much worse. In some forms of migraine headache (called the classic migraine), the person may see blind spots, light flashes, or other visual changes before the start of the headache.

How is it prevented?
Avoid emotional upset, destress your life, and get plenty of rest. Alcohol and certain foods may trigger a migraine, so eliminate them if you feel they are a factor in the problem.

What is the conventional treatment?
Aspirin or nonsteroidal anti-inflammatory drugs (NSAIDs) help some people, but others must rely on prescription medications such as vasoconstrictors, lidocaine nasal drops, cardiovascular drugs, antidepressants, and antiseizure drugs (Imitrex).

What are some alternative treatments?
- **Herbal therapy**—feverfew
- **Homeopathy**—belladonna LMI (homeopathic deadly nightshade), calcarea carbonica (homeopathic calcium carbonate from oyster shell)
- **Hydrotherapy**—a cold cloth or ice pack to the head, splash face with cold water
- **Mind/body treatments**—music therapy, relaxation response, progressive muscle relaxation

■ **Nutritional therapy**—elimination diet (avoid food triggers such as coffee, preservatives, wine, cheese, nitrites, monosodium glutamate, and yeasts)

The basics

1. *What's been proven to work?* Eliminating triggers is the first line of defense, followed by treating the headache pain as soon as you feel the first symptom. A new drug called Amerge (naratriptan) provides relief within four hours of treatment, and the relief lasts up to 24 hours. Another drug called Zomig (zolmitriptan) also helps a migraine and the nausea that accompanies it. Imitrex (sumatriptan), which has been proven to give rapid relief, now is available in a nasal spray.

2. *How long until treatment works?* Using medications such as these, you may find relief within 20 minutes.

3. *How much does it cost?* The newer medicines cost around $100 to $125 for nine tablets.

Although many new migraine drugs seem like miracle cures, there are reported side effects. For example, many patients have side effects of flushing, sweating, chest tightness, an unpleasant taste in the mouth, and a narrowing of already diseased coronary arteries. Ask your doctor before taking any of these medications.

Whole-body disorders

Whole-body disorders include very serious, chronic problems such as AIDS, cancer, and diabetes. The outlook for these diseases used to be poor, but with the breakthroughs in scientific research, today's

"
After suffering with migraine headaches since childhood, I've learned to take my medication at the first sign of headache pain. If I wait even 30 minutes, it takes much longer to get relief.
—Linda, 53, administrator
"

outlook is positive. For most of these ailments, treatment can allow you to live a very normal life. The bottom line is early detection and early treatment. Check out the following diseases to see whether new methods of treatment might help you or a loved one.

AIDS (acquired immune deficiency syndrome)

AIDS is a major failure of the body's immune system (immunodeficiency disease). It decreases the body's ability to fight infection and to suppress multiplication of abnormal cells such as cancer cells. It is caused by a virus named Human Immunodeficiency Virus (HIV). This virus attacks the body's cells, especially cells in the blood called T4 Helper cells. These cells are important in the body's defense against infection and tumors. When the T4 Helper cells are diminished or crippled, the body's ability to defend itself against infection is lowered. Mild infections, which may not affect those not infected with AIDS(HIV), can cause severe disease in people with AIDS. Respiratory diseases, particularly lung infections, are the major causes of illness and death.

How is it prevented?

The disease is spread through sexual contact, exposure to infected needles, or contact between AIDS-infected blood and an easily infected area such as a sore or open wound.

The majority of people who have been diagnosed with AIDS are homosexual or bisexual men, but people who receive transfusions, intravenous drug users, and those who engage in unprotected sexual intercourse (men and women alike) also are at an increasingly high risk. To prevent AIDS, you must avoid situations that create risk.

What is the conventional treatment?

Current treatments for AIDS include AZT, DDI, DDC, D4T, 3TC, and Saquinavir, usually in combination with AZT or DDC. Although these drugs delay the onset and slow the progress of AIDS, they may only have short-term effects for some people.

What are some alternative treatments?

- **Ayurvedic medicine**—spirituality, Transcendental Meditation, yoga

- **Homeopathy**—silicea

- **Nutritional supplements**—vitamins A, C, and E (antioxidants), B-complex vitamins

- **Nutritional therapy**—indoles, allylic sulfide, limonene, saponins, flavonoids, green tea, low-fat diet, soy foods, eating a well-balanced diet high in phytochemicals and antioxidants

- **Mind/body treatments**—art, music, dance, laughter therapies, social support, counseling, psychotherapy

The basics

1. *What's been proven to work?* Some people believe the homeopathic medicine silicea has strong effects on stimulating the body's immune system, but there is still no cure for AIDS in sight. Treating the opportunistic infections that occur (for example, with antibiotics) can help stop problems early on before they go into full-blown AIDS.

2. *How long until it works?* There are no studies that specify a guaranteed period of time before this medicine works.

3. *How much does it cost?* Silica costs from $7 to $15. Until a cure for AIDS is discovered, prevention

Bright Idea
There is no cure for AIDS yet, but keeping your body as healthy as possible is important to avoid complications. Use the mind/body methods of treatment to destress and eat a nutrient-dense diet to boost immune function.

is the only protection. Use latex condoms when you have sex, avoid sex with people who are at high risk for contracting AIDS, don't share needles with anyone (even for steroids or insulin), and don't share personal items that could have blood on them (such as razors). If you've been diagnosed with HIV or AIDS, make sure you are under the care of an HIV specialist.

Cancer

Cancer is a malignant tumor capable of causing destruction or death, and it tends to invade surrounding tissue. It is difficult to identify the agents that cause cancer. It rarely develops after a single exposure to a carcinogen. Cancer usually requires many exposures over long periods of time, and it is usually many years after exposure that the cancer becomes apparent. For example, the risk of lung cancer is directly related to smoking. It is rare to develop cancer in less than 20 years of smoking, yet not all smokers develop lung cancer. It takes 7 to 10 years after you stop smoking to notice a reduction in the risk of lung cancer. Some of the greatest cancer risk factors include:

- Hereditary factors
- Smoking
- Alcohol
- Radiation
- Chemicals
- Hormone treatment
- Sunlight
- Diet

The symptoms of cancer can range from unusual bleeding, difficulty swallowing, or a painless lump to a change in the color of moles, skin changes, or an unexplained cough or pain. Sometimes there are no visible symptoms, and the condition is discovered through a routine laboratory test.

What is the conventional treatment?

Cancer can be treated with surgery, chemotherapy, radiation, any combination of these three, or all three.

What are some alternative treatments?

- **Detoxification**—quit smoking, reduce alcohol intake

- **Environmental medicine**—avoid toxins and contact with chemicals and carcinogens

- **Nutritional supplements**—vitamins A, C, and E (antioxidants), selenium

- **Nutritional therapy**—indoles, allylic sulfide, limonene, saponins, flavonoids, green tea, phytochemicals, low-fat diet, soy foods

The basics

1. *What's been proven to work?* If you have cancer, seek medical treatment. If you want to prevent cancer, watch what you eat . . . and what you don't eat. Nutrition is one of your best defenses against this disease. In countries such as Japan and Norway—where diets are rich in beta-carotene—the populations have a low incidence of lung, colon, prostate, cervical, and breast cancer. A recent study at the University of Arizona Cancer Center found that three to six months of daily beta-carotene pills dramatically reduced precancerous mouth lesions in 70 percent of the patients.

Watch Out!
Be aware of the latest cancer diagnostic tests, and ask your doctor if they would help you to stay cancer-free. Also tell your doctor about any family history of cancer or if you have been exposed to a known carcinogen.

According to the National Cancer Institute, a diet high in fiber cuts the risk of colon cancer by up to 70 percent. The American Dietetic Association's recommendation for adults is 20 to 35 grams of fiber daily. Studies show that omega-3 fatty acids (found in salmon, sardines, tuna, and bluefish) have anti-carcinogenic benefits, and olive oil is linked to reduced breast cancer risk. Soy foods are associated with a reduction in breast and prostate cancer. Perhaps an even greater discovery is that tea contains cancer-fighting polyphenols and may also increase the level of good enzymes that metabolize carcinogens.

2. *How much does treatment cost?* Adding cancer-fighting foods to your diet will not cost more if you substitute them for unhealthy food choices.

3. *How long until it works?* Fighting cancer is a life-long project, but it starts working the moment you watch what you feed your body and mind.

Not only is prevention important with a nutritious diet, exercise, and vitamin supplements, early detection is crucial to stopping cancer. The earlier cancer is detected and treated, the less likely the disease will be fatal. Conventional medical examinations such as breast examinations, Pap tests, mammograms, rectal examinations, and PSA tests, among others, can be lifesavers.

Diabetes

Diabetes is caused by abnormally high levels of glucose in the blood. The actual cause is not known, and no cure is available. Risk factors for this disease include obesity, age, and family history. There may be no symptoms at all, or you may have one or more of the following:

- Change in vision
- Weight loss
- Severe fatigue
- Frequent urination of large amounts
- Increased thirst
- Frequent infections
- Severe illness
- Burning in hands and feet

How is it prevented?
Stay at a normal weight and maintain a regular exercise program.

What is the conventional treatment?
Type I diabetes is insulin-dependent; this means you must add insulin to the body to keep blood sugar levels normal. Type II diabetes often can be controlled with diet and weight loss. Good control decreases the chance of complications. In some cases, type II diabetes will progress to insulin-dependent diabetes, a more serious form.

What are some alternative treatments?
- **Nutritional supplements**—chromium, antioxidant vitamins (vitamins A, C, and E)
- **Nutritional therapy**—eat more soluble fiber, complex carbohydrates, and foods rich in magnesium, potassium, and calcium; avoid alcohol and high-fat foods

The basics
1. *What's been proven to work?* Obesity is a risk factor for 80 to 90 percent of all type II (adult-onset) diabetes. Weight loss—even 10 pounds—can greatly reduce the risk. Exercise helps to keep blood sugar levels stable.

66
With diabetes running in my family, I have to work extra hard to change its course in my life. I get my blood-glucose tested periodically, avoid eating a diet high in sugar, and exercise daily. I think I can beat this!"
—Kevin, 33, attorney
99

Watch Out!
A U.S.
Department of
Agriculture study
found that
chromium helps
normalize glu-
cose insulin lev-
els in people
with diabetes. If
taken in amounts
of 1,000 mil-
ligrams daily,
however, too
much chromium
can cause ane-
mia and kidney
damage. Ask your
doctor before
administering
this treatment.

2. *How much does treatment cost?* Exercise and a reduced-calorie diet are free.

3. *How long until it works?* If you watch your calorie and fat intake and increase expenditure of calories through exercise, you should enjoy weight loss of about half a pound per week. You can lose 10 pounds in about two and a half months, if your diet and exercise are consistent.

There are 16 million Americans with diabetes. About 15 million have type II, which is usually triggered by a combination of obesity, lack of exercise, high blood pressure, and family history. Prevention is crucial and the steps are easy—reduce the risk factors and stay diabetes free.

Just the facts

- Most chronic diseases are caused by specific risk factors, many of which you can control or change.

- Increasing exercise, stopping smoking, losing weight, and destressing all are healthy lifestyle choices that will reduce your risk of heart disease.

- A diet high in carotenoids has been found to give protection against cancer.

- Staying at a normal weight and increasing exercise are important factors in avoiding type II diabetes.

GET THE SCOOP ON...

How mind/body treatments can help you relax ▪ The herbal cure for insomnia ▪ How your over-the-counter pain or headache remedy may be keeping you awake all night long ▪ The herbal cure for depression that millions are now taking

Neurological and Psychological Disorders

Chapter 15

Neurological and psychological disorders are very complicated afflictions. They are not as easy to diagnose or to treat as other physical problems described in this section. Many times, problems such as alcoholism, anxiety, or depression can stem from a biochemical imbalance. Quite often, professional help is needed to maintain, control, and cure these problems. While many excellent prescription drugs and many medical protocols can assist greatly, a host of mind/body treatments also may help. Look at the following ailments and treatments to see if some may help your situation.

Alcoholism

Psychological and physiological dependence on alcohol is brought about by negative emotional stresses such as anger, mania, depression, or introversion, and by genetic and family influences, especially alcoholic or divorced parents and pressure to drink within social atmospheres. Symptoms include the need for alcohol at the beginning of the day or at times of stress, a preoccupation with purchasing alcohol more than usual, and hiding and drinking from family and friends.

How is it prevented?

Moderate your alcohol intake. Know your limits. Don't drink alone. Seek professional help; alcoholism generally can't be self-cured.

What is the conventional treatment?

First you need to admit there is a problem; then seek professional counseling or join a support group such as Alcoholics Anonymous (AA). Detoxification and reassessment of your lifestyle are helpful. In some cases, your doctor may prescribe medications such as Antabuse to help alleviate withdrawal symptoms.

What are some alternative treatments?

- **Ayurvedic medicine**—Transcendental Meditation
- **Chinese medicine**—acupuncture, tai chi, yoga
- **Nutritional therapy**—an elimination diet (no sugar, white flour, additives, or preservatives)
- **Mind/body treatments**—counseling, prayer, meditation, and social support

The basics

1. *What's been proven to work?* Millions of people have successfully ended problems with alcohol using support groups such as Alcoholics Anonymous. This particular program is based on a 12-step plan that focuses on lifestyle issues and faith.

2. *How long until it works?* Although it takes years to end an abusive relationship with alcohol, giving

up alcohol is a day-by-day process. Getting the proper support is key to successfully overcoming this disease.

3. *How much does treatment cost?* Alcoholics Anonymous is free, and meetings are held in many convenient locations. The medication Antabuse costs about $40 per month.

Alternative methods such as social support, faith in something greater than self, prayer, and meditation have helped millions break destructive habits with alcohol. Seek professional guidance if this is a concern.

Anxiety

Anxiety is a physical and emotional reaction to stress. It is caused by constant stressful situations or by worrying about a situation. Alcohol and drug problems often are causes of anxiety. Symptoms include restlessness, headaches, nausea, sweating, fatigue, sleeplessness, trembling hands, rapid heart rate and breathing, and terrifying dreams.

How is it prevented?

Recognize the problem and its symptoms and then try to alleviate what is creating the anxiety. Eliminate stimulants such as caffeine from your diet and learn to prioritize your time to avoid overcommitment and added stress.

What is the conventional treatment?

Manage thoughts of stressful situations and work to overcome fears and phobias. Physical exercise, meditation, and other forms of stress management also are helpful for prevention and treatment. Serious anxiety may require counseling and medications such as Xanax.

Watch Out!
Being obsessive with your fears—focusing on what may happen—will make it difficult to move in a positive direction in life. It is far better to recognize your fears and to redirect your energy toward optimistic behaviors. Worrying about what cannot be changed will only make you more anxious.

What are some alternative treatments?

- **Ayurvedic medicine**—Transcendental Meditation, yoga

- **Chinese medicine**—tai chi

- **Bach Flowers**—Rescue Remedy

- **Bodyworks**—therapeutic massage for relaxation

- **Herbal therapy**—chamomile, kava kava, valerian, and St. John's wort

- **Mind/body treatments**—autogenic therapy, music therapy, deep abdominal breathing, and the relaxation response

- **Nutritional supplements**—essential fatty acid (EFAs), B-complex vitamins (especially B_6), vitamin C, folic acid, zinc

- **Nutritional therapy**—serotonin-boosting foods that provide a calming effect such as pasta, bagels, and sherbet

The basics

1. *What's been proven to work?* The first remedy is to reduce your stress. Figure out what is causing you to be in overload and eliminate overcommitment. Use alternative treatments to gain control of your diet and your lifestyle. If this does not work, seek professional counseling.

2. *What does treatment cost?* Most alternative methods to reduce anxiety are free. Herbal therapies such as kava kava or valerian cost about $10 for a 30-day supply.

3. *How long until it starts working?* If you take control of your lifestyle with a nutritional diet, regular exercise and sleep, and alternative measures to reduce your stress, you should

notice a difference in your anxiety level within five days to two weeks.

A certain amount of anxiety is both normal and healthy. Yet if you have deep, continuing anxiety that keeps you from living a normal routine, seek professional help.

Attention deficit hyperactivity disorder (ADHD)

ADHD is a pattern of behavior that includes a short attention span, impulsivity, and hyperactivity. ADHD affects about 10 percent of school-aged children. Adults also can be affected. Actual causes of ADHD are unknown, although it is speculated that there is a biological connection. Symptoms include inability to remain seated, impatience, and disruptive behavior.

How is it prevented?

There currently is no way to prevent ADHD.

What is the conventional treatment?

A psychological evaluation is given to the child and then a diagnosis is made. Although most of the symptomatic signs of ADHD are common in children, when diagnosing the disorder, a criteria of many of the symptoms usually must be met. A change in diet or a structured environment may help alleviate ADHD, although severe cases may require stimulant medications such as Ritalin. Some adults benefit from antidepressants such as Wellbutrin, which help them stay attentive to the task at hand.

What are some alternative treatments?

- **Environmental medicine**—avoid chemical additives in foods

Watch Out!
If you or your child has been diagnosed with ADHD, ask your doctor if a food elimination diet may help. Sometimes a food allergy causes symptoms that mimic attention deficit disorder.

- **Nutritional therapy**—an elimination diet (avoid sugar, white flour, preservatives, and colorings)
- **Mind/body treatments**—biofeedback

The basics

Watch Out!
Although psychostimulants seem to have a calming affect on children with ADHD, there is also a host of potential side effects such as sleep disturbances, depression, headaches, stomach aches, loss of appetite, and stunted growth. Weigh your options and then treat this disorder carefully.

1. *What's been proven to work?* Most people rely on medications to control symptoms of ADHD, although new reports suggest that behavioral modification therapies using biofeedback can help in some cases to exert a new control over brain waves. This treatment is based on a certain sort of electrical activity in the brain that produces alpha waves. Experts, however, feel it may be experimental or the placebo effect.

2. *How long until it works?* If the medication works, you should see or feel a difference within days. With behavioral therapies, it may take several weeks or months to see any change.

3. *How much does it cost?* Medications can vary from $20 to $60 a month, depending on the type and whether the drug is generic or name brand. Biofeedback costs about $60 to $100 per session.

Scientists are revealing that behavioral and cognitive therapies can focus on strategies that alter an undesired behavior. A combination of these techniques, along with medications such as Ritalin, appears to work best for controlling the symptoms.

Chronic fatigue syndrome

Chronic Fatigue Syndrome (CFS) is extreme fatigue that persists for longer than six months, even after extensive bed rest and relaxation. The cause is unknown, but an atypical immune system could be a factor. Epstein-Barr virus has also been implicated. Symptoms include fatigue, low-grade fever, painful lymph glands, sore throat, muscle weakness, headaches, sleep disturbances, joint pain, psychological problems, and sometimes vision changes.

How is it prevented?
There currently is no cure or prevention for CFS.

What is the conventional treatment?
Maintain a positive outlook on life and either seek psychotherapy or join a local support group. Maintain good nutrition and a set day-to-day schedule.

What are some alternative treatments?
- **Ayurvedic medicine**—yoga
- **Herbal therapy**—echinacea, garlic, ginkgo biloba, ginseng
- **Nutritional supplements**—vitamins A, C, and E (antioxidants), B-complex vitamins, iron (if needed)
- **Nutritional therapy**—healing foods high in phytochemicals and antioxidants

The basics
1. *What's been proven to work?* A combination of destressing, getting more rest, and building the immune system with diet and supplements.

2. *How much does treatment cost?* Virtually nothing except for nutritional supplements such as vitamins (about $20 for one month's supply) or echinacea.

3. *How long until it works?* Chronic fatigue is a mystery. Some people will find that symptoms ease within weeks; others report unrelenting fatigue for months on end.

Bright Idea
Depression is very debilitating and is common in both men and women of all ages. Check out the following symptoms to see whether you have these feelings. If you do, check with your health care provider and seek treatment.

Disturbed sleep patterns

Loss of interest in usual activities

Weight loss or gain (more than 5 percent of body weight)

Fatigue

Thoughts of death or suicide

Irritability

Mood swings

Avoiding social contact

Reduced or increased appetite

Difficulty concentrating

Because chronic fatigue is a vague but debilitating illness, it's imperative to check with your doctor to review all options for treatment.

Depression

Depression is a condition in which you feel sadness, hopelessness, dejection, and guilt. Many factors can cause depression such as excess stress, personal loss, the death of a loved one, hormone imbalances, personal failures, or chronic illness, among many others. Manic depression can be inherited.

Symptoms include loss of appetite, loss of libido, insomnia, fatigue, and boredom. A drug or alcohol problem also can contribute to the onset of depression. Headaches and stomach cramps with no signs of an illness may be found in people with depression.

How is it prevented?

Depression is prevented through significant life changes and through gaining control of contributing factors. Controlling anger and moderating or minimizing stress also are good ways to fight and beat depression.

What is the conventional treatment?

Exercise, medications, and counseling are used to treat minor depression. For severe cases of depression, psychotherapy and hospitalization might be recommended.

What are some alternative treatments?

- **Aromatherapy**—rosemary essential oil used topically (contains the compound cineole, which stimulates the central nervous system)

- **Herbal therapy**—St. John's wort, ginkgo, Siberian ginseng, valerian, skullcap, hops, or California poppy

- **Homeopathy**—Pulsatilla, Natrum muriaticum, Sepia, Ignatia amara, Aconite, Arsenicum

- **Nutritional supplements**—essential fatty acid (EFAs), B-complex vitamins (especially B_6), vitamin C, folic acid, zinc

- **Nutritional therapy**—spinach, foods that increase serotonin (complex carbohydrates)

The basics

1. *What's been proven to work?* The National Institutes of Health is studying St. John's wort and its effect on depression. This common herb is the most widely prescribed treatment for depression in Germany and has been found to improve sleep quality. Siberian ginseng acts like an antidepressant in some people and may help improve well-being. New pharmaceuticals such as Paxil, Zoloft, Wellbutrin, and Prozac are helping millions fight this dark cloud in their lives, but some of these medications have problematic side effects.

2. *How much does treatment cost?* St. John's wort costs from $15 to $25 for one month's supply, depending on the brand and place of purchase.

3. *How long until it works?* You should notice a difference within one to two weeks.

Almost everyone has a bad day or a low moment, but no one should have to feel depressed for a long period of time—if they seek help. Many herbal treatments and pharmaceuticals can help lift depression and help you feel positive again.

Insomnia

Insomnia is a sleep disorder characterized either by difficulty or inability to fall asleep or by falling

Watch Out!
If you are pregnant, treat St. John's wort as you would any pharmaceutical—do not use it. In addition, if you are taking a prescribed antidepressant, ask your doctor before making the herbal substitution.

asleep but constantly waking up. It can be caused by depression, stress, significant changes in lifestyle or daily schedule, drugs and alcohol, or medical conditions. Arthritis, heart conditions, and asthma all can cause insomnia due to the nature of the illness. Symptoms include restlessness at bedtime, sleeplessness, waking up at early hours in the morning (between 2:30 and 4:30 a.m.) and not being able to fall back asleep.

How is it prevented?

Maintain a written schedule of your day-to-day events. Plan ahead, stay on schedule, and make sure you go to sleep at the same time every night and wake up around the same time every morning.

What is the conventional treatment?

Many people use over-the-counter sleeping pills or prescription medications such as Halcion or Ambien. Some antihistamines such as Benadryl also are used to bring about sleep.

66

Taking a warm bath scented with lavendar essential oil is my sleep tonic each night. Also, I keep my bedroom lights low in the evening and the air temperture cool to make it conducive for sleep.
—Susan, 46, author

99

What are some alternative treatments?

- **Aromatherapy**—lavender essential oil

- **Bodyworks**—Swedish massage

- **Herbal therapy**—kava kava, lemon balm, or valerian

- **Hydrotherapy**—passive heating (a warm bath three hours before bedtime)

- **Mind/body treatment**—music therapy, relaxation response, or visualization

- **Nutritional supplements**—melatonin

- **Nutritional therapy**—soothing complex carbohydrates that boost serotonin levels

The basics

1. *What's been proven to work?* A combination of alternative therapies will help you get over insomnia and get healing sleep. A report in *The Lancet*, a well-respected medical journal, revealed that lavender oil was associated with reduced symptoms of insomnia in the elderly and, therefore, could reduce the need for hypnotic drugs. Valerian may work because it contains valepotriates, valeranone, and kessyl and bornyl esters, which provide a sedative effect.

2. *How long until it works?* You should notice a difference in two to four nights.

3. *How much does treatment cost?* Most alternative therapies are virtually free. Kava kava, valerian, or melatonin cost about $12 for one month's supply. For melatonin, use the smallest dose possible and only take it for a few nights unless you check with your doctor.

Relaxation and meditation will help relieve stress, and listening to soothing music will help ease a racing mind. Make sure your bed is comfortable and that the room is not too hot or cold. Most importantly, avoid caffeine after noon each day. Many common medications are loaded with caffeine (see Table 16.1).

Moneysaver
Consider trying alternative sleep therapies before you fill any type of prescription. It will save you money!

Panic disorder

Panic disorders are extreme, impulsive anxiety attacks that cause the nervous system to physically respond to the situation at hand. Although many medical disorders can mimic a panic attack (drug withdrawal, complications from seizures, heart problems), panic disorders usually are caused by a struggle with an unresolved event that caused

TABLE 16.1   CAFFEINE CONTENT OF COMMON MEDICATIONS

Brandname	Amount	Milligrams of Caffeine
Anacin, Empirin, Midol	2 tabs	64
Excedrin	2 tabs	130
No Doz	2 tabs	200
Dexatrim	1 tab	200

Timesaver
Before you invest in hours of psychotherapy, try some of the mind/body relaxation techniques listed in this book. Many times, learning how to shut down the anxieties and worries of the day will ease your nervousness and reduce panic.

extreme emotional stress. Stress, fatigue, and drug abuse also can bring on panic disorders. Symptoms include nervousness in the stomach (butterflies), trembling of the extremities, muscle spasms, fear of dying, and a sense that something is wrong or will soon go wrong.

How is it prevented?

Psychotherapy and medications (such as tranquilizers) are two ways to alleviate the severe impact a panic disorder can have on the human body. Talk about the situation with a friend and explain your anxiety about the situation.

What is the conventional treatment?

Possible treatments include medication, support groups, counseling, exercise, and dietary changes.

What are some alternative treatments?

- **Aromatherapy**—patchouli, orange, berry
- **Ayurvedic medicine**—Transcendental Meditation
- **Bach Flowers**—Rescue Remedy
- **Herbal therapy**—chamomile, kava kava, or valerian
- **Mind/body treatments**—autogenic therapy, biofeedback, dance therapy, or the relaxation response

- **Nutritional supplements**—calcium, essential fatty acid (EFAs), B-complex vitamins (especially B_6), vitamin C, folic acid, zinc
- **Nutritional therapy**—calming foods high in serotonin, an elimination diet (avoid caffeine)

The basics

1. *What's been proven to work?* Use a combination of conventional and alternative treatments to destress your life and to make necessary lifestyle changes that will help you avoid anxiety-producing situations. Prescription medications such as Xanax (generic) should be used only for a short period of time because they are addictive. Some antidepressants such as Paxil have been found to help reduce panic attacks. The relaxation response brings about the opposite of the fight or flight mode, as explained in Chapter 8. Once you learn this, you can automatically go into this relaxation mode during stressful times to avoid panic.

2. *How long until it works?* If you work on all areas of your life to reduce anxiety, in addition to taking medication or going to therapy, you should notice a difference within one to three weeks.

3. *How much does treatment cost?* Medication for reducing panic costs about $15 to $30 for two weeks.

It's important to change the way you view life. Your body reacts to what your mind tells it. If your mind perceives life's challenges as impossible, your body will be super-charged and go into fight or flight mode. Learn how to relax ahead of time so that, when interruptions hit, you can calm the red-alert signals your body sends.

Watch Out!
The symptoms of stress can surprise you and can mimic more serious problems. You may experience a rapid, pounding heartbeat, facial flushing, or even dilated pupils after experiencing chronic stress. Understanding the signs and symptoms is important so you know when to take control of life's stressors.

Bright Idea
Keep valerian tea around for those days when the phone won't quit ringing and the kids won't quit whining. Have a cup of tea after dinner and experience the calming effect.

Stress

Stress is anything that disturbs a person's healthy mental or physical well-being. What causes it? Life! Symptoms include increased heart rate and blood pressure, chest pains, insomnia, nervousness, feelings of panic, and difficulty concentrating, among many others.

How is it prevented?

Realize what stressors cause negative symptoms and get in control of them by prioritizing your life. Avoiding overcommitment and eliminate stressors you can control.

What is the conventional treatment?

Treatments can include lifestyle changes, counseling, and medication such as Xanax or Valium. Sometimes antidepressants such as Prozac, Paxil, or Zoloft may be prescribed.

What are some alternative treatments?

- **Aromatherapy**—patchouli, orange, berry
- **Ayurvedic medicine**—Transcendental Meditation
- **Bach Flowers**—Rescue Remedy
- **Bodyworks**—therapeutic massage for relaxation
- **Herbal therapy**—chamomile, kava kava, valerian, and St. John's wort
- **Mind/body treatments**—autogenic therapy, music therapy, deep abdominal breathing, and the relaxation response
- **Nutritional supplements**—essential fatty acid (EFAs), B-complex vitamins (especially B_6), vitamin C, folic acid, zinc

- **Nutritional therapy**—serotonin-boosting foods that provide a calming effect such as pasta, bagels, and sherbet

The basics

1. *What's been proven to work?* You can reduce stress by making major lifestyle changes to prioritize time and commitments and by using destressing techniques to lower your heart rate and blood pressure. The relaxation response (pages 153–54) also is excellent for reducing stress—even in the midst of anxiety-producing situations.

2. *How long until it works?* After re-evaluating your life and priorities, you will feel relief within one to three weeks.

3. *How much does treatment cost?* Treatment is free (see Chapter 8).

While occasional stress is normal and even helps us to increase productivity, chronic or daily stress can cause a negative immune response, which can lead to illness. Learn effective coping techniques such as mind/body treatments to make stress work for you instead of against you.

Just the facts

- Alcoholism is best controlled using a combination of detoxification, nutritional therapy, and mind/body treatments.

- St. John's wort is a treatment for depression now being studied by the National Institutes of Health.

- Valerian and kava kava have been found to ease sleep problems associated with stress.

Unofficially . . .
According to the American Institute of Stress, 89 percent of adults report having high levels of stress. In fact, at least 50 percent complain of this intense stress level at least once or twice a week, and more than 25 percent say they are stressed on a daily basis.

- Stress is a major cause of many visits to the physician and can lead to symptoms that mimic a heart attack such as rapid heart rate and chest pains.

Ear, Eye, Nose, and Throat Disorders

Chapter 16

Everyone experiences respiratory breathing difficulties from time to time. For most people, the symptoms eventually subside, and they can move on with their lives. But when debilitating symptoms such as coughing, sneezing, stuffy nose, breathlessness, and wheezing are relentless, you experience a poor quality of life. Many people claim breathing problems have ruined much of their lives, but with today's treatment options, it does not have to be this way. Read on to find out the latest in alternative and conventional treatment.

Allergy

Allergies are exaggerated or abnormal reactions—such as sneezing, bronchial spasms, skin rashes, or itching—to substances, situations, or physical states that do not occur in the average person. They're brought on by an overreaction by your immune system to an ordinarily harmless substance called an *allergen* (see Table 16.1). Allergens are substances that trigger the body's allergic reactions.

Unofficially . . .
An estimated 60 million Americans suffer from allergies including skin reactions. If you have allergies, you have a hypersensitivity to substances known as allergens, which trigger these reactions.

TABLE 16.1   COMMON ALLERGENS, IRRITANTS, AND PHYSICAL CHANGES THAT TRIGGER ALLERGIC RESPONSES

Animal dander
Cockroaches
Cold air
Exercise
Feathers
Foods (chocolate, shellfish, milk, citrus, eggs, nuts, corn)
Food additives or colorings (sulfites or preservatives)
Gases
Hormones
Household dust (dust mites)
Industrial chemicals
Insect stings
Medications (aspirin, anti-inflammatory drugs, penicillin, beta-blockers)
Molds and mildew
Perfumes or inhalants
Plant pollens
Respiratory infections
Smoke
Tree pollens
Weather changes

Uncontrollable sneezing, coughing, wheezing, nasal stuffiness, malaise, fatigue, itchy eyes, and rashes are just a few of the symptoms.

How is it prevented?
Histamine is the substance that causes nasal stuffiness and dripping in a cold or hay fever, bronchoconstriction in asthma, and itchy spots in a skin allergy. An *antihistamine* is a medication that counteracts the histamine in the body. To prevent allergy, avoid known allergens and take an antihistamine before you come in contact with the trigger.

What is the conventional treatment?

There are many conventional treatment methods, starting with allergy testing and desensitization with immunotherapy (allergy shots). Other treatments include avoidance of known allergens, antihistamines (which reduce drainage from the nasal cavity), decongestants (which constrict blood vessels in the nose and are designed to dry up nasal secretions to increase drainage from the nasal cavity), inhaled nasal steroids, nasal saline sprays, and oral steroids (which reduce inflammation). Spray decongestants containing pseudoephedrine or phenylpropanolamine are faster and more effective, but they are irritating to the nose and may cause rebound congestion.

What are some alternative treatments?

- **Environmental medicine**—remove known triggers from the home and workplace

- **Herbal therapy**—anise seed, bee pollen, echinacea, eucalyptus, goldenseal, garlic, ginger, or dandelion

- **Homeopathy**—quercetin or bromelain

- **Nutritional supplements**—vitamins A, C, and E (antioxidants), calcium, magnesium, vitamin B-complex, potassium, zinc, and coenzyme Q10 (to counter histamine)

- **Nutritional therapy**—elimination diet (avoid foods known to cause allergy)

The basics

1. *What's been proven to work?* Antihistamines do not cure your allergy or congestion, but they do block the effects of histamine and help relieve annoying symptoms such as sneezing, itching,

66

My allergies were horrible until I did the elimination diet. This involved removing foods from my diet that most people are allergic to, then slowly, one at a time, adding them back. I was able to add milk and wheat to my diet, but when I started eating corn, my throat began to tickle, my nose itched, and I could not stop sneezing. Now I avoid corn products like the plague and breathe better because of this.
—Ashley, 32, architect

99

congestion, discharge, and other skin and eye conditions. These drugs work best when taken before symptoms begin. The most common side effects of antihistamines are sedation, drowsiness, and dry mouth. You may want to take any sedating antihistamine at night before bedtime to avoid feeling sluggish during the day. Some prescription antihistamines, such as loratadine (Claritin), fexofenadine (Allegra), and certirizine (Zyrtec), also are highly effective and are unlikely to cause drowsiness or deleterious side effects. Removing airborne allergens from your home or workplace is another way to improve breathing.

2. *How much does treatment cost?* Over-the-counter antihistamines cost about $5 to $7 for one week's supply. Prescription products cost about $25 to $40 per month. Quercetin costs about $15 to $20 per bottle, and echinacea costs from $8 to $15 for 10 days.

3. *How long until it works?* You should feel relief within one to three hours.

Antihistamines work best if they can build up in the blood for three to four days to provide a protective effect. Instead of putting a Band-Aid on your allergy problem, however, consider allergy testing to find the source of your running nose and itchy eyes. Immunotherapy (allergy shots) may help reduce your body's reaction to the particular allergen.

Asthma

Asthma is a chronic inflammatory disease of the airways. It is caused by twitchy airways that become inflamed when they meet stimuli such as allergens or cold air. Spasms of the bronchial muscles, along with swelling of the mucous membranes lining the bronchi or excessive amounts of mucus, contribute to airway narrowing. Consequently, the airway resistance and the work of breathing increase to cause wheezing and shortness of breath. You also may experience coughing, chest tightness, and production of mucus.

How is it prevented?

Avoid triggers that cause airway inflammation and bronchospasm. Common triggers include pollen, dust, mold, animal dander, weather changes, and stress.

What is the conventional treatment?

You can use oral and inhaled bronchodilators to open up the bronchial tubes, inhaled and oral steroids to reduce inflammation, and mucus thinners (guafinesin) to increase expulsion of mucus.

What are some alternative treatments?

- **Ayurvedic medicine**—brown mustard oil, ginger, fennel, cumin, and ghee (an Indian product made from clarified butter to help regulate the digestive forces); herbal tonics including shatavari, bala, licorice, triphala, and chavanprash (a tonic for the respiratory system made from the amla fruit mixed with cinnamon, cardamom, honey, and herbs); breathing exercises called pranayama

- **Chinese medicine**—qigong, tai chi

- **Herbal therapy**—anise, fennel, coffee, coltsfoot, elderberry, ginger, ginkgo, slippery elm, mullein

- **Mind/body therapy**—relaxation response and other destressing tools

Bright Idea
Zafirlukast (Accolate by Zeneca) and montelukast sodium (Singulair by Merck) are new asthma drugs that keep bronchial tubes from constricting. Some researchers have found that these new medications may be almost as effective as steroids but without the side effects.

▪ **Nutritional supplements**—fish oil capsules, flaxseed or evening primrose oil, vitamins A, C, and E

The basics

1. *What's been proven to work?* Steroids, both oral and inhaled, have become the first-line treatment for asthma and may play a role in other lung diseases. In fact, recent studies support the use of inhaled steroids early in the course of disease. Steroids are anti-inflammatory medications that suppress airway inflammation. Commonly used inhaled steroids include triamcinolone (Azmacort), flunisolide (Aerobid), beclomethasone (Vanceril or Beclovent), and fluticasone (Flovent). To relieve symptoms, short-acting inhaled beta2-agonists such as albuterol (Proventil, Ventolin) can be used as necessary. A longer-acting inhaled beta2-agonist called salmeterol (Serevent) also can help. This inhaler is used only twice per day (two puffs each time). Unlike the short-acting inhaled beta2-agonist, which is a *reliever medication* for acute attacks, salmeterol is a *controller medication*. Its effect on the airways is not immediate, and it should never be used in an acute attack.

2. *How much does treatment cost?* Albuterol costs about $15 to $25 per month, salmeterol costs about $25 to $30 per month, and inhaled steroids cost about $25 per month. Fish oil capsules to reduce inflammation cost from $7 to $12. Mullein tea costs about $5.

3. *How long until it works?* Albuterol works immediately to relieve asthma symptoms. You should notice a difference in 5 to 15 minutes. It takes approximately one hour for salmeterol to take

action in the body. Inhaled steroids take two to three weeks to fully take effect; oral steroids may ease symptoms within 2 to 12 hours.

Asthma is an inflammatory disease of the airways, and it needs to be treated as such. Although relieving symptoms is crucial, preventing symptoms by keeping inflammation at bay with inhaled steroids is the main treatment method.

Bad breath

Bad breath, or *halitosis*, is an offensive odor that comes from the mouth. It usually is caused by bacteria on the back of the tongue that produce sulfur compounds that smell bad. Periodontal (gum) disease also can cause bad breath.

How is it prevented?

Brush and floss teeth daily and scrape the very back of the tongue. Keep your mouth moist to wash away food debris and bacteria. Use nasal saline sprays to wash away postnasal drip and see your dentist regularly.

What is the conventional treatment?

Your dentist may prescribe chlorhexidine gluconate mouthwash to use in combination with tongue scraping.

What are some alternative treatments?

- **Ayurvedic medicine**—brush tongue in the morning
- **Herbal therapy**—anise, cardamom, parsley, basil, and cilantro

The basics

1. *What's been proven to work?* Brushing the tongue and flossing the teeth keep food and bacteria out of the mouth. The herb cardamom is the

richest source of cineole, an antiseptic that kills bad breath. Chew a few cardamom seeds after lunch and then spit them out.

2. *How long until it works?* You will have cleaner breath within minutes after brushing, flossing, and using cardamom seeds.

3. *How much does it cost?* Cardamom seeds cost about $5 for one week's supply.

Brush your teeth after every meal and before bedtime, floss daily, and focus on scraping the back of your tongue to remove any bacteria from food and sinus drainage.

Bronchitis

Bronchitis is a respiratory illness caused by a viral or bacterial infection or by environmental pollutants that attack the mucous membranes in the windpipe or the air passages of your respiratory tract. If you have bronchitis, you may have a cough with production of sputum, which may be thick and yellow or occasionally blood streaked. You also can have a fever and fatigue, wheezing, and shortness of breath. If your bronchitis is severe, it can progress into pneumonia, which is an inflammation of the lungs.

How is it prevented?

Stop smoking, avoid second-hand smoke and other known allergens, and avoid air pollution or chemical irritants. Also avoid exposure to cold, wet weather.

What is the conventional treatment?

You can use oral or inhaled bronchodilators (medicines that open up the bronchial passages) and antibiotics to kill bacteria. Sometimes expectorants such as guafinesin are used to help thin mucus.

Bright Idea
Some people claim that eating hot, spicy foods can help alleviate the symptoms of bronchitis. In fact, ginger tea is said to help loosen thick phlegm, while hot pepper sauce can help bring up bronchial secretions.

What are some alternative treatments?

- **Aromatherapy**—anise seed, comfrey, chaparral, horehound, fennel seed

- **Chinese medicine**—acupuncture (helps contracted muscular walls to dilate)

- **Bodywork**—*tapotement*, a percussion-type movement that includes hacking, tapping, and clapping with the hands or fingertips to break up congestion

- **Herbal therapy**—astragalus, cat's claw, cayenne, echinacea root, elderberry, eucalyptus, garlic, ginger, ginseng, horehound, licorice (to relieve symptoms of bronchitis); hyssop, mullein (to loosen phlegm in the lungs and throat)

- **Homeopathy**—arsenicum, belladonna, hepar, sulphur, kali bic, pulsatilla, bryonia, and spigella

- **Hydrotherapy**—breathe a mist of steam

- **Nutritional supplements**—vitamin C (at least 1,000 milligrams per day) and vitamins A and E; chicken soup, which is said to have antibacterial properties

The basics

1. *What's been proven to work?* For a mild case of bronchitis, herbal therapy may help open clogged breathing passages and allow mucus to flow freely. Licorice is filled with antiviral compounds, acts as an expectorant, and soothes tissues and mucous membranes. Cayenne also helps heal irritated tissues and promotes drainage, and mullein has been endorsed by Germany's Commission E because it stops the muscle spasms that trigger coughs. For more

> 66
> *Gerard's Herball,* written in 1597, states that a "decoction of Hyssope made with figges, water, honey, and rue and drunken, helpeth the old cough."
> 99

serious cases of bronchitis or for chronic bronchitis, depend on conventional medical treatments such as bronchodilators.

2. *How much does treatment cost?* Herbal therapy
costs about $15 a week. Bronchodilators cost
$30 to $50 for one month's supply.

3. *How long until it works?* An inhaled bronchodilator should open clogged passages within 5 to 30
minutes. Herbal therapy may take several hours
to receive benefit.

Don't fool around with breathing problems.
Although prevention is crucial—keeping mucus
thin, avoiding viruses and allergens, and keeping
the immune system boosted—medication is necessary to provide optimum relief during a coughing or
wheezing spell.

Common cold

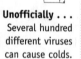

Unofficially . . .
Several hundred
different viruses
can cause colds.

The common cold is a viral illness that affects the
airways, sinuses, throat, voice box, and bronchial
tubes. Discomfort in your throat followed by symptoms such as clear, watery nasal discharge, sneezing,
a tired sensation (malaise), and sometimes fever
indicates that you've been bit by a cold bug.
Postnasal drip causes the sore throat and cough that
accompany colds.

How is it prevented?

Avoid fatigue or stress, both of which tear down
immune function. Stay away from people who have
a cold virus and wash your hands frequently.

What is the conventional treatment?

Over-the-counter decongestants, antibiotics, and
acetaminophen or ibuprofen can help ease symptoms. No matter what you take, colds usually last

from three to seven days. Sometimes antibiotics are necessary if you also have a bacterial infection.

What are some alternative treatments?

- **Aromatherapy**—essential oils of eucalyptus, tea tree, and peppermint

- **Chinese medicine**—astralgus (huang qi) tea

- **Herbal therapy**—astralgalus, cayenne, dandelion root, ma huang, licorice, ginseng, or mullein (to help ease cold symptoms); echinacea or purple coneflower (to fight off colds by increasing the activity and number of immune cells); one cup of tea three times a day

- **Homeopathy**—aconitum napellus, natrum muriaticum, allium cepa, nuxvomica, eupatorium pefoliatum

- **Hydrotherapy**—a humidifier (to add moisture to dry, hot air) and a hot, steamy bath (to help reduce swelling of clogged passages)

- **Nutritional supplements**—zinc lozenges, increased intake of vitamin C (which has an antihistamine effect in the body)

The basics

1. *What's been proven to work?* Studies from Dartmouth College reported that students who took zinc lozenges at the onset of a cold had only five days of symptoms compared with nine days for students who received placebos. This may be because zinc has an antiviral effect in the mouth and nose. Echinacea can help prevent colds and flu and can boost your production of T lymphocytes (a type of white blood cell). If taken when symptoms first appear, this herbal therapy works to reduce the symptoms

66
Last year I religiously took my daily vitamins, including an antioxidant supplement (vitamins A, C, and E). I also intentionally reduced situations in my life that caused stress. Call it coincidental or the result of my healthy efforts, but I didn't have one cold the entire year.
—Phil, 43, business owner
99

and duration of a cold. Echinacea loses its healing power after taking it for eight weeks.

In a double-blind study at the University of Wisconsin, researchers concluded that vitamin C actually can reduce the severity of a cold. Of 16 college students—half took 2,000 milligrams of vitamin C daily and the rest received a placebo—13 caught colds when exposed to cold viruses. The students who had taken 2,000 milligrams of vitamin C had much milder symptoms and recovered faster. Research continues about the actions of ginger and chili peppers as expectorants, which cause the sneezing and coughing that help work cold viruses out of the body.

2. *How much does treatment cost?* You'll spend about $6 for enough zinc lozenges to last the duration of your cold. Echinacea costs about $5 a week to prevent colds. Vitamin C supplements cost about $6, and ginger and chili peppers probably are already in your kitchen cabinet.

3. *How long until it works?* You should notice a difference in two to four days.

Colds are a fact of life, and there is no cure. You might as well shorten the time you are miserable by using zinc gluconate lozenges—if you can stand the taste. Some lozenges, however, are flavored with lemon and taste better than straight zinc. Depend on echinacea to keep your immune system strong enough to ward off colds on its own. It also wouldn't hurt to add some herbs with bioflavonoids (feverfew, spearmint, or yarrow), which may prevent histamine from forming in the first place.

Flu

Influenza, or flu, is an acute respiratory infection that mimics a cold. It is caused by a flu virus, and symptoms can include sudden onset of muscle aches and soreness, headache, fatigue, coughing, sore throat, runny nose, and fever.

How is it prevented?

Flu viruses enter your body through the mucous membranes of the nose, eyes, or mouth. Keep hands germ-free with frequent washing and get an annual flu shot.

What is the conventional treatment?

Newer prescription antivirals, such as rimantadine and amantadine, can help prevent and treat the influenza-A virus, although they must be used within the first 48 hours of symptoms.

What are some alternative treatments?

- **Aromatherapy**—essential oils of eucalyptus, peppermint, or tea tree

- **Ayurvedic**—one teaspoon of *amla*, a gooseberry jam (to build the immune system and to fight the virus)

- **Chinese medicine**—astragalus (huang qi) tea, acupuncture

- **Herbal therapy**—cat's claw, cayenne, echinacea root, licorice, garlic, gingerroot, ginseng, and mullein

- **Homeopathy**—oscillococcinum or gelsemium (yellow jasmine), belladonna, baptista, bryonia

- **Hydrotherapy**—a warm steam bath, a humidifier with a few drops of eucalpytus (to soothe nasal passages)

Bright Idea
Annual flu epidemics have caused more than 10,000 deaths since 1957. An annual flu vaccine, called Fluvax, is one way to prevent the flu altogether. Talk to your doctor to determine which month is best for receiving this vaccine.

- **Mind/Body treatments**—laughter therapy
- **Nutritional supplements**—vitamins A, C, and E (antioxidants), bioflavonoids, zinc lozenges
- **Nutritional therapy**—oranges, grapefruit, garlic, onions

The basics

1. *What's been proven to work?* Unless you have a secondary infection, the best remedy for the flu is to get in bed, to rest, and to ride it out. Drink plenty of liquids, increase vitamin C, and use a humidifier to keep nasal passages from drying out. Zinc lozenges may help shorten the duration of the flu, and echinacea—especially in liquid form—has been found to stimulate the production of infection-fighting white blood cells. You also might consider laughter therapy—at least 30 minutes throughout the day. Studies at Loma Linda University School of Medicine in California found that students had activated T cells, natural killer cells, and antibodies (the body's defense against viruses and infections) after watching an hour-long comedy.

2. *How much does treatment cost?* Remedies for the flu can cost as much as $10 a day if you use nutritional supplements, juices, and zinc lozenges. Liquid echinacea costs about $12 to $15 for a seven-day supply. Laughter is free!

3. *How long until it works?* It depends on how weakened your immune system is, whether you had a flu shot, and the exact strain of flu that hit.

Prevention is crucial to avoid the flu. Work on strengthening your immune system, use a combination of alternative therapies, and get an annual flu shot. Stay away from anyone who has the flu and wash your hands—at least 30 seconds each time—frequently throughout the day. Perhaps most importantly, work on your social network. Studies show that people who enjoy social activities with a strong circle of friends have greater resistance to colds and flu.

Hay fever

While allergies result in symptoms from itchy eyes and wheezing to hives and skin rashes, *hay fever* or *rhinitis* is the term for disorders of the nose. Allergic rhinitis is the single most common chronic disease experienced by humans, affecting more than 40 million people in the United States alone. It is caused by antibodies that induce your body's immune cells to release histamines in response to contact with allergens. If you are experiencing hay fever, you may feel a constant runny nose, ongoing sneezing, swollen nasal passages, excess mucus, weepy eyes, and a scratchy palate and throat. Common results of rhinitis include infected ears, fluid in the ears because of blocked eustachian tubes, and unending fatigue.

How is it prevented?
Avoid known *allergens* (see Table 16.2).

What is the conventional treatment?
Over-the-counter antihistamines such as Chloratrimeton (Chlorpheniramine meleate) help reduce swelling and have a drying effect. Prescription antihistamines such as Claritin and Allegra do not cause drowsiness.

What are some alternative treatments?
- **Aromatherapy**—anise seed, comfrey, chaparral, horehound, fennel seed

Watch Out!
Medication rhinitis is the result of chemical irritation from using over-the-counter decongestant nasal sprays for a prolonged period of time. These sprays relieve nasal congestion by reducing the blood flow to the lining of the nose. Be sure not to use these sprays longer than three to five days, or they might worsen your nasal swelling and discharge.

TABLE 16.2   COMMON ALLERGENS

Common Outdoor Allergens
Environmental pollution
Grass
Industrial pollution
Mold spores
Pollen
Ragweed
Trees
Weather changes (cold air, fronts, wind, humidity)
Common Indoor Allergens
Aerosols
Cosmetics
Dander from pets
Dust
Feathers
Foods
Fumes
Mold
Smoke
Wool

- **Environmental medicine**—remove known triggers of allergy in home and workplace

- **Herbal therapy**—coffee, bee pollen, echinacea, goldenseal, garlic, ginger or dandelion, quercetin or bromelain

- **Homeopathy**—belladonna, nux vomica, allium cepa, natrum muriaticum

- **Nutritional supplements**—vitamins A, C, and E (antioxidants), calcium, magnesium, vitamin B-complex, potassium, zinc, coenzyme Q10 (to counter histamine)

- **Nutritional therapy**—elimination diet (avoid foods known to cause allergy)

The basics

1. *What's been proven to work?* If antihistamines make you drowsy or dull, you may try a hot cup of java to relieve hay fever symptoms. Realizing that caffeine is a stimulant and that it acts as a bronchodilator in asthmatics, researchers have been studying its effect on other respiratory conditions. In one study at Harbor-UCLA Medical Center, researchers gave hay fever sufferers a tablet containing 400 milligrams of caffeine (equal to the amount in about 18 ounces of coffee). Other sufferers were given a placebo tablet. All abstained from caffeine for two days prior to the study. Four hours after taking the caffeine tablets, the group reported a 51 percent improvement. The group taking the placebo reported only a 19 percent improvement.

2. *How much does treatment cost?* Over-the-counter medications cost about 50 cents a day. Two cups of coffee in the morning or when needed costs about 10 cents, if brewed at home.

3. *How long until it works?* Medications usually take about one to two hours to have an effect on symptoms. If caffeine works for you, you will notice a difference within 30 minutes.

Talk with your doctor and find out what is best for your individual allergy situation. Prevention of allergies—before they take over your life—is crucial. If you start using them prior to hay fever season, some of the new steroid nasal sprays can keep symptoms at bay and can let you breathe easier.

Hiccups

Hiccups are a spasm in the back of the throat caused by a tightening of the diaphragm from swallowing air, from drinking too much liquid, or from eating too fast. An upset stomach also may lead to hiccups. The brain fires off the nerve impulses that start the spasm.

What is the conventional treatment?

Hold your breath, breathe into a paper bag, or swallow a teaspoon of sugar fast.

What are some alternative treatments?

- **Hydrotherapy**—ice water gargle
- **Nutritional therapy**—suck on a slice of lemon or lime

The basics

1. *What's been proven to work?* Because a hiccup is a nerve action, the best way to end it is to break that action. Swallowing something textured or gargling with ice water may do the trick.

2. *How much does treatment cost?* Treatments can cost just pennies.

3. *How long until it works?* Once the nerve receptors in the back of the throat are stimulated, relief should be felt soon.

The key to resolving hiccups is to distract your brain. Whether someone scares you or you suck on a lemon, find what works for you.

Pneumonia

Pneumonia in an inflammation in the lung that can be caused by a virus, bacteria, fungi, or noninfectious causes. If you have pneumonia, you may have a cough—which can be either unproductive (dry) or productive (with yellow, green, or bloody phlegm)—shortness of breath, fever, and sometimes sharp pains in the chest when you take a deep breath.

How is it prevented?
Immunization for pneumonia is available and is effective in lowering the risk of this infection.

What is the conventional treatment?
The usual treatment is antibiotic therapy.

What are some alternative treatments?

- **Bodywork**—*tapotement,* a percussion-type movement that includes hacking, tapping, and clapping with the hands or fingertips to break up congestion (see page 79).

- **Herbal therapy**—astragalus, cat's claw, cayenne, echinacea root, elderberry, eucalyptus, garlic, ginger, ginseng, horehound, or licorice (to relieve symptoms of bronchitis); hyssop and mullein (to loosen phlegm in the lungs and throat)

- **Homeopathic remedies**—arsenicum, belladonna, hepar, sulphur, kali bic, pulsatilla, bryonia, and spigella

- **Hydrotherapy**—breathe a mist of steam

- **Nutritional supplements**—vitamin C (at least 1,000 milligrams a day) and vitamins A and E; chicken soup (said to have antibacterial properties)

The basics
1. *What's been proven to work?* Pneumonia can be deadly, so don't fool around with self-medicaton. See your doctor for an accurate diagnosis and treatment.

Bright Idea
To avoid getting pneumonia, ask your doctor about the pneumococcal vaccine (Pneumovax or Pneu-Immune 23).

TABLE 16.3   ANTIBIOTICS FREQUENTLY USED FOR RESPIRATORY INFECTIONS

Brand Name	Generic Name
Embezzle	Amoxicillin
Augmentin	Amoxicillin-potassium clavulanate
Bactrim, Septra	Trimethoprim-sulfamethoxazole
Biaxin	Clarithromycin
Ceclor	Cefaclor
Cipro	Ciprofloxacin
Floxin	Ofloxacin
Omnipen	Ampicillin
Pen-Vee K	Penicillin and potassium
Sumycin	Tetracycline
Vibramycin	Doxycycline
Zithromax	Azithromycin

2. *How much does treatment cost?* Antibiotics for pneumonia cost about $25 to $40 per week (see Table 16.3).

3. *How long until it works?* You should notice a difference in three days to one week. If symptoms worsen, call your doctor immediately.

If you get pneumonia, do not administer treatment. Get an accurate diagnosis because some types of pneumonia are difficult to treat and can lead to serious illness.

Sinusitis

A sinus infection (*sinusitis*) is an inflammation of the mucous membranes that line the sinus cavities. It is caused by irritants, air pollution, smoke and fumes, a viral or bacterial infection, allergic rhinitis (hay fever), chronic rhinitis, a deviated nasal septum, polyps, or anything that causes inflammation of the mucous membranes lining the sinus cavities. If you are experiencing sinusitis, you may feel a headache, pain in the sinus area, upper molar tooth pain, nasal obstruction, postnasal drip, cough, sore throat, thick yellow or green nasal drainage, high fever (102 degrees F and above), and tenderness or dull pain around the eyes and cheek bones.

How is it prevented?

Treat sinus infections early in the illness, avoid irritants, and keep mucus flowing with the use of nasal saline sprays and decongestants.

What is the conventional treatment?

An antibiotic is the standard treatment for sinus infections if you have an increased amount of thick mucus or mucus that is colored (yellow, green, or brown). The antibiotic will get to the root of the problem, which usually is infection caused by bacteria.

Oral nasal decongestants can open the mucous membranes in the nose and can help drain inflamed sinuses and reduce congestion. Commonly used decongestants include phenylpropanolamine, pseudoephedrine, and phenylephrine. These all work in the same way to reduce swelling and congestion. Decongestant nasal sprays such as oxymetazoline (Afrin) and phenylephrine (Neo-Synephrine) can provide immediate relief to swollen sinuses. Unlike oral decongestants, however, you only can use decongestant nasal sprays for three to five days to avoid rebound or recurrent congestion.

An *expectorant* or *mucokinetic agent* is a drug that helps to thin mucus, making it easier to flow. Many experts feel water is most beneficial to help liquefy

> 66
> The best way to keep my sinuses running clear is to use saline sprays, which can be purchased at any drug or grocery store. The salt water helps to break up congestion and toughens the nasal passages.
> —Amelia, 31, pharmacist
> 99

Moneysaver
You also can create a homemade nasal wash by mixing eight ounces warm water, one-half teaspoon salt, and one pinch baking soda. Pour this mixture into a plastic bottle. You then can pour a small amount of this liquid into your cupped hands, or you can use a large rubber-bulb syringe filled with the mixture to get liquid into the nose. Gently swish around, and be sure to blow the nose carefully after each cleaning.

mucus, but you also can use medications such as guaifenesin (Robitussin Expectorant or HumiBid).

What are some alternative treatments?

- **Aromatherapy**—anise seed, comfrey, chaparral, horehound, fennel seed

- **Chiropractic**—helps sinuses to drain properly

- **Herbal therapy**—echinacea, garlic, and goldenseal

- **Hydrotherapy**—Nasal saline solutions are a form of hydrotherapy. They are used to restore moisture to your sinuses and may help lessen the inflammation of nasal membranes. If used regularly, they can help decrease postnasal drip and can cleanse your passages, removing bacteria. These agents are mild and safe to use. Some over-the-counter nasal saline sprays include Ocean and NaSal sprays.

The basics

1. *What's been proven to work?* Decongestants and antibiotics are therapies proven to end sinusitis and sinus infections. You also might try a tea made with two teaspoons of thyme steeped in boiling water for 15 minutes. This alternative therapy has been found to relieve congestion.

2. *How much does treatment cost?* An over-the-counter decongestant costs about $6 for one week's supply. A nasal decongestant spray costs about $5, and antibiotics cost $15 to $30 for 10 days.

3. *How long until it works?* In adults, decongestant nasal sprays can provide relief in one to three hours. An oral decongestant can help open clogged passages within one to two hours.

Nonetheless, it can take several days for antibiotics to work on sinus infections because of the poor blood supply in the sinuses. If you are not finding relief within a few days for any respiratory tract infection, check back with your doctor to see whether the antibiotic is working for your particular infection. Certain bacteria have become resistant to some antibiotics in some locations, and stronger medications may be necessary.

You may find excellent relief with short-term decongestant, saline, or steroid nasal sprays. These can significantly reduce the swelling in your nasal passage and sinuses and can help ease the problem. *Expectorants* are useful if your mucus is thick and hard to expel. This medicine liquefies mucus so it can drain easily, which can help reduce swelling and pain. The key is to understand the treatment, including the effect and side effects, and then trust your doctor to make the best decision with your overall health in mind.

Snoring

Snoring is a loud or constant sound from the throat during sleep. It is caused by changes in the upper airway from the back of the nose to the base of the tongue. The muscles supporting the opening of the upper airway relax during sleep. Extra tissue in the palate and the uvula—the fleshy piece between the tonsils—vibrates with each breath. Thus, there is a tendency for the airway to close at any point along this pathway. Some risk factors for snoring include:

- Sleeping on your back
- Being overweight, especially people with thick necks

Watch Out!
Snoring is
caused by the
vibration of the
soft parts of
the throat while
inspiring air dur-
ing sleep, and
the noise may be
either continu-
ous with almost
every breath or
intermittent with
breath-holding
spells. These
periods of sus-
pension of
breathing are
called *apneas,*
and they are due
to obstruction of
the upper airway
at the level of
the uvula or the
base of the
tongue.

- Cigarette smoking and heavy alcohol drinking
- Allergy, sinusitis, or asthma
- Facial shape
- Narrowed airways due to nasal obstruction, deviated septum, and polyps

Snoring not only robs you of restful sleep, it often can be related to:

- Hypertension, arrhythmias, heart disease, stroke, and even brain damage
- Personality changes, irritability, and hormonal imbalances
- Impotence and morning headaches
- Night sweats, heartburn, or nerve damage
- Sinusitis, bronchitis, lung disease, and some stomach diseases

People who snore not only have disturbed sleep and awaken fatigued, they also may have headaches, high blood pressure, dry mouth, sore throats upon awakening, depression, and concentration problems.

How is it prevented?
Don't drink alcohol or take medications that are sedating, keep nasal passages clear, sleep on a pillow, and avoid sleeping on your back.

What is the conventional treatment?
The U.S. Patent Office has more than 300 would-be snoring remedies, but most are not helpful. Specially made dental appliances such as the Herbst prosthesis may be used to pull the mandible (jaw-bone) forward to widen the airway space at the base of the tongue. Some people have found excellent results with nasal dilators purchased at any grocery

or drug store, combined with a nasal decongestant spray to open blocked airways. For sleep apnea, the most effective treatment is nasal *continuous positive airway pressure (CPAP)*. This is a custom-fitted nasal mask worn during sleep that is attached to a quietly functioning pump. The pump delivers room air at a positive pressure, serving as a pneumatic splint to prevent collapse of the airway. There also are medications that improve upper-airway muscle strength or tone during sleep, including medroxy-progesterone (a form of the female hormone progesterone) for postmenopausal women and anti-depressant drugs (protriptyline) for people with mild obstructive sleep apnea.

What are some alternative treatments?

- **Herbal therapy**—garlic, mullein, horehound, licorice, ephedra

- **Nutritional supplements**—vitamin C

- **Nutritional therapy**—weight-loss diet

The basics

1. *What is proven to work?* The best remedy for snoring is the laser-assisted uvulaopalatoplasty (LAUP). This is a 15- to 30-minute office procedure to trim and reshape the uvula and soft palate. It requires only a local anesthetic and has a success rate of curing snoring in about 95 percent of cases.

2. *How long until it works?* It may require three to five visits—with one month of healing time in between.

3. *How much does it cost?* LAUP costs around $1,500 to $2,000 in most parts of the nation.

Bright Idea
Try one of the new nasal strips to help you breathe better at nighttime. These strips of tape are placed over the bridge of the nose. The plastic strip springs back and helps gently open your nasal passages, reducing airflow resistance. Some people believe these strips help reduce snoring.

LAUP cures snoring in most cases. It is an outpatient office procedure in which you remain
upright and awake, and you leave with no stitches
and only a minor sore throat. People who have had
laser surgery say it is comparable to the amount of
time and stress experienced with having a cavity
filled.

An old wives' tale suggested that primitive men
defended their women at night by making horrible
sounds to scare off predators. We now know, however, that snoring may be an early warning sign for
various medical problems, especially for obstructive
sleep apnea (OSA). If you snore, it is time to take
this sleep-time malady seriously. See your doctor and
ask whether an evaluation at a sleep disorders clinic
would help find a solution.

Eyes and ears

The information in this section cannot replace good
medical care, but it offers a streamlined and under-
standable wealth of information about some common eye and ear problems. Knowing these facts,
along with the best alternative and conventional
treatments, you can take charge of your health and
can avoid future problems.

Conjunctivitis

Conjunctivitis (also known as pink eye) is an inflammation of the eyelid's underside and the white part
of the eye. It is caused by a viral or bacterial infection; an allergic reaction to airborne pollen, dust,
mold spores, and animal dander; or a partially
closed tear duct. Symptoms include a pus-like
discharge, eye pain, swelling of the eyelids, a gritty
feeling in the eye, and intense itching (allergic
conjunctivitis).

How is it prevented?

Keep your hands clean and away from your eyes. Wash your hands frequently with soap and warm water and avoid exposure to eye irritants. Make sure children are protected from exposure in day care settings.

What is the conventional treatment?

Your doctor may prescribe antibiotic or antiviral eye drops, sulfa eye drops, or ointment to fight infection. In more severe cases, oral antibiotics may be given. Along with these drops, warm compresses can provide relief.

What are some alternative treatments?

- **Hydrotherapy**—warm, moist compresses

The basics

1. *What's been proven to work?* If you have allergic conjunctivitis, finding the trigger or allergen and removing it will help solve the problem temporarily. Keep the eye clean and soothed with warm, wet compresses. If you have bacterial conjunctivitis, antibiotic drops or oral antibiotics are warranted.

2. *How much does it cost?* Polytrim (antibacterial drops) costs about $30 for 10 days.

3. *How long until it works?* When treated correctly, bacterial conjunctivitis will clear up in two to three days, but you should continue to use the medicine as prescribed by your doctor. Viral conjunctivitis is a complication of a cold or the flu. This type has less discharge but more tearing than the bacterial form. Antibiotics don't work. Viral conjunctivitis can take 14 to 21 days to clear up.

If the infection does not improve in two to three days, it may be caused by an insensitive bacteria, virus, or allergy. At this point, an ophthalmologist may need to culture the conjunctivae or make special studies to determine the cause of the conjunctivitis. If left untreated, conjunctivitis may spread and damage the cornea permanently, impairing vision.

Earache

Bright Idea
To avoid ear infections, try to reduce ear pressure in the middle ear. Gently but firmly blow through your nose while holding both nostrils closed until you hear a pop. You can do this several times a day.

Pain that occurs in the inner, middle, or outer ear (an *earache*) can be caused by a build-up of fluid in the ear from sinus or nasal congestion, injury, or serious diseases. Symptoms include severe and piercing or mild and throbbing pain in the ear.

How is it prevented?

Avoid infections by watching out for warning signs such as fever, slight pain in the ears, plugged ears, or head congestion. When you get a cold or congestion, take a decongestant to reduce fluid buildup. After swimming, use an over-the-counter product such as Swim-Ear or Auro-Dri to prevent swimmer's ear, if you are susceptible to this problem. Try an over-the-counter product such as Debrox or Murine Ear Drops to remove earwax buildup. Chew gum while flying or in high elevations to keep the ear canals open.

What is the conventional treatment?

Your doctor may prescribe antibiotics, allergy medications (usually decongestants), or prescription pain medications (both oral and ear drops). Other treatments include ear wax removal, draining fluid out of the ear, and correcting dental problems.

What are some alternative treatments?

- **Aromatherapy**—warm mullein essential oil or tea tree oil in ear

- **Chinese medicine**—forsythia, gentian, and honeysuckle (use in tea or sprinkle herbs on yogurt)

- **Herbal therapy**—echinacea, garlic, goldenseal

- **Homeopathy**—echinacea spp., baptisia tinctoria, galium aparine

Watch Out!
Never ingest essential oils unless directed to do so. Tea tree oil, even a small amount, may be fatal if taken internally.

The basics

1. *What has been proven to work?* Decongestants and NSAIDs are great for ear pain associated with congestion. Try to reduce the pain by applying heat to the infected ear using a heating pad; a warm, dry towel; or a covered hot water bottle to reduce pain. An unopened plastic bag of frozen vegetables wrapped in a towel may bring relief from inflammation. Take an analgesic to reduce pain or fever, if you experience any.

2. *How long until treatment works?* Depending on the cause of the ear pain, you may feel relief within one hour to two days. If the ear pain is sharp or severe, or if you have a fever, call your doctor.

3. *How much does it cost?* Decongestants cost about $5 for one week's supply.

Heed the old saying "Never put anything smaller than your elbow into your ear." This includes cotton-tipped swabs and your smallest finger. Doing so could damage either the delicate skin that lines the ear canal or your eardrum. When you blow your nose, do so gently and keep congestion to a minimum using decongestants.

Watch Out!
People in their forties and older are at risk for glaucoma, a disease in which the fluid pressure inside the eye rises. This rise in pressure can lead to partial vision loss or blindness if not treated. Most people don't experience any symptoms; the only way to identify and treat glaucoma before it does damage is through regular examinations.

Stye

A *stye* is an infected gland on the eyelid. This occurs when eyelid hair follicles become clogged by the body's oils. These follicles become infected and cause inflammation on the eyelid. Symptoms include itching and then pain and swelling of the eyelid.

How is it prevented?

Keep bacteria out of the eye and keep the eyelid clean with daily washing (just like flossing the teeth).

What is the conventional treatment?

Use moist heat to reduce swelling, clean the eye with a skin cleanser such as Cetaphil, and take antibiotics to normalize the eye glands' fatty-acid secretions. This will help reduce the glands' clogging.

What are some alternative treatments?

- **Herbal therapy**—a poultice of raspberry leaf tea and warm water (to wash inflamed skin)

- **Hydrotherapy**—wash with warm water (dilates the glands in the eyelids, helping to liquefy and remove bacteria and secretions)

- **Nutritional supplements**—zinc, copper, selenium, lactobacillus, folic acid, B-complex vitamins, and vitamins A, C, and E (antioxidants)

The basics

1. *What's been proven to work?* Use a combination of alternative and conventional treatments—daily warm water washes using Cetaphil will keep bacteria out of the hair follicle and will help keep styes at bay. For stubborn problems, you may have to use the antibiotic tetracycline.

2. *How long until it works?* Using the combination of treatments, you will feel relief within two days to one week.

3. *How much does it cost?* Skin cleansers cost about $8 to $12. Tetracycline will cost about $15 to $30 for several weeks' dosage.

Prevention is the best way to avoid styes. If your stye problem is persistent, check with your doctor to make sure nothing more serious is wrong. Sometimes skin cancers can start out with swelling and inflammation.

Tinnitus

Tinnitus is a constant humming, buzzing, or ringing noise. In most cases, the cause is unknown, although it is linked to loud sounds that damaged hearing, aging (which often is accompanied by hearing loss), medications, hypertension, hypothyroidism, Meniere's disease, cardiovascular problems, ear infections, head trauma, and allergies. Although tinnitus is not fully understood, the nerve is believed to transmit impulses that originate inside the head or within the ear itself. Occasionally, something more serious such as a tumor can cause tinnitus. Symptoms include a constant noise heard even when there is no environmental noise. This may be a persistent sound, high or low pitched, and can even keep rhythm with your heart rate.

How is it prevented?

Avoid constant loud noise, keep blood pressure in check, reduce stress, and don't smoke.

What is the conventional treatment?

Hearing aids can sometimes help, and distraction sounds can sometimes mask the sounds of tinnitus.

Bright Idea
Turn your radio to a nonstation and keep it low. Sometimes this white noise can help distract you enough to sleep at night without hearing the tinnitis noise.

Auditory habituation trains the auditory system to ignore internal sound.

What are some alternative treatments?

- **Aromatherapy**—lavender
- **Bach Flowers**—Rescue Remedy
- **Chinese medicine**—acupressure, acupuncture, shiatsu
- **Herbal therapy**—ginkgo biloba
- **Mind/body therapy**—relaxation response, music therapy, progressive muscle relaxation, visualization
- **Nutritional supplements**—niacin (a B vitamin), melatonin
- **Nutritional therapy**—elimination diet (avoid any product with caffeine)

The basics

1. *What's been proven to work?* There is evidence that the B vitamin niacin may ease tinnitus, and some studies show that melatonin also may have a helpful effect. Destressing helps many people, but researchers are finding that some people with tinnitis are wired differently.

2. *How long until treatment works?* Tinnitis is a tough problem because there is no cure or perfect remedy. You really need to try different treatments to find the one that works best for you.

3. *How much does it cost?* A bottle of B-complex vitamins costs about $6 for one month's supply. Melatonin costs about $10 for one month.

See an Ear, Nose, and Throat specialist (ENT) to find out more about tinnitis. There are no easy answers.

Mouth

Nothing is more painful than a cut or sore in your mouth, especially when you eat something salty that penetrates the open wound. You want treatment—and fast! This section describes some common mouth ailments as well as conventional and alternative therapies. Read carefully to see what can help the next time your mouth is screaming for relief.

Cold sores

Cold sores are painful blisters usually found inside the mouth or on the lips or face. They are caused by the herpes simplex virus, which is related to the virus that causes genital herpes. Cold sores can be brought on by stress, sun, or windburn, or they can be the result of an illness that weakens the body's immune system. For women, they are more likely to occur during monthly menstrual periods. Symptoms include a tingling or burning sensation at the place where the cold sore is about to develop, often accompanied by itching. Within a couple of hours, the sore is noticeable. It appears first as small, red bumps that fill with watery fluid. The bumps may join together to form one large blister. The blister is painful and itchy. Sometimes a fever develops or the lymph nodes in the neck begin to swell. In about a week the blister usually dries out, forms a scab, and heals over, usually without leaving any obvious scarring.

How is it prevented?

Keep your immune system strong, decrease stress, and protect yourself from sun or windburn. If you have a cold sore, change your toothbrush frequently to avoid reinfection, and always change it at the end of an attack because the virus can live on a toothbrush for several hours.

What is the conventional treatment?

The typical cold sore will heal on its own, usually within two weeks. For regular cold sore sufferers, a doctor may recommend an antiviral medication such as acyclovir, which is available in capsule and ointment form or by injection.

What are some alternative treatments?

- **Herbal therapy**—echinacea, lemon balm, mint

- **Hydrotherapy**—ice pack (applied to the cold sore at the first sign of symptoms to reduce inflammation), keep area clean with frequent washing

- **Nutritional supplements**—vitamin C, zinc, and lysine tablets (to prevent sores from erupting)

The basics

1. *What's been proven to work?* Lemon balm or melissa has been found to have antiviral and antiherpes properties, and echinacea can keep your immune system boosted if you take it when you first notice an eruption. The antiviral medication should be taken immediately after noticing the first symptoms of a cold sore.

2. *How long until treatment works?* The antiviral medication will reduce healing time by two to three days.

3. *How much does it cost?* Acyclovir costs about $90 for a five-day supply.

The key to treating cold sores or any herpes-type blisters is to be aggressive as soon as you notice the first reddening or eruption.

Gingivitis

Gingivitis is an inflammation or infection of the gums caused by plaque, illness, poor nutrition, or ignored teeth and gums. Symptoms include swollen, tender, red, and bleeding gums, occasionally accompanied by bad breath and fever. Untreated gingivitis may lead to periodontitis, an advanced stage of gum disease that can lead to bone loss and loosening of teeth.

How is it prevented?

Keep your teeth clean, floss at least once a day, and eat a healthy diet. Sometimes the risk increases with pregnancy or illnesses such as diabetes.

What is the conventional treatment?

If measures such as regular cleaning and flossing do not work, your dentist may prescribe antibiotics to fight infection and may suggest a fluoride mouthwash. Surgery may be necessary to remove infected gum tissue.

What are some alternative treatments?

- **Herbal therapy**—aloe, echinacea, myrrh, and goldenseal (excellent for treating gum problems); tea tree oil (a potent antiseptic that can be toxic if swallowed); toothpaste such as Viadent that contains sanguinariae, a compound found in bloodroot (reduces dental plaque)

- **Nutritional supplements**—vitamin C (to help maintain connective tissue and to fight infection) and zinc (to stimulate the immune system and to reduce oral bacteria)

The basics

1. *What's been proven to work?* Brush your teeth carefully at least three times a day. Carefully floss between teeth twice daily to remove plaque and to rid your mouth of toxins. Cut down on acidic

foods, eat more fibrous and crunchy foods, and chew sugar-free gum to help remove food between meals.

2. *How long until it works?* Using a toothpaste that contains sanguinariae will show results within one week.

3. *How much does it cost?* Brushing and flossing your teeth daily costs about $5 per week.

You can prevent gingivitis by keeping your teeth and gums healthy. Avoid candy, sweet drinks, and sweet snacks because sugar stimulates the production of acid, which attacks normal teeth. See your dentist at least twice a year for regular cleaning and exams.

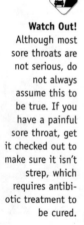

Watch Out!
Although most sore throats are not serious, do not always assume this to be true. If you have a painful sore throat, get it checked out to make sure it isn't strep, which requires antibiotic treatment to be cured.

Sore throat

A *sore throat* is an irritation, tickle, or inflammation of the back of the throat. It can be caused by a cold or another virus, a bacterial infection such as strep, sinus drainage, inflamed tonsils, or overuse. Symptoms include bright red, inflamed skin in the back of the mouth, pain upon swallowing, thickness in back of throat, and swelling of the tonsils. Sometimes white spots may appear on the tonsils.

How is it prevented?

Take allergy medication at night so sinus secretions do not irritate the back of your throat while you are sleeping. Avoid overusing your voice and keep your immune system boosted so bacterial infections stay away.

What is the conventional treatment?

If a sore throat is caused by allergy, over-the-counter antihistamines or decongestants may help. If it is caused by strep, your doctor will take a culture of the throat and will treat the strep with penicillin.

What are some alternative treatments?

- **Herbal therapy**—eucalyptus, licorice, slippery elm (made into teas); horehound drops
- **Hydrotherapy**—gargle with warm salt water
- **Nutritional supplements**—vitamins A, C, and E (antioxidants)

The basics

1. *What's been proven to work?* For sore throats caused by sinus drainage, gargling with warm salt water frequently can help heal irritated and inflamed tissues. For strep throat, penicillin is necessary to end the bacterial infection.

2. *How long until it works?* Antibiotics work within three days to one week. Gargling with warm salt water for an irritated throat should help within hours to two days.

3. *What does the treatment cost?* Gargling with warm salt water costs just pennies. Antibiotics cost about $15 to $40, depending on the type and your location.

Don't fool around with a sore throat. Although many times it is just a tickle, an irritation, or the first sign of a cold, if you have fever with the sore throat, it could indicate a strep infection.

Temporomandibular joint syndrome (TMJ)

TMJ is pain and inflammation in the temporomandibular joint—the joint on either side of the jaw that opens and closes the mouth—and its adjoining muscles. TMJ is caused by injury or faulty alignment between the upper and lower jaws, inflammation, or disease. Stress, popping of the jaw, clenching the jaw, chewing hard foods, and some types of arthritis also can cause this problem. Symptoms include dull, aching pain on one side of the jaw (below the ear) that radiates to the temples, the back of the head, and along the jaw line; tenderness of the muscles used to chew; clicking or popping sounds when opening the mouth; inability to open the jaw completely; and headaches or toothaches.

How is it prevented?

Reduce stress, relax your muscles, and don't grind your teeth. Learn techniques for relaxing muscles and relieving tension, such as biofeedback, meditation, and exercise.

What is the conventional treatment?

Treatment often is a combination of stress management, reducing inflammation, pain control, and correction of the bite using orthodontic devices. A dentist may fit you for a night-guard prosthesis—a plastic splint that fits inside the mouth over the tops of the teeth to eliminate incorrect biting pressure.

What are some alternative treatments?

- **Chinese medicine**—acupressure (points on your ears and scalp reduce tension in the jaw)

- **Bodywork**—massage (destresses tight muscles)

- **Hydrotherapy**—moist heat applications on inflamed tissues

- **Mind/body therapy**—relaxation response, biofeedback, hypnosis, visualization, meditation

The basics

1. *What's been proven to work?* Destressing is the best prevention for TMJ. The higher your anxiety, the more likely you are to tense your jaw and cause pain. NSAIDs help with inflamed tissues and pain, and moist heat also provides excellent relief. Avoid hard or crunchy foods and don't

chew gum. If necessary, talk to your dentist about a night-guard prosthesis.

2. *How long until treatment works?* You will notice a difference in a few days with regular applications of moist heat and using NSAIDs. Destressing takes time as you learn mind/body relaxation therapies. The night-guard prosthesis is a long-term treatment, and it may take several weeks to work and to keep tension at bay.

3. *How much does it cost?* A prosthesis can cost from $200 to $400. A combination of acupressure, massage, moist heat applications, and stress reduction costs just pennies a day. NSAIDs cost about $5 to $10 for seven days.

TMJ is easily avoidable if you use the alternative treatments listed in this book. Remember, your body reacts to what you feed it, so carefully feed it soothing, calming thoughts.

Toothache

A sharp or throbbing pain coming from the teeth can be caused by infection, a broken tooth, a chipped filling, or an erupting new tooth. Symptoms include sensitivity to hot or cold, pain, swelling, or inflammation of the skin around a tooth. Sometimes you might have a headache, a jaw ache, or swollen glands due to infection.

How is it prevented?

Schedule regular visits with your dentist to catch problems ahead of time.

What is the conventional treatment?

Depending on the cause of the toothache, you might need antibiotics for infection, a new filling, a crown to protect the tooth, or a root canal if there

❝
If you want to save your teeth, avoid chewing ice and eating hard candy. Take it from me, I lost two teeth recently that cracked in half while chewing ice. The ice freezes the tooth, then when you crunch down, you do not realize how hard you are actually chewing. It's an expensive, bad habit that only you can stop!"
—Bob, 48, engineer
❞

Timesaver
Can't remember to floss your teeth? Keep dental floss next to your favorite relaxation spot, whether it's a favorite chair near the TV, next to your home computer, or on the night stand by your bed. Whenever you pause for some much needed R&R, take a minute to floss those pearly whites. Remember, they are the only set you get!

is root involvement. Over-the-counter pain relievers such as Advil or Tylenol may help as you drive to your dentist's office.

What are some alternative treatments?

- **Herbal therapy**—clove oil (a strong anesthetic and antiseptic containing the chemical eugenol, which dentists use) and ginger

- **Hydrotherapy**—moist heat on the jaw

The basics

1. *What's been proven to work?* Go to your dentist with any toothaches; this is a warning sign that something is amiss.

2. *How long until treatment works?* It depends on the cause. If the tooth is infected, your dentist will start you on antibiotics and may give you a prescription for pain pills. If the tooth has a broken filling or needs a crown, your dentist can take care of the pain immediately by resolving the problem.

3. *How much does it cost?* A trip to the dentist will cost about $50 to $150, if X-rays are taken. A root canal can cost $400 to $600, and a crown will cost from $500 to $700, depending on your location.

Brush and floss your teeth each day and make sure you see your dentist at least every six months. Prevention is far better than a toothache!

Just the facts

- There is evidence that the B vitamin niacin may help people who suffer from tinnitis.

- Reducing the inflammation that causes asthma is the key to treatment; several alternative remedies can help do this.

- Snoring often can be treated by losing weight, avoiding alcohol, and sleeping on your side, but laser surgery provides the cure in most cases.

- Many ailments such as toothaches, TMJ, and even sore throats can easily be avoided by taking aggressive preventive measures ahead of time.

Know Your Rights

PART IV

GET THE SCOOP ON...
Stumbling blocks you may face while getting
insurance providers to pay for alternative care ▪
What you can do to fight your provider for
payment ▪ What insurance companies look for
before they grant payment for experimental
therapy ▪ How to evaluate your policy to see
whether alternative therapies are covered

Facing Legal and Insurance Issues

Chapter 17

U sing a combination of conventional medical treatments and alternative therapies, we do our best to avoid major health problems. We eliminate the risk factors for disease that we can control, eat a low-fat diet packed with fruits and vegetables, get preventive tests, and make time daily to exercise our mind, body, and spirit. Yet, in spite of our efforts, sometimes we still get sick.

Reducing risk factors, eating right, and exercising are only part of the wellness equation. To achieve optimum health, you also need to understand your health care policies and know what is legal and what is not.

Self-care, managed care, or no care?

In the past, people who sought alternative therapies were thought to be uneducated or gullible. Conversely, today's studies reveal that the educated, middle- or upper-middle-class consumer is the most health conscious and seeks full participation in self-care.

Four out of 10 adults in the U.S. (42 percent) used some type of complementary treatment this past year, and holistic health coverage is in great demand. According to a survey conducted by Landmark Health Care and InterActive Solutions, two-thirds of Americans consider access to alternative medicine to be a key factor in choosing a health plan. Responding to this outpouring demand, more than half of Health Maintenance Organizations (HMOs) will cover alternative medicine therapies by the end of 1998.

Providing holistic therapies is not new to some insurers. For years, two specific alternative medicine therapies, chiropractic and acupuncture, have been covered by some insurers. At this time, at least 41 state governments require chiropractic coverage, and 6 require acupuncture coverage. Still, most alternative medicine therapies are considered experimental, and a quick check of many policies reveals that, even when they cover chiropractic, sometimes it is just for one particular ailment such as lower-back pain instead of for whole-body treatment.

That is why it is crucial for you to be a savvy consumer when you study your policy: Investigate the extras it provides, ask pertinent questions ahead of time, and even push your provider to pay if the therapy seems reasonable and works in your specific situation.

Due to public demand, competition for market share, and perceived cost savings, managed care organizations (MCOs) are becoming more open to alternative medicine therapies. In 1997, Oxford Health Plans, Inc., a large national health care company in Norwalk, Connecticut, was the first to provide full coverage for alternative medicine therapies. Under Oxford's alternative medicine rider, premiums are reportedly 3 percent higher than standard rates, but members receive full coverage for acupuncture, chiropractic, and naturopathic medicine. Even with the higher premium, this coverage is consistent with what Americans want in health care. The Landmark Report on Public Perceptions of Alternative Care found that 45 percent of people surveyed said they would be willing to pay more each month to have alternative care, and most people (67 percent) believe the availability of alternative care is an important factor when choosing a health plan. Other survey findings include:

- 80 percent of people surveyed use massage therapy
- 80 percent of people surveyed use vitamin therapy
- 75 percent use herbal therapy
- 73 percent use chiropractic

Oxford also has partnered with Harvard Medical School to perform clinical outcome studies on its alternative medicine program.

Most companies that offer coverage for alternative medicine therapies are located on the West Coast, including:

- Prudential (pays for acupuncture treatment)
- Blue Cross of Washington and Alaska (provides access to acupuncturists, homeopaths, and naturopaths)
- Health Net of California (offers chiropractic, acupuncture, acupressure, and Chinese herbal medicine)

Timesaver
If you are not sure what treatment is covered by your policy, call your insurance company. If the person taking your call seems unsure about the treatment, ask to speak to a supervisor until you find someone who really understands the coverage policies.

- American Western Life of Foster City, California (pays for various alternative medicine therapies)

- PacifiCare of Colorado and Kaiser Permanente (offer chiropractic riders)

- Sloans Lake Managed Care of Colorado (will begin offering an alternative medicine rider)

In 1996, the state of Washington required all health insurance policies to cover licensed, unconventional practitioners such as acupuncturists, naturopaths, and midwives. This controversial Washington law, the only such mandate in the United States, was invalidated by a federal judge in 1997.

Paying through the nose

How much would you be willing to pay if you could use conventional or alternative practitioners? Costs vary, depending on a variety of factors:

- The type of alternative medicine therapy covered

- Whether the payment is based on capitation or fee for service

- Co-pays or deductibles

PacifiCare's chiropractic rider costs $1 to $2 per member every month. Blue Cross of Washington and Alaska had only a small increase (1 percent) in costs. American Western Life of Foster City, California, estimates that premiums for alternative plans are 15 to 20 percent lower than premiums for traditional medical plans; in 1994, the company's holistic health hotline yielded $250,000 in savings. Sloans Lake Managed Care's rider costs $7 per member per month, and these costs will cover a variety of alternative therapies up to $500 a year with $20 co-payments.

Getting through the gatekeepers

MCOs (Managed care organizations) typically require patients to obtain referrals from primary care physicians (known as *gatekeepers*) before seeing a specialist. Some plans consider alternative health practitioners to be specialists and require referrals from the patient's primary physician. With these plans, the MCO does not have to pay for the service if you do not have a valid referral. Most plans covering alternative medicine therapy opt to use a fee-for-service payment method that does not require a referral.

Legally speaking

As public support for alternative medicine grows, managed care organizations MCOs, insurers, and other third-party payers are confronted with legal issues regarding coverage, costs, and payments.

Assessing your insurance contract

An MCO or insurer's obligation to provide and pay for alternative medicine therapy, a plan member's right to alternative medicine therapy treatment for covered services, and a provider's right to receive payment for alternative medicine therapy services or treatment are based, for the most part, on the contractual obligations. These are contained in the managed care plan or insurance policy, the alternative medicine therapy provider's participating provider agreement (in the case of a managed care plan), or the patient's insurance policy (in the case of insurance). As discussed more thoroughly in the following sections, many MCOs or insurers

Watch Out!
If you feel your claim has been unjustifiably denied, file a complaint with your state insurance commission. This agency watches over the insurance industry and resolves disputes with policy holders.

Moneysaver
Was your claim denied even though it helped your health problem? Consider going to small claims court and fighting your insurer. You do not need a lawyer for small claims court, and if your claim seems reasonable, the judge may rule that you get reimbursement.

specifically exclude coverage for experimental or investigational treatments or, as an alternative, adopt the Medicare treatment of such services or treatments.

What's experimental, what's not?

Alternative medicine therapies are difficult to measure for effectiveness due to their subjectivity. Remedial success often depends on patient participation. Traditional research protocols are not appropriate for measuring the effectiveness of alternative therapies. As a result, alternative medicine therapies often are classified by insurers as experimental or investigational. Subsequently, the managed care industry is struggling with the question: When is an alternative medicine therapy no longer considered experimental?

For many MCOs and other third-party payers, how this question is answered determines whether the therapy will be covered or excluded.

Conventional wisdom would suggest that any treatment that has undergone clinical trials showing it to be safe and cost-effective should no longer be considered experimental or investigational. Because the term *experimental* is inexact and has many meanings, however, classification often appears to be more of a financial decision than a scientific one. Under some plans and policies, chiropractic and acupuncture still are considered experimental and coverage is denied, even though both modalities have scientific studies to back them up. The reality is that any plan or policy can classify an alternative medicine therapy as experimental and deny coverage.

There is little consistency among managed care organizations when determining which treatments are experimental and, therefore, excluded from coverage. What is deemed experimental by one plan may be standard to another. Hence, many insurers look to Medicare to design their coverage.

Assessing medicare's coverage

Medicare bases its coverage determinations on whether the services are reasonable and necessary. Reasonable and necessary services are defined as services that are safe, effective, appropriate, and not experimental. This may include many of the alternative treatments discussed in this book. For government-funded programs (such as food stamps and WIC), the U.S. Food and Drug Administration (FDA) determines what technologies meet this criteria.

On the private side, the national Blue Cross Blue Shield Association reportedly has developed an objective process for determining whether a technology should no longer be considered experimental. The guidelines include:

- The technology must have final approval from the appropriate government regulatory bodies.

- Scientific evidence provides conclusions related to alternative medicine therapies' effect on health outcomes.

- The alternative medicine therapy must improve health outcomes.

- These improvements must be achievable outside the research setting.

While most health plans and insurers traditionally have relied on scientific or medicinal research studies to determine whether an alternative medicine therapy will be covered, an increasing number now require approval from a medical association

> 66
> For three years I fought my insurance company to pay for acupuncture for chronic pain. When the National Institutes of Health agreed that acupuncture was an acceptable means of treatment for some pain, I took this release to small claims court, along with my previously paid bills. My insurer was required by the judge to reimburse me for treatment. It does pay to be persistent.
> —Kim, 39, homemaker
> 99

and/or an independent board of physicians before providing coverage for an experimental treatment. This may be where the snags occur. How many conventional doctors want to see their patients receive treatment elsewhere, especially from practitioners who did not "pay their dues" with years of medical school training?

To recap, exclusionary clauses in contracts are one way insurers can deny coverage for what they consider to be expensive treatments. The drafting of excluded benefits is a legal challenge for MCO lawyers. Exclusionary clauses preclude coverage of experimental or investigational treatments.

The alternative "legal" cure

In the midst of insurance companies telling you what they will or won't pay, there are still some checks and balances that put the final decision back in your court.

Denying coverage

Denying coverage for a specific treatment can expose an organization to antitrust, contract, and tort liability. Antitrust issues prohibit two or more health plans from actions that may constitute a boycott of a particular therapy or treatment. For example, MCO A and MCO B cannot legally agree to exclude aromatherapy from coverage. Such conduct could constitute an illegal boycott or restraint on trade. MCOs must be very careful with regard to the process used to determine excluded services. Even the hint of impropriety can lead to antitrust liability.

This does not mean health plans cannot share scientific research studies. Health plans have a legitimate right to make informed decisions regarding coverage of services. Legal problems arise when documentation and correspondence fail to accurately reflect how they reached the decision.

MCOs can review one another's scientific analysis and can decide to exclude a particular therapy based on this evidence. It must be carefully documented, however, that the analysis was reviewed and that this decision was independently determined to be appropriate.

The best way for an MCO to avoid the risk of antitrust liability is for the documentation and correspondence to be reviewed by the MCO lawyer.

Concerning the contract

Contract issues primarily focus on the clarity of the language of the insurance policy or managed care plan. The policy or plan is a contract between the policyholder and the insurance company or MCO. The policyholder agrees to pay the required premiums, and the insurance company agrees to reimburse for health care costs listed in the contract. Litigation usually focuses on ambiguous words in the policy that could be interpreted in more than one way. Courts will look to the specific language of the policy in resolving conflicts. If the exclusionary clause is ambiguous, the policyholder may prevail. If it is clear, the court determines whether it will be construed to exclude an alternative medicine therapy as experimental. In many cases involving ambiguous language in contracts, courts have ruled in favor of coverage because the insurer or MCO had control over writing the contract provisions. Case law regarding nonreimbursement issues has been inconsistent, mainly because the language in managed care contracts varies significantly between companies.

Bright Idea
Before you file your claim, get a copy of your alternative practitioner's license, certification, or educational degree(s). Attach these to your claim and include a cover letter explaining the purpose of the treatment. It also helps to get a stamp of approval from your primary care medical doctor.

Courts generally will require insurers to provide coverage when the contract fails to define experimental treatment or when it bases the exclusion on unspecified criteria. Some courts have upheld exclusions if the insurer can prove that the treatment is experimental or is not medically necessary. Due to the increase in litigation, many HMOs are developing specific scientific guidelines for determining whether a procedure will be covered. They also are using clear, specific language in the exclusionary clauses.

Tort claims

Tort claims primarily are based on theories of negligence or intentional violations of a duty of care (for example, negligent administration of benefits, intentional negligence, misleading advertising, or fraud). The purpose of tort law is to compensate an injured party for the harm suffered. This compensation also acts as a deterrent for the negligent party to prevent the situation from occurring again. Every state has a legitimate interest in protecting the health, safety, and welfare of its residents. Since alternative medicine therapies, on the whole, remain stigmatized in the medical and business communities, courts can be expected to closely scrutinize cases involving patient injuries from alternative medicine therapy. In a recent case, an alternative medicine practitioner recommended that a patient forego chemotherapy and radiation treatment for cancer and instead undergo an alternative medicine therapy, which included a special diet and six coffee enemas a day. The patient sued after her cancer recurred causing blindness and severe back problems. The Supreme Court of New York ruled that the practitioner was 51 percent at fault and the patient 49 percent. The jury awarded more than $4 million in damages.

Quality control

Even in cases without a patient injury, the courts have sanctioned physicians for use of alternative medicine therapy as a departure from the standards of acceptable medical practice. In North Carolina, a physician's departure from standards of acceptable and prevailing medical practice, even though it did not pose a threat to the patients or to the public, was enough justification to revoke his medical license. Each state regulates the practice of medicine differently. There is no universal definition of the practice of medicine. Although the practice of medicine is expanding to include various alternative medicines, most state medical boards still consider allopathic medicine to be the standard of acceptable medical practice. Each state passes statutes to protect the public from the unlicensed practice of medicine. Alternative medicine therapy practitioners often are licensed by the state so the quality of their care can be regulated by licensing boards and disciplinary committees. Unfortunately, this regulatory system is not well suited to alternative medicine, in which patients share responsibility with the practitioner for their health outcome. Instead of protecting the patient from harm, the regulations impose arbitrary restrictions on alternative medicine therapy. As acceptance of alternative medicine therapy grows in the medical community, regulations will adapt to meet their unique needs.

Covered or not?

How do you know whether a treatment is covered and whether you can expect a fight over its coverage? Take out your policy and read it—line for line.

Go through your plan and see whether the following therapies are covered treatments:

- Acupuncture
- Ayurvedic medicine
- Biofeedback
- Birthing centers and midwives
- Bodywork and therapeutic massage
- Chelation therapy
- Chinese medicine
- Chiropractic
- Colonic irrigation
- Conventional or alternative medical care
- Dental services
- Detoxification
- Environmental medicine
- Herbal remedies
- Homeopathic remedies
- Hospital of choice
- Hospital services
- Hydrotherapy
- Light box therapy
- Magnet therapy
- Major medical coverage
- Maternity/reproductive
- Mental health services
- Mind/body treatments
- Naturopathy
- Nutritional supplements
- Nutritional therapy

- Osteopathy
- Oxygen therapy
- Prescription drugs
- Preventive care
- Specific alternative therapies
- Worldwide coverage
- X-ray/lab tests

Questioning your coverage

Once you have assessed the specific therapies covered, you need to determine whether any condition is covered under each therapy or only specific diagnosed conditions are covered. While you are doing this, write down any questions—no matter how trite they may seem—and ask your provider. Your policy may cover acupuncture, for example, but it may only list coverage for fibromyalgia, chronic headaches, and back pain. This means that, if you are seeking acupuncture for chronic nausea or neck pain, you will not be reimbursed.

While you are reading your policy, find out how much is paid for a particular treatment, what the standard deductible is, and whether this treatment must have a referral through your gatekeeper. Many HMOs will not touch a treatment unless your gatekeeper or primary care doctor on the HMO's plan has referred you and unless the specialist to which you are referred also is listed on the plan. Sometimes insurers will only pay part of the bill for alternative therapies (such as 50 percent), if any at all.

Even if you are told over the phone that a specific treatment is not covered, it is important to know that alternative medicine is big business. More than $11 billion is spent out-of-pocket on alternative therapies annually, and money can talk. Continue up the chain of authority in your insurance company until you are satisfied that you have spoken with someone who understands your policy. If you still feel you have a case to seek payment, document this and go to small claims court. Nevertheless, to avoid headaches and hassles regarding payment for services, check it out ahead of time—before you need the therapy—to ensure the greatest success in using alternative medicine.

What about the natural pharmacy?

Most alternative therapists will not be writing you a prescription for the neighborhood drugstore. Rather, the naturopathic practitioner will recommend that you take a natural remedy such as an herbal therapy, vitamin supplement, or homeopathic elixir, among others. These botanical agents, vitamins, amino acids, enzymes, and homeopathic therapies can be costly. Even though you may be healed of what ails you, insurance companies can refuse to reimburse you. In a survey by Blue Cross of Washington and Alaska to analyze their AlternaPath pilot project, it was determined that 39 cents of every benefit dollar was spent on natural products. That means an enormous portion of health care dollars are being spent on health care not yet reimbursed.

Alternative medicine takes center stage

Because most alternative practitioners focus on creating health rather than treating symptoms, many believe that the time has come to recognize alternative medicine in its own right. Why wouldn't an insurance provider want clients to stay well while saving billions in major medical expenses?

Watch Out!
An herb may seem like it is helping, but is it effective or a fraud? Send for a copy of the National Consumer's League brochure about alternative medicine. Mail your request plus $1 for shipping and handling to NCL, 1701 K Street NW, Suite 1200, Washington, DC 20006 or call 202-835-3323.

By removing alternative medicine from the list of experimental or investigational treatments, reimbursement issues would be resolved. CPT codes could be created for the various therapies, and each therapy could be regulated through its particular state license board. Legal action and judicial and regulatory scrutiny are likely to play key roles in speeding this process along.

Just the facts

- There is an outpouring demand from Americans for alternative treatments to complement conventional medical care.

- No matter what benefit you receive from alternative therapies, MCOs are not likely to cover any therapies not listed in your policy.

- Each state defines what the practice of medicine should be, and most states define it as allopathic or conventional medical care.

- If you are refused coverage and you fully believe the alternative treatment is helpful, go to small claims court and fight your case.

Navigating Through the Drugstore and the Health Food Store

PART V

What's Available?

There is something about the earthy, grainy smell of a natural food store that sets it apart from any other retail outlet. If you are a health-conscious shopper or an advocate of natural food stores, perhaps you can recognize and distinguish the varying odors that are often masked by incense, flower essence oils, and the strong smell of natural vitamins and supplements.

Judging by the olfactory sense alone, it is apparent that health food stores have more to offer than trendy vitamins and bins of granola. In fact, many natural food stores offer cooking utensils, cosmetics and beauty aids, natural fiber clothing and accessories, topical reading material about a myriad of health issues, and shelves of homeopathic, herbal, and dietary supplements. It is not unusual today to find a vegetarian-based café or a natural juice bar with an attendant waiting to mix a power-packed smoothie.

What kind of consumer are you?

Have you always gone to health food stores for your vitamin and mineral supplies? Or are you a

Chapter 18

405

bargain-hunting, health-conscious consumer? A new study released by Nutrition Business International, Inc., in San Diego, California, places the size of the U.S. nutrition industry at $17.2 billion annually. Of this total, dietary supplements (vitamins, minerals, herbs, and natural medicines) make up 52 percent of natural product sales ($8.9 billion), natural foods and beverages represent 36 percent of sales ($6.2 billion), and natural care and beauty products fill the remaining 12 percent of sales ($2 billion).

While natural food stores may be the preferred place to shop (receiving 44 percent of natural products sales), about one-fourth (26 percent) of all consumers are starting to use drugstores and grocery stores. You may be surprised to know that many chain discount drugstores and grocery stores are in strong competition with these "natural" establishments. Although mass-market retail outlets carry the same or similar supplements and supplies, they usually are at great discounts. In fact, studies show that herbal products rang up a healthy $1.6 billion in sales last year, making botanicals the fastest-growing category in drugstores.

Alternative health provides many choices. With natural therapies, you can choose where to shop, what to buy, and how much you spend. This is why a thorough understanding of what's available and what's not—in both health food stores and the local drugstore—is helpful before you make your list and head out on your herbal hunt.

Sifting through pills, powders, pollen, and potions

Before we discuss the bargains at chain discount drugstores, let's take a stroll through a typical mall health food store. If this is a new experience, it may seem overwhelming. You are greeted by shelf after shelf of colorful bottles, jars, cans, and bags of new and often very foreign products. A host of vitamins, minerals, amino acids, and enzymes are available to the average consumer who is seeking a natural boost for the immune system. As you continue down the aisles toward the back of the store, you also may find a complete line of body-building products, energizers, weight-reduction aids, and special training equipment for the avid weight lifter.

The soothing music you hear, the tray of natural food samples, and the smells of granola add to the appeal of wellness, good health, and self-care. Imagine, all this right at your fingertips—and all at a hefty price!

From rage to ridiculous

With the major boom in natural medicine, count on your health food store to be in the forefront with trendy treatments. For example, you may find popular homeopathic cough syrups, zinc lozenges, herbs to relieve nausea, elixirs to calm PMS, and guaranteed insomnia cures. Shelves are filled with safe allergy-relief capsules, supplements to end prostate problems, and even an all-natural vaginal moisturizer. Some of these natural cures are safe, effective, and appropriate—keep reading, though, because some are downright ridiculous.

Take the rage of herbal colon cleansing. This method of detoxification often consists of a variety of pills and capsules swallowed or taken as hot tea. Proponents of inner-cleansing claim it takes at least a three-day fruit, vegetable, and juice fast or a three-month intestinal cleanse with supplements to really detoxify the colon, ridding it of harmful toxins. This may seem reasonable to you. Nonetheless, as you

Timesaver
No time to shop for vitamins and herbs? Look on the Internet for discounted suppliers or use catalogs to make purchases by phone. It is estimated that more than 5 percent of all natural products are sold by mail order. Check out the Resource Directory on page 433 for a listing of suppliers and Internet sites.

move on down the aisle, you will soon come to methods that seem questionable. You might find a costly natural enema bag and rubber hose that claims to provide the "quickest solution to chronic constipation and disease." That's fine if you want rubber tubing passed up your rectum pumping water in and out. But does quickest also mean safest?

Next to this conglomeration of rubber tubing, you will find neatly packaged bottles of coffee, lemon, and distilled water that are labeled as detoxifying ingredients. This means that you can use the coffee and the distilled water in the enema for personal colon cleansing.

Colon cleansers available in pill form include psyllium seed husks, garlic, and cranberry. Most display on their labels that they may cause indigestion, stomach pain, or diarrhea. Acidophilus, a culture found in most yogurts, is another intestinal cleanser said to kill bacteria without causing an uncomfortable feeling.

Rage or ridiculous? That's for you to decide.

Pump me up!

Another trendy product offered at natural food stores is energy supplements. Thousands of varieties of pills, powders, and liquids available for purchase claim to increase one's energy, endurance, and youthfulness. The ingredients range from royal jelly, ginseng (of which there are several different forms), bee pollen, creatine, and protein (egg, whey, or vegetable). Even though these products are expensive, most are quite harmless.

There are, however, some potentially dangerous or even deadly products containing caffeine and ephedrine that also claim to increase energy. Several energy promises will include vitamins and/or cleansing herbs in their formulas. Not only will you be pumped up, you also will get detoxified and nourished—all in one pill. Rage or ridiculous? Again, you decide.

Calm me down

On a more relaxing note, chamomile, valerian root, melatonin, lavender, rose hips, hops, and the ubiquitous St. John's wort usually are in a special section of products that have a calming effect. Next to a variety of sleepy time aids, you will find powders, pills, and magic potions to help you lose or gain weight. Across the aisle, you may even find products intended for the family Fido or feline.

Lotions and lather

When it comes to personal care of the body, most natural food stores have an extensive (and expensive) line of natural products to replace your soap, shampoo, conditioner, and lotion. Some stores even carry natural toothpaste, deodorant, makeup, shaving cream, oil, and hair color.

Again, it is wise to compare the ingredients of all products. Although natural ingredients such as chamomile, aloe, honey, tea tree oil, vitamins A and E, and lavender are popular ingredients in many of these products, some products make claims that simply are not true. Antacids, mouthwashes, masks, mineral baths, and sunscreen all are available in a more natural form, and your quest for the world's greatest all-natural lip balm may end at your local health store.

Incense and oils

The most delightful area of the natural food store is designed to be sensual and to soothe a tired body and a weary soul. The complete line of

Watch Out!
For people with sensitive, dry, or oily skin, it may not be wise to use these natural skin products. Many of them contain rich oils or exfoliants; some even contain alcohol and other chemicals.

Bright Idea
Organic foods are a $3.5 billion industry, yet there have been no uniform standards to ensure quality until now. The U.S. Department of Agriculture will oversee a certification program that will hold organic-food producers, packagers, and producers to scrupulous guidelines by law. What are the rules?

▪ The soil for organic crops must be untouched by synthetic herbicides and pesticides for at least three years.

▪ Livestock must be able to roam the outdoors and must be raised on organic feed.

▪ Products cannot be altered genetically.

▪ Canned goods and processed foods cannot contain any additives, artificial coloring, or flavors.

aromatherapy candles, essential oils, and incense is delightful for cleansing, changing, blessing, and making your personal space sacred. Some stores offer or have connections to oil manufacturers so you can custom blend your own scent. Or you may want to pick up oil while you are at the store.

Essential oils can be wonderful when used as body oil (dilute it in a natural oil base, as suggested on page 104), potpourri refresher, or massage oil or when diffused through the air. Oil diffusers usually are available at these stores. Herbs and oils are quite similar in their uses sometimes, and both can be diffused throughout the air for healing purposes.

Naturally expensive

Another bonus provided by a natural food store is a food market. Stocked with dried, fresh, and often organic products, the natural food market is a common choice for shoppers interested in a healthier life—even if these choices are overpriced.

Many health-food suppliers offer dietary staples such as whole-grain fresh breads, pastas, cereals, crackers, and rice. Flavored and natural oils and vinegar are sold, as well as a large selection of natural salad dressings, condiments, and sweeteners. Organic flour, granola, and baked goods are widely available, as are organic soups and juices. It is possible to purchase non-irradiated and organic cooking herbs and spices.

The vegetarian diet is largely respected at these places; few offer meat other than frozen selections. Other frozen products include ethnic dinners, veggie burgers, tofu/non-dairy ice cream, and non-dairy meatless pizzas. This also is a good place to buy organic dairy and egg products, tofu, and other meatless protein products.

If you are following a diet recommended by an Ayurvedic or Chinese-medicine practitioner, a health food store is the place to go. You will find foods from around the world, international and organic coffees and teas, and a variety of nuts, beans, and seeds grown in the U.S. and in far-away lands.

Nourish your mind

For people interested in a more spiritual, holistic lifestyle, there are many books on healing, nutrition, and meditation. If a person is struggling with family issues, reading material about parenting, relationships, and psychology can be found. Books about homeopathy, cooking, ecology, and herbs also are available. You also can find books about yoga, reflexology, massage, and other physical nurturers. Some stores sell comfortable, natural cotton clothing for exercising or relaxing, and shoes and handbags made from natural fiber fabrics.

Checking out the drugstore

Compared with the soothing ambiance of a natural food store, the discount drugstore is a wake-up call that brings you back to the real world. The bright fluorescent lights, harried shoppers pushing metal carts, and periodic "blue-light specials" can be distracting. If you are truly bargain-hunting, however, this store may meet your needs.

Most discount drugstores offer a comprehensive array of vitamins and minerals—both name brands and generic brands—along with some herbs and dietary supplements. Because these supplements are bought in bulk for hundreds of stores across the U.S., you will be able to take advantage of lower costs and, sometimes, discount coupons.

If you are used to purchasing natural woven clothing or freshly squeezed carrot-kiwi juice at your natural food store, chances are your trip to the discount drugstore will be disappointing. But, based on the selection at several large chain stores, you will be able to purchase:

- Vitamins

- Minerals

- Dietary supplements, such as DHEA, melatonin, creatine, flaxseed and evening primrose oil supplements, and omega-3s (fish oil supplements)

- Herbs, such as St. John's wort, garlic, valerian, saw palmetto, kava kava, senna, black cohosh, dong quai, milk thistle, echinacea, goldenseal, ginseng, and ginkgo

- Candles, incense, and essential oils as well as some natural creams, lotions, hair products, and cosmetics

- Detoxifying tools such as an enema bag and hose, natural loofas, and mineral water (for liquid fasts)

- Weight loss and energizing products (some containing ephedra)

- Power bars, body-building powders and pills, and amino acids

- Popular books and magazines about natural healing, herbal therapies, vitamins and minerals, and disease prevention

Although most discount drugstores are limited to the preceding selections, your local large-chain grocery store will probably be able to complement these choices with organic foods, soy foods, canned juices, recycled-paper products, fat-free and reduced-fat products, reduced-salt products, wheat- and gluten-free foods, grains, granolas, dried fruits, nuts, fresh fruits and vegetables, and a host of ethnic foods.

Comparing expensive apples to discount oranges

"But the bottle is so big, it seemed like a bargain!" That's what most people think when they step into a health food store. If you are going to make alternative healing part of your lifestyle, however, you will have to become a savvy consumer. The best way to do this is to read labels—yes, even the fine print.

Finding lots of bargains at a health food store is not unusual, such as "buy one, get one free" specials in the vitamin section. That seems like a deal until you find out that 100 multivitamin tablets cost $12.99. Well, you might say, that means you get 200 tablets for $12.99, which is closer to a deal. Not quite. Compare the vitamins in the bottle—line for line—with the generic vitamins you can buy at your local chain drugstore. You will find that you can get 200 tablets with exactly the same vitamins and minerals for $4.99. Just think, you could buy almost 600 vitamins at your local drugstore for what the health food store is charging.

Watch the advertising

While roaming the aisles at the health food store, you need to check out the advertising and the promised claims. Remember, if something sounds too good to be true, it probably is. Keep this truth in mind while you read all the advertised claims.

You will find tiny capsules that claim to help you lose 20 pounds in two weeks, elixirs that supposedly make you feel younger instantly, and thick protein

Moneysaver
If you think you have a bargain, buyer beware! Check out the information on the side of the bottle. Read all the ingredients, the amount of the ingredient in each pill or capsule, and the number of pills in each bottle. You may think you have a bargain, but it often takes four to six tablets to provide the nutrient information listed on the side of the bottle— not just one.

Watch Out!
On a more serious note, bottles of pills that promise the consumer heightened energy or rapid weight loss may contain ephedrine or ephedrine-elated substances that can cause serious problems, even death. Other pills may contain herbs and other substances that can cause allergies or digestion problems. If you have any chronic health problems, check with your doctor before taking any product with unfamiliar ingredients. Products that provide instant energy for some people, may lead to stroke or heart attacks in others. Especially stay away from products containing pennyroyal, comfrey, yohimbe, kola nut, and ma huang (ephedra).

powders that claim they will make you energetic, more vital, and alert—all at once. Don't believe it! Then again, if you would like to try the placebo effect, buy it and see how you feel.

What about credentials?

At a drugstore, you can always ask the pharmacist about a particular product. One of the gravest concerns about natural food stores is often the people giving advice—the clerks that wait on customers. If you ask a clerk for health advice, make sure you first ask for her credentials. Studies have shown that employees of health food stores sometimes recommend potentially dangerous products without warning about their side effects. Although these same employees claim to have studied nutrition, not many have the scientific background to understand drug-drug or drug-food interactions, especially when supplements are taken along with strong prescription pharmaceuticals.

In one study reported in the *Southern Medicine Journal* (1995), employees suggested combinations of different products to help an AIDS patient. The Chinese herb ginseng was the single item mentioned most often. Other remedies they endorsed were echinacea, aloe, shark cartilage, and garlic. The same employees also recommended dietary changes and megavitamins—alternative treatments that cost up to $147 for a month's supply. Sadly, not one of the workers warned the AIDS patient about the potential side effects of these remedies (high blood pressure, respiratory failure, diarrhea, asthma, and other serious conditions if the substances are taken in high doses or in certain combinations).

Checking out herbal cures

Both health food stores and drugstores are notorious for offering a wide variety of herbal and medicinal cures for everything from the common cold, flu, or headache to anxiety, depression, or insomnia. While medicinal cures are regulated by the FDA, herbal cures are not. Whether packaged as a pill, capsule, elixir, powder, ground pollen, dried root, or fresh flower, you can rest assured that some type of flower-power cure exists for what ails you. Again, some of these cures are reasonable, and proponents claim they really work. For example, you may regularly use either valerian tea to ease anxiety and to promote restful sleep or cascara to help alleviate constipation. These commonly used herbs appear to have no harmful side effects. To be a discerning consumer, however, you need to go further and find out:

- How much can be taken safely to remedy the problem?
- What are the instructions for taking the herbal cure?
- How should this treatment be stored?
- Can the herbal cure safely be taken indefinitely or is there a specific window of time in which they are considered to be safe?
- Can this be taken with my medications?

Be discerning

Always examine all the ingredients of an herbal product, read background information from a reputable resource, and ask your medical doctor or pharmacist about any product with unknown properties. Remember, the FDA does not regulate the herbal industry, and a product usually is not proven hazardous until it has been on the shelves for months. This became a reality when a 37-year-old San Francisco woman died after drinking an herbal "dieter's tea" over a period of several months. This tea contained a laxative (senna) and a diuretic (uva ursi). Both senna and uva ursi can deplete the body of a key electrolyte, potassium, needed to regulate the heartbeat. There were no warnings on the label, however, nor did the package directions give an upper limit for consumption. On a less dangerous note, while some herbal products taste pleasant on their own, others (like valerian) can have a bitter, bland, or even unpleasant taste. When possible, ask for a sample at the store to prevent an unsatisfactory and expensive purchase.

Finding the store for you

How can you begin to know where to shop for your alternative therapies? For starters, you may want to divide your health purchases into several categories: supplements, food, and personal care. It's not news that the discount drugstore will give you the best bargains on vitamin and mineral supplements and will provide some herbal remedies or dietary supplements, such as melatonin, omega-3s, and creatine. If you are a devout natural healing advocate, you already know that, although the drugstore has the best prices, it also is limited in selection.

To find the widest selection of herbal concoctions, homeopathic remedies, vitamins, minerals, and dietary supplements, along with the most thorough selection of organic foods and natural products, you must turn to the natural food store. Expensive? Yes. Expect to pay more than you would at your local chain drugstore. When you weigh options with cost, however, it may be worth it to you.

Is it what the doctor ordered?

It is important to research all your options when choosing natural therapies. If you feel uncomfortable researching this on your own, consult with your medical doctor, pharmacist, certified nutritionist, or naturopathic doctor. Remember, the staff at a health store may seem knowledgeable, but they are not licensed or qualified to prescribe any products. Most importantly, know yourself and your body's needs. This is the first and safest step in choosing effective alternative treatments as you formulate a natural prevention plan that leads you to optimum health.

Just the facts

- The Internet is an excellent resource for purchasing discounted nutritional supplements, including vitamins, minerals, herbs, and homeopathic remedies.

- Choose a natural food store if you like to shop for an array of products, including organic foods, fresh and dried herbs, and natural fiber clothing and accessories.

- Choose a discount drugstore or grocery store if you are looking for standard vitamin, mineral, and herbal supplements at reduced cost.

- Check out the credentials of anyone who recommends a natural treatment to cure what ails you. Always ask your medical doctor if you are unsure about drug-drug or drug-food combinations.

Glossary

Absolute oil   A highly concentrated liquid taken from a plant and extracted by alcohol.

Acupressure   A Chinese medical therapy similar to acupuncture except it relies on the hands for massage and touch instead of needles.

Acupuncture   Ancient stress reliever that uses needles to puncture the skin at certain points on the body. Acupuncture helps to stimulate the body's natural defenses and to alter the activity of the immune system. The National Institutes of Health has approved acupuncture as effective relief for nausea.

Alexander technique   Technique developed in the late 1800s by Frederick Matthias Alexander, an actor who realized that the way he tensed his body negatively affected the relationship between his head, neck, and back and greatly affected his voice. The techniques he developed are said to release painful muscle tension, to improve posture, and to reduce stress and fatigue through reeducation of the kinesthetic sense.

Allopathic medicine   Focuses on defining disease based on measurable symptoms and then eliminating those signs.

Aloe   Extract from an aloe plant used externally for skin irritations, minor burns, sunburn, cuts, skin irritations, rashes, canker sores, cold sores, ulcers, acne, frostbite, poison ivy, vaginal dryness, and skin abrasions. Take internally to relieve constipation, gastritis, and stomach ulcers.

Angelica   (dong quai) Available in dried herb, supplement, or tincture. Said to relieve menstrual discomfort, minimize symptoms of menopause, boost production of red blood cells, and treat weakness and fatigue.

Antibiotic   A drug that kills or slows down the reproduction of bacteria. In doing so, antibiotics help the body's own immune defenses, such as white blood cells and various antibodies, to clear bacteria from the body.

Aromatherapy   Alternative medicine therapy that relies on chemical scents from natural herbs and extracts to relieve symptoms and to boost immunities.

Astragalus   Stimulates the immune system, boosts white blood cell activity, and increases the production of interferon. Take to promote urination, to speed healing of burns, and to bolster resistance to disease.

Ayurveda   Holistic medical practice focusing more on the balance of mind and body than on specific symptoms or disorders. Ayurvedic medicine was formed in India around 3,000 years ago.

Bee pollen   Balances the endocrine system, helping to relieve menstrual or prostate problems. Also helps to counteract the effects of aging and to strengthen the body's natural immunity against illness. Use as an antidote during allergy season to relieve bronchitis, sinusitis, and colds.

Beta-carotene Beta-carotene—found in apricots, carrots, cantaloupe, pumpkins, and spinach—is converted to vitamin A in the body. Protects from the damaging effects of the sun's ultraviolet rays and protects the membranes of mouth, nose, throat, and lungs, thereby reducing susceptibility to infections.

Biofeedback Physical and mental control over the responses of the voluntary and involuntary systems of the body to prevent or alleviate medical problems.

Black cohosh root Acts similarly to estrogen, the female-produced chemical, and has been prescribed for women going through menopause. Black cohosh may help treat fatigue, a sore throat, arthritis, and rattlesnake bites. It contracts the uterus and increases menstruation.

Black currant seed oil Contains essential fatty acids (EFAs). EFAs are not manufactured by the body but are essential to cardiovascular health and normal brain development.

Bodywork The alternative term used to describe the techniques of massage, touch, and movement.

Burdock root A detoxifying herb that promotes healthy kidney function and helps to prevent water retention; it also helps to heal arthritis and rheumatism and is used as a blood purifier and cleanser.

Capsaicin Effective in preventing muscle aches and arthritis pain. Capsaicin reduces the levels of prostaglandins, chemical messengers that inflame joints.

Carbunkle A cluster of boils that occurs when infection spreads.

Cayenne pepper Helps relieve symptoms of bronchitis. Also helps heal irritated tissues and promote drainage.

Chamomile   A destressor used to relieve insomnia and to promote relaxation.

Chelation   Chelation therapy is an expensive and highly controversial regimen that is said to help clear arteries clogged by arteriosclerosis. A chelating chemical is injected into the body to find toxins in the blood. The acid binds with, or "chelates," certain minerals (particularly calcium) and removes them from the body through the urinary tract.

Chiropractic   Manipulation of the spine to alleviate symptoms and to promote healing of all sorts of medical disorders as well as muscular and bone injuries.

Choline   A brain chemical that is important for recall and memory.

Chromium   An important trace mineral that helps cells break down sugar into energy for the body. Supplements can help regulate blood sugar, fat, and carbohydrate metabolism.

CoEnzyme Q10   An antioxidant that helps to lower cholesterol levels and to reduce oxidative damage to blood vessels.

Colonic irrigation   A detoxification therapy in which a rubber tube is inserted into the rectum and then passed for a distance of up to 20 or 30 inches. Warm water is gently pumped in and out through the tube a few pints at a time, typically using 18 to 22 or more gallons.

Cranberry   Helps to prevent and alleviate symptoms caused by urinary tract infections.

Creative visualization   *(See Guided imagery)*

Dandelion root   Helps to support the body's potassium levels and to detoxify the system. Improves enamel of teeth when eaten as a food. The juice from the stem is used to treat acne, blisters, and corns.

Detoxification   The act of cleansing the body of toxins. Purification of the human body, mind, and spirit.

DHEA   An antiaging hormone sometimes called the mother hormone because the body converts it into estrogen and testosterone. DHEA raises sex hormones and is said to make you feel younger and sexy.

Dong quai   *(See Angelica)*

Echinacea   Stimulates the immune system and helps to ward off colds or the flu. Heals wounds and has an anti-inflammatory, antiviral, and antibacterial effect on the body.

Elderberry   Helps relieve symptoms of bronchitis.

Enema   The act of cleansing and detoxifying the colon by injecting water or other fluids into the rectum *(for more information, see Colonic irrigation)*.

Environmental medicine   Focuses on the removal of harmful chemicals and toxins from your workplace.

Essential fatty acids (EFAs)   Not manufactured by the body, EFAs are essential to cardiovascular health and normal brain development. Found in fish oils and in plant oils such as evening primrose, black currant, and borage.

Essential oils   An essential oil is an extract or essence that's been distilled—usually by steam—from the seed, leaves, stem, flower, bark, root, or another part of a plant.

Evening primrose oil   Contains gamma linolenic acid (GLA), an essential nutrient that creates substances called prostaglandins, which help keep blood running smoothly.

Fasting   Detoxifying the body by not eating and by drinking only water, juices, or clear liquids.

Feldenkrais method A type of subtle touch to help release compulsive habits. Also attempts to improve the efficiency of the motor nervous system.

Fen-Phen A once popular but now controversial weight-reduction medicine.

Feverfew May inhibit inflammation and fever, slow the blood vessel reaction to vasodilators such as prostaglandins, and act similar to aspirin. Also used to treat arthritis and chronic or migraine headaches.

Fiber Can be *insoluble* or *soluble*. *Insoluble fiber* does not dissolve in water. It includes the woody, tough parts of plants such as the bran coating around grains, fruits, and vegetable skins. Insoluble fiber passes through the digestive tract mostly unchanged. *Soluble fiber* dissolves in water. It is abundant in beans, oats, broccoli, and many fruits and has the consistency of gel. As it absorbs water, it gives a feeling of fullness and accelerates food transit through the digestive tract.

Flower essences A combination of flowers used to change negative feelings such as anger, worry, jealousy, and fear into optimism, joy, and hopefulness.

Garlic Has antimicrobial and immunostimulating properties and may provide some relief from symptoms of colds or upper respiratory problems by stimulating the mucus-producing vagus nerve reflexes. Garlic may lower blood pressure and prevent cancer and blood clots.

Gerson therapy Utilizes diet, detoxification, and therapeutic supplementation to reactivate and strengthen the immune system and to restore the body's essential defenses.

Ginger Helps to fight nausea and improve digestion, soothes aching joints and upset stomach, which helps to fight cold viruses and provides an anti-inflammatory effect, and stimulates the production of interferon.

Ginkgo biloba Relaxes and opens up blood vessels, may increase male sexual performance and counteract male impotence, and protects cell membranes from free radical damage, improving concentration and memory.

Ginseng Used to increase energy and to relieve stress. May stimulate special enzymes that promote elimination of toxic foreign substances and may increase the immune response by stimulating the number of antibodies in the body.

Glutathione Found in the pulpy part of watermelon and in cruciferous vegetables. Also has been found to strengthen the immune system.

Gotu-kola Used as brain food to promote memory, to alleviate mental fatigue, and to normalize blood pressure. Considered to be a nerve tonic.

Green tea A powerful antioxidant that may help prevent liver, pancreatic, breast, lung, esophageal, and skin cancers. It has also been found to help reduce the risk of cardiovascular disease and stroke. Some new studies indicate it may help prevent osteoporosis.

Guided imagery Alternative stress-reduction technique that uses visualization to help synchronize the bodies' mental and physical components.

Hawthorn berries Used to strengthen the muscles and nerves to the heart. May help to regulate high or low blood pressure and battle arteriosclerosis, hypoglycemia, and heart disease.

Herb A plant or a part of a plant that can be used in medicine or seasoning.

HMO Abbreviation for a Health Maintenance Organization, a managed-care planner.

Homeopathy A naturopathic form of medicine that helps reduce allergic rhinitis, hay fever, migraine headaches, trauma, gastritis, allergic asthma, acute childhood diarrhea, fibromyalgia, and influenza.

Hydrotherapy Any rehabilitative therapy that involves soaking in water, usually warm whirlpool baths.

Hypnotherapy A mind/body technique that provides a temporary condition of altered attention in which the brain shuts out external events. This intense state of concentration is used to control pain or stress or to alter negative behaviors.

Isoflavones Phytonutrients found in soy that are converted into phytoestrogens. They can be used for cancer prevention and estrogen therapy.

Kelp Provides energy and endurance, helps relieve nervous tension, and promotes circulation to the brain and reduction of high blood pressure.

L-Lysine A cold sore preventer that may also be effective against herpes.

Lavender Used to prevent dry and cracked skin, inflammation, and sleeplessness and for aromatherapy.

Lemon Used as an astringent and germicide. Also may increase mental alertness.

Licorice root Is filled with antiviral compounds and acts as an expectorant, soothing tissues and mucous membranes.

Light therapy Light therapy involves using natural or artificial light to cause physiological changes in the human body.

Macrobiotics A semivegetarian diet that is said to improve health and to prolong life. It is based on the need to keep the principles of yin (the force of expansion) and yang (the force of contraction) balanced in the body.

Meadowsweet An herb that eases the pain of arthritis or rheumatism.

Medicine Any substance taken into your body for therapeutic (cure) or preventive value.

Meditation A stress releaser that seeks to integrate the mind, body, and spirit through intentionally focusing on the silent repetition of a focus word and peaceful thoughts.

Melatonin A natural hormone secreted from the pineal gland in the brain that has a major influence on the human body's inner clock, which governs the sleep-wake cycle and other biological functions.

Milk thistle An herb that increases levels of glutathione, the main vehicle of detoxification in the body. Also bolsters the immune system, supports the liver's ability to maintain normal liver function, and stimulates production of new liver cells to replace old, damaged ones.

Mind/body medicine Medicine based on the influence of the mind in healing the body.

Minerals These substances, which help set off chemical reactions in cells, are required for normal growth and development and the maintenance of good health.

Mullein Used as a bone, flesh, and cartilage builder, it works as an expectorant to relieve respiratory problems such as asthma, bronchitis, and sinus congestion. It is applied externally to heal ulcers, hemorrhoids, and tumors.

Natural Not artificial. A product that comes from nature.

Naturopathy Preferring to avoid drugs and surgery and trying to rely on the body's natural healing capacity.

Nutritional therapy Therapy relying on foods that contain essential nutrients to help prevent disease and heal the body.

Omega-3 acids Found in fish oil, these acids are believed to have several therapeutic properties including use as anticarcinogens.

Osteopathy Using manual adjustments of the muscles, joints, and spine before using drugs and surgery.

Papaya A fruit that can be mashed to treat various insect bites.

Parsley A common herb that can be used as a skin treatment.

Passionflower A common herb frequently used as a mild tranquilizer or to ease insomnia, stress, and anxiety. Also relieves shingles, hiccups, and asthma.

Peppermint An herb containing oils that can soothe the digestive track.

Phenylalanine An amino acid that produces norepinephrine, keeps you alert, improves memory, and reduces hunger.

Phytochemical A nutrient that boosts the immune system and keeps the body well.

Placebo effect A reaction that refers to the mysterious and uncharted mechanisms by which the power of suggestion can result in a physiological change. Usually refers to case studies in which participants are given sugar pills rather than the studied product.

Psychotherapy Behavioral treatment that allows you to change your own biology without invasive treatment or medications. Psychotherapy will let you identify and then verbalize inner conflicts as you learn positive coping skills.

Qigong A Chinese self-healing method that increases the delivery of oxygen to the tissues, that enhances the elimination of waste products and the transportation of immune cells through the lymph system, and that shifts the chemistry of the brain and the nervous system.

Quercetin   A nutrient found in citrus fruits, red and yellow onions, and broccoli. Quercetin reduces inflammation associated with allergies, can inhibit the growth of head and neck cancers, and may reverse transcriptase, the method HIV uses to replicate itself.

Red clover   Promotes new skin growth.

Reflexology   An alternative technique to relieve stress and to promote healing by systematically probing the feet.

Rolfing   A method of bodywork that promotes natural healing by realigning the body's underlying structure. The practitioner, or rolfer, uses fingers, knuckles, and elbows to sculpt the client's body into correct alignment.

Saw palmetto   Used as a treatment for benign prostatic hypertrophy or an enlarged prostate, it relieves the main symptom of frequent urination. Also relieves nasal congestion, asthma, and bronchitis.

Selenium   A nutrient that can help your body stay cancer-free or, if you have cancer, can boost your health.

Shaman   A member of certain tribal societies that mediates between the visible and invisible spirit worlds for healing purposes and to control natural events.

Shark cartilage   A supplement said to have cancer-fighting properties.

Shiatsu   A Chinese medicine therapy that draws on the Chinese notion of qi—energy that flows along meridians throughout the body. Firm, rhythmic pressure is applied for 3 to 10 seconds on specific points. This pressure is given to wake up the meridians, or healing channels of the body.

Siberian ginseng   An herb said to reduce blood pressure and to increase concentration. It is available in health food stores in liquid or capsule form.

Spinal manipulation   This type of therapy used exclusively by chiropractors may help correct imbalances in the body and give relief to back pain.

St. John's wort   A popular herb taken internally to relieve depression without the serious side effects of prescription antidepressants. Use externally to aid in wound healing.

Supplement   Substitutions for a diet weak in essential nutrients, vitamins, and minerals. Available in different forms such as capsules, caplets, and pills.

Support group   Any group or member organization that brings together individuals who have a common problem, disease, or disorder.

Suppository   An ointment in a solid but easily melted form (usually medicated) that is inserted into the rectum for lubrication.

Tai chi   An ancient Chinese defensive martial art similar to shadow boxing. In tai chi, you follow a series of slow, graceful movements that mimic the movements you do in daily life.

Tea tree oil   A potent antiseptic that can be toxic if swallowed.

Therapeutic touch   The act of physically touching a patient to promote healing.

Toxins   Any chemical the human body naturally rejects to when absorbed.

Trans-fatty acids   Compounds found in margarine, snacks, fast-food products, crackers, pastries, and many processed foods that can lead to many types of cancer, obesity, and even heart disease.

Tryptophan A natural relaxant that can alleviate insomnia and can help in treatment of migraines.

Valerian An herb that helps to relax tense muscles and to destress the body.

Vegan A person that eats a strict plant-based diet with no animal byproducts such as milk or honey.

Yoga A type of Ayurvedic medicine that can help stretch tightened muscles and can ease the tension causing the pain.

Resource Directory

Acupressure

Acupressure-Acupuncture Institute, Inc.
10506 N. Kendall Dr.
Miami, FL 33176
Phone: 305-595-9500
Fax: 305-595-2622

Acupressure Institute
1533 Shattuck Ave.
Berkley, CA 94709
Toll free: 800-442-2232 (outside California)
Phone: 510-845-1059 (in California)

Acupuncture

American Academy of Medical Acupuncture
5820 Wilshire Blvd., Suite 500
Los Angeles, CA 90036
Toll free: 800-521-AAMA
Phone: 213-937-5514
Web site: www.medicalacupuncture.org

American Association of Acupuncture and Bio-Energetic Medicine (AAABEM)
2512 Manoa Rd.

Honolulu, HI 96822
Phone: 808-946-2069
Fax: 808-946-0378

American Association of Acupuncture and Oriental
Medicine
4101 Lake Boone Trail, Suite 201
Raleigh, NC 27607
Phone: 919-787-5181

American Association of Oriental Medicine
433 Front St.
Catasauqua, PA 18032
Phone: 610-266-1433
Fax: 610-264-2768

National Certification Commission for Acupuncture
and Oriental Medicine
1424 16th St. NW, Suite 501
Washington, DC 20036
Phone: 202-232-1404
Web site: www.nccaom.org

National Commission for the Certification of
Acupuncturists
Phone: 919-787-5181

Alternative insurance companies
Alternative Health Insurance Services
Toll free: 800-966-8467

Bienestar Gold
Toll free: 888-692-4363

Group Health Insurance Services
Toll free: 800-358-8815 (individual)
Toll free: 800-542-6312

Kaiser Foundation Health Plan
Phone: 510-596-1120

Oxford Health Plans
Personal Freedom Plan
Toll free: 800-444-6222

Alternative medicine advocates

The Alternative Medicine Connection
Healthsavers Press
P.O. 683
Herndon, VA 22070
Phone: 703-471-8465

Alternative Medicine Political Action Committee, Inc.
1718 M St., #205
Washington, DC 20036

Office of Alternative Medicine Clearinghouse
P.O. Box 8218
Silver Spring, MD 20907-8218
Toll free: 888-644-6226
TTY/TDY: 888-644-6226
Fax: 301-495-4957
Web site: altmed.od.nih.gov

Alternative therapies associations

American Botanical Council
P.O. Box 2016601
Austin, TX 78720

American Herbal Products Association
P.O. Box 2410
Austin, TX 78768
Phone: 512-320-8555

The Herb Growing and Marketing Network
P.O. Box 245
Silver Spring, PA 17575-0245
Phone: 717-393-3295

International Herb Association
1202 Allanson Rd.
Mundelein, IL 60060
Phone: 708-949-4372

Life Extension Foundation
P.O. Box 229120
Hollywood, FL 33022-9120
Toll free: 800-841-5433

Aromatherapy

International Federation of Aromatherapists
204 Chiswick High Rd.
London, W4 England

National Association for Holistic Aromatherapy
P.O. Box 17622
Boulder, CO 80308-0622
Phone: 303-258-3791

National Oils Research Association
894H Route 52
Beacon, NY 12508
Phone: 914-838-4340

Ayurveda

American School of Ayurvedic Sciences
10025 NE 4th St.
Bellevue, WA 98004
Phone: 206-453-8022

Ayurvedic Foundations
1550 East 3300 South
Salt Lake City, UT 84106
Phone: 801-466-8324

Ayurvedic Institute
11311 Menaul NE, Suite A
Albuquerque, NM 87112
Phone: 595-291-9698

Ayurvedic practitioners

California College of Ayurveda
135 Argall Way
Nevada City, CA 95959
Phone: 916-265-4300

Vinayak Ayurveda Center
2509 Virginia NE, Suite D
Albuquerque, NM 87110
Phone: 505-296-6522
Fax: 505-298-2932

Biofeedback

Association of Applied Psychophysiology and
Biofeedback
10200 W. 44th Ave., Suite 304
Wheat Ridge, CO 80033-2840
Phone: 303-422-8436

Biofeedback Certification Institute of America
10200 W. 44th Ave., Suite 304
Wheat Ridge, CO 80033
Phone: 303-420-2902
Web site: www.bcia.org

Bodywork/therapeutic massage

Alexander Technique
1692 Massachusetts Ave., 3rd Floor
Cambridge, MA 02138
Phone: 617-497-2242
Fax: 617-497-2615

American Massage Therapy Association
820 Davis St., Suite 100
Evanston, IL 60201-4444
Phone: 847-864-0123
Fax: 847-864-1178
Web site: www.amtamassage.org

Associated Bodywork and Massage Professionals
Toll free: 800-458-2267
Web site: www.abmp.com

International Massage Association
Phone: 202-387-6555
Web site: www.imagroup.com

Catalogs and mail order

Alternative Approach Pty. Ltd.
(Buteyko method for stopping asthma)
A.C.N. 076 259 124
P.O. Box 41
Annerley Q.L.D. 4103
Australia
Phone: 61-7-38479750
Fax: 61-7-33973832
E-mail: pathein@gil.com.au

Austin Nutritional Research
(Vitamins and nutritional supplements)
4815 W. Braker Ln.
Building 502, Suite 180
Austin, TX 78759
Phone: 512-267-7644
Fax: 512-267-4448
Web site: www.realtime.net/anr/catalog.html

B & A Exportrade AB
(Ecological hair- and skin-care collection)
Rullagergatan 9
P.O. Box 367
SE-401 25 Gothenburg
Sweden
Phone: +46-31-727-5154
Fax: +46-31-727-5155
E-mail: b.a.exportrade@bigfoot.com

Biotone
(Massage lubricants and essential oils)
4757 Old Cliffs Rd.
San Diego, CA 92120
Toll free: 800-445-6457
Fax: 800-664-7567

BodyBridge: The Back Solution
(Natural approach to back health and equipment to relieve pain)
6281 S. Park Ave.
Tucson, AZ 85706
Phone: 800-326-2724
Web site: www.bodybridge.com

Buteyko Method
(Alternative method of asthma control)
Buteyko Online
Phone: 646-878-0101
Fax: 646-878-0103
E-mail: buteyko@voyager.co.nz
Web site: www.buteyko.co.nz

Diamond Herpanacine Associates
(Vitamins and nutritional supplements)
P.O. Box 544
Ambler, PA 19002
Phone: 215-542-2981
Fax: 215-542-2983
E-mail: herpana@aol.com

Enzymatic Therapy
(Vitamins and supplements)
825 Challenger Dr.
Green Bay, WI 54311-8328
Phone: 920-469-4419
Fax: 920-469-8390

Fernwood Herb Farms
P.O. Box 332
Fernwood, ID 83830

Herbal Valley
(Herbs and essential oils)
1664 N. Cedar St., #85
Laramie, WY 82072
Toll free: 800-644-2482

Homeocare
ELS International, Inc.
(Homeopathic products)
P.O. Box 630115
Riverdale, NY 10463
Phone: 888-HOMEOCARE
Fax: 718-796-7292
Web site: homeocare.com

Homeopathic Educational Services
(Complete homeopathic supplies)
2124 Kittredge St.
Berkeley, CA 94704
Phone: 800-359-9051
Fax: 510-649-1955
Web site: www.homeopathic.com

Hoosier Herbal Remedies
(Herbal remedies and energy supplements)
6816 Pebblebrook Ct.
Brownsburg, IN 46112
Phone: 317-852-4997
Web site: www.ezlinks.com/herbal

Jurlique International Pty. Ltd.
(Skin care, aromatherapy, environmental medicine,
herbal therapy)
Toll free: 800-854-1110
Phone: 770-643-6999

Fax: 770-643-4999
Web site: www.jurlique.com

Kushi Cuisine
Toll free: 800-490-0044

New England Herbal Supply Co.
299 Jagger Ln.
Hebron, CT 06248
Toll free: 800-742-0631
Phone: 860-228-9705
Fax: 860-228-9705
E-mail: NEHerbalSupply@Sprintmail.com

North American Herbal Company
Nature's Solutions
(Drinkable herbal supplements)
P.O. Box 2945
Plattsburg, NY 12901-0269
Phone: 800-644-5587
Web site: www.natures-solutions.com

The Pressure Positive Company
(Hands-on massage tools to relieve muscular pain)
128 Oberholtzer Rd.
Gilbertsville, PA 19525
Phone: 800-603-5107
Fax: 610-754-6327

Robyn's Nest Products
P.O. Box 20331
Cheyenne, WY 82003
Phone: 307-637-2307
Fax: 307-637-2307

Chinese medicine

American Association of Oriental Medicine
433 Front St.
Catasauqua, PA 18032
Phone: 610-266-1433

Chiropractors

American Chiropractic Association (ACA)
1701 Claredon Blvd.
Arlington, VA 22209
Toll free: 800-986-4636
Phone: 703-276-8800
Web site: www.amerchiro.org

International Chiropractors Association (CA)
1110 N. Glebe Rd., Suite 1000
Arlington, VA 22201
Toll free: 800-423-4690
Phone: 703-528-5000
Web site: www.chiropractic.org

Dance therapy

American Dance Therapy Association
2000 Century Plaza, Suite 108
Columbia, MD 21044-3263
Phone: 410-997-4040

Dental

Holistic Dental Association
Holistic/Alternative Dentistry
P.O. Box 5007
Durango, CO 81301

Government agencies

National Institute of Mental Health Public Inquiries
5600 Fishers Ln., Room 7C-02, MSC 8030
Bethesda, MD 20892-8030

Office of Alternative Medicine Clearinghouse
P.O. Box 8218
Silver Spring, MD 20907-8218
Toll Free: 888-644-6226
TTY/TDY: 888-644-6226
Fax: 301-495-4957

USDA Foreign Agricultural Service
(For foreign herb information)
Information Division, Room 5074-S
Washington, DC 20250-1000
Phone: 202-720-7115
Fax: 202-720-3229

USDA National Agricultural Library (NAL)
10301 Baltimore Blvd., Room 304
Beltsville, MD 20705-2351
Phone: 301-504-6559

Herbalists

AMERICAN HERBAL PHARMACOPOEIA™
P.O. Box 5159
Santa Cruz, CA 95063
Phone: 408-461-6317
Fax: 408-438-7410
E-mail: herbal@got.net

The American Herbalists Guild
P.O. Box 1683
Sequel, CA 95073

Herb Society of America
9019 Kirtland-Chardon Rd.
Kirtland, OH 44094
Phone: 216-256-0514
Fax: 216-256-0541

International Herb Association
P.O. Box 317
Mundelein, IL 60060-0317
Phone: 847-949-4372
Fax: 847-949-5896

Medical Herbalism
Bergner Communications, Inc.
P.O. Box 20512
Boulder, CO 80308

Phone: 303-541-9552
E-mail: bergner@concentric.com

National Institute of Medical Herbalists
56 Longbrook St.
Exeter, Devon EX4 6AH
England
Phone: 01392-426022
Fax: 01392-498963

Revitalizing our Herbal Traditions
P.O. Box 746555
Arvada, CO 80006
Phone: 303-423-8800
Fax: 303-402-1564
E-mail: ahgoffice@earthlink.net

Western Reserve Herb Society
11030 East Blvd.
Cleveland, OH 44106

Homeopathy

Homeopathic Educational Services
2124B Kittredge St.
Berkeley, CA 94704
Phone: 510-649-0294
Fax: 510-649-1955

International Foundation for Homeopathy
2366 Eastlake Ave. East, Suite 325
Seattle, WA 98102
Phone: 206-776-4146

National Center for Homeopathy
801 N. Fairfax St., Suite 306
Alexandria, VA 22314
Phone: 703-548-7790
Web site: www.homeopathic.org

Hypnosis

The Society of Clinical and Experimental Hypnosis
3905 Vincennes Rd., Suite 304
Indianapolis, IN 46268

Society of Clinical Hypnosis
2200 E. Devon Ave., Suite 291
Des Plaines, IL 60018

Insurance providers—alternative medicine

Alliance for Alternatives in Healthcare, Inc.
P.O. Box 6279
Thousand Oaks, CA 91359
Phone: 805-494-7818
Fax: 805-494-8528

Alliance for Natural Health
P.O. Box 4035
Hammond, IN 46324
Phone: 708-974-9373
Fax: 708-974-6002

Alternative Health Insurance Services, Inc.
P.O. Box 6279
Thousand Oaks, CA 91359-6279
Toll free: 800-966-8467
Fax: 805-379-1580
E-mail: AltHlthIns@AOL.com

Group Health Cooperative
Toll free: 888-901-4636
Phone: 206-901-4636
Fax: 206-901-4612

St. Anthony's Alternative Medicine Integration & Coverage
11410 Isaac Newton Sq.
Reston, VA 20190

Internet resources

Ayurvedic Foundation: www.ayur.com

Ayurvedic Health Center: www.ayurvedic.org

Ayurvedic Newsgroup: alt.health.ayurveda

Chiropractic Online: www.amerchiro.org/

Dr. Andrew Weil's Web Site: www.drweil.com
Get the facts on H.R. 1055—a proposal to have the federal government spend more money on alternative medicine research: www.naturalhealth village.com/townhall/federal

Healthy World Online: www.healthy.net

Herb Providers: www.frontierherb.com/ homepage.html

Herb Research Foundation: www.herbs.org/ index.html

Herb Resources on the Internet: www.herbnet.com/

Internet Mental Health: www.mentalhealth.com

Mental Health Net: www.cmhc.com

National Institutes of Health: www.nih.gov

National Library of Medicine: www.nlm.nih.gov/

Office of Alternative Medicine: altmed.od.nih.gov/oam/

Massage

American Massage Therapy Association
820 Davis St., Suite 100
Evanston, IL 60201-4444
Phone: 847-864-0123

International Association of Infant Massage
1720 Willow Creek Circle, Suite 516
Eugene, OR 97402
Toll free: 800-248-5432

Magazines

Alternative Medicine Digest
Toll free: 800-333-HEAL
Web site: www.alternativemedicine.com

Delicious! Magazine
New Hope Communications
1301 Spruce St.
Boulder, CO 80302

First Peace
P.O. Box 123
Stourbridge West Midlands
DY12 0WL
UK

Health
Two Embarcadaro Center, Suite 600
San Francisco, CA 94111
Phone: 415-248-2700

Journal of Herbs, Spices & Medicinal Plants
Haworth Press, Inc.
10 Alice St.
Binghamton, NY 13904-1580

Journal of Naturopathic Medicine
10 Morgan Ave.
Norwalk, CT 06851

National Journal of Homeopathy
Web site: 208.129.23.180.njh/

Prevention
P.O. Box 7319
Red Oak, IA 51591-0319
Toll free: 800-813-8070
Web site: www.healthyideas.com

Protocol Journal of Botanical Medicine
Natural Health
P.O. Box 57320
Boulder, CO 80322-7320

Walking
9-11 Harcourt St.
Boston, MA 02116
Phone: 617-266-3322
E-mail: letters@walkingmag.com

Yoga Journal
2054 University Ave.
Berkeley, CA 94704
Phone: 510-841-9200

Medical and alternative associations

American Academy of Pain Management
13947 Mono Way #A
Sonora, CA 95370
Phone: 209-533-9744

American Association of Alternative Medicine, Inc.
1000 Rutherford Rd.
Landrum, SC 29356

American Association of Naturopathic Physicians
2601 Valley St., Suite 105
Seattle, WA 98102

American Chronic Pain Association
P.O. Box 850
Rocklin, CA 95677
Phone: 916-632-0922

American College for Advancement in Medicine
23121 Verdugo Dr., Suite 204
Laguna Hills, CA 92653

American Holistic Medical Association
4101 Lake Boone Trail, Suite 201
Raleigh, NC 27607

American Preventive Medical Association
459 Walker Rd.
Great Falls, VA 22066
Phone: 703-759-0662

Anxiety Disorders Association of America
6000 Executive Blvd., Suite 513
Rockville, MD 20852
Phone: 301-231-9350

Arthritis Foundation
1314 Spring St.
Atlanta, GA 30309
Toll free: 800-283-7800

Arthritis Society
250 Floor St. East, Suite 901
Toronto, Ontario
M4W 3P2
Canada
Phone: 416-967-1414

Fibromyalgia Association
P.O. Box 21988
Columbus, OH 43221-0988
Phone: 614-457-4222
Fax: 614-457-2729

Fibromyalgia Network
5700 Stockdale Highway, Suite 100
Bakersfield, CA 93309
Phone: 805-631-1950

Help for Incontinent People
P.O. Box 544
Union, SC 29379

National Arthritis & Musculoskeletal & Skin
Diseases Information Clearinghouse
1 AMS Circle
Bethesda, MD 20892-3675
Phone: 301-495-4484

The National Association of Certified Natural Health Professionals
810 S. Buffalo St.
Warsaw, IN 46580

National Chronic Fatigue Syndrome and Fibromyalgia Association
3521 Broadway, Suite 222
Kansas City, MO 64111
Phone: 816-931-4777

National Headache Foundation
Toll free: 800-843-2256

National Medical Association (NMA)
1012 10th St. NW
Washington, DC 20001
Phone: 202-347-1895

National Rehabilitation Information Center
8455 Colesville Rd., #935
Silver Spring, MD 20910-3319
Toll free: 800-346-2742
Phone: 301-588-9284
Fax: 301-587-1967

Mental health

Internet Mental Health
601 W. Broadway, Suite 902
Vancouver, B.C.
V5Z 4C2
Canada

National Foundation for Depressive Illness
Toll free: 800-239-1263

National Institute of Mental Health Public Inquiries
5600 Fishers Ln., Room 7C-02, MSC 8030
Bethesda, MD 20892-8030

National Mental Health Association
Toll free: 800-969-6642

Naturopaths

The American Association of Naturopathic
Physicians
601 Valley St., Suite 105
Seattle, WA 98109
Phone: 206-298-0126
Fax: 206-209-0129
Web site: www.naturopathic.org

Organizations

American Chronic Pain Association
P.O. Box 850
Rocklin, CA 95677
Phone: 916-632-0922
Fax: 916-632-3208

Back Pain Association of America
P.O. Box 135
Pasadena, MD 21122
Phone: 410-255-3633
Fax: 410-255-7338

National Institute of Arthritis and Musculoskeletal
and Skin Diseases Information Clearinghouse
1 AMS Circle
Bethesda, MD 20892-3675
Phone: 301-495-4484

North American Spine Society
6300 N. River Rd., #115
Rosemont, IL 60018-4231
Phone: 708-698-1630
Fax: 708-823-8668

Vermont Rehabilitation Engineering Research
Center for Low Back Pain
1 S. Prospect St.
Burlington, VT 05401
Toll free: 800-527-7320

Phone: 802-656-4582 (voice/TDD)

Fax: 802-660-9243

Osteopaths

American Academy of Osteopathy (AAO)

3500 DePauw Blvd., Suite 1080

Indianapolis, IN 46268

Phone: 317-879-1881

Web site: www.aao.medguide.net

American Osteopathic Association

142 E. Ontario St.

Chicago, Illinois 60611

Toll free: 800-621-1773

National Osteopathic Foundation

5775G Peachtree-Dunwoody Rd., Suite 500

Atlanta, GA 30342

Psychotherapy

American Psychiatric Association

Phone: 202-682-6000

The American Psychological Association

Phone: 202-336-5700

The National Association of Social Workers

Phone: 202-408-8600

Research

Herb Research Foundation

1007 Pearl St., Suite 200

Boulder, CO 80302

Phone: 303-449-2265

Fax: 303-449-7849

Support groups

Allergy and Asthma Network

Mothers of Asthmatics

3554 Chain Bridge Rd., Suite 200

Fairfax, VA 22030
Phone: 703-385-4403

American Academy of Environmental Physicians
Phone: 913-642-6062

American Allergy Association
P.O. Box 7273
Menlo Park, CA 94026

American Dietetic Association
Toll free: 800-366-1655

American Lung Association
Toll free: 800-586-4872

American Natural Hygiene Society
P.O. Box 30630
Tampa, FL 33630
Phone: 813-855-6607

American Self-Help Clearinghouse
St.Clares-Riverside Medical Center
25 Pocono Rd.
Denville, NJ 07834
Phone: 210-625-7101

American Sleep Disorders Association
1610 14th St. NW, Suite 300
Rochester, MN 55901

Asthma & Allergy Foundation of America (AAFA)
1125 15th St. NW, Suite 502
Washington, DC 20005
Toll free: 800-624-0044 or 800-7-ASTHMA

Asthma Explorers Club
Toll free: 800-982-3902

Asthma Zero Mortality Coalition
Toll free: 800-777-4350

Celiac Disease Foundation
13251 Ventura Blvd., Suite 3

Studio City, CA 91604-1838
Phone: 818-990-CELIAC

Cystic Fibrosis Foundation
6931 Arlington Rd.
Bethesda, MD 20814
Toll free: 800-344-4823

Food Allergy Network
10400 Eaton Pl., Suite 107
Fairfax, VA 22030-2208
Phone: 703-691-3179

International Society for Orthomolecular Medicine
16 Florence Ave.
Toronto, Ontario
M2N 1E9
Canada
Phone: 416-733-2117

Macrobiotic Center
61 E. 81st St., Suite 65
New York, NY 10028
Phone: 212-505-1010

Manitoba Lung Association
629 McDermot Ave.
Winnipeg, Manitoba
R3A 1P6
Canada
Phone: 204-774-5501

National Association of Managed Care Professionals
(NAMCP)
4435 Waterfront Dr., Suite 101
Glen Allen, VA 23060
Toll free: 800-722-0376

National Institute on Aging Information Center
P.O. Box 8057
Gaithersburg, MD 20898-8057
Phone: 800-222-2225

North American Vegetarian Society
P.O. Box 72
Dolgeville, NY 13329
Phone: 518-568-7970

Vegetarian Resource Group
P.O. Box 1463
Baltimore, MD 21203
Phone: 410-366-VEGE

Recommended Readings

Alternative Advisor. (By the editors of Time-Life Books)

Ashley, Martin. *Massage: A Career at Your Fingertips.* (Enterprise Publishing)

Balch, James F., M.D. and Phyllis A. Balch, C.N.C. *Prescription for Nutritional Healing.* (Avery)

Benson, Herbert, M.D. *The Relaxation Response.* (Avon Books)

Bianchi, Eugene, Ph.D. *Aging as a Spiritual Journey.* (Crossroad Publishing)

Borysenko, Joan. *Minding the Body, Mending the Mind.* (Addison-Wesley)

Bruce, D.F. *Bone Boosters.* (Kensington)

Chan, Pedro. *Finger Acupressure.* (Ballantine Books)

Crayhon, Robert. *Nutrition Made Simple.* (M. Evans and Company)

Cummings, Stephen and Dana Ullman. *Everybody's Guide to Homeopathic Medicines.* (Jeremy P. Tarcher/Putnam Publishing)

Fisher, Jeffrey A. *The Chromium Program.* (Harper)

Friedan, Betty. *The Fountain of Age.* (Simon & Schuster)

Hall, Nicholas. *Mind-Body Interactions and Disease and Psychoneuroimmunological Aspects of Health and Disease.* (Health-Dateline)

Hoffmann, David. *The Herb User's Guide.* (Thorson's)

Hoffmann, David. *The Holistic Herbal.* (Findhorn Press)

Johnson, Joan. *The Healing Art of Sports Massage.* (Rodale Press)

Krohn, Jacqueline, M.D. *The Whole Way to Allergy Relief and Prevention.* (Hartley and Marks)

Lockie, Andrew, M.D. and Nicola Geddes, M.D. *The Women's Guide to Homeopathy.* (St. Martin's Press)

McIlwain, Harris. *The Fibromyalgia Handbook.* (Henry Holt)

McIlwain, Harris. *The Osteoporosis Cure.* (Avon Books)

Marti, James E. *Alternative Health Medicine Encyclopedia.* (Visible Ink Press)

Mitchell, Susan, and Cathy Christie. *I'd Kill for a Cookie.* (Dutton)

Null, Gary, Ph.D. *The Woman's Encyclopedia of Healing.* (Seven Stories Press)

Smolley, Laurence. *Breathe Right Now.* (W. W. Norton)

Tierra, Michael. *Planetary Herbology.* (Lotus Press)

Weed, Susun. *Healing Wise.* (Ash Tree Publishing)

Weed, Susun. *Menopausal Years The Wise Woman Way.* (Ash Tree Publishing)

Weil, Andrew. *Spontaneous Healing.* (Fawcett)

Weiss, Rudolph Fritz. *Herbal Medicine.* (Beaconsfield Arcanum)

Wood, Matthew. *Seven Herbs: Plants as Teachers.* (North Atlantic Press)

A

The *Unofficial Guide*™ Reader Questionnaire

If you would like to express your opinion about alternative medicine or this guide, please complete this questionnaire and mail it to:

The *Unofficial Guide*™ Reader Questionnaire
Macmillan Lifestyle Group
1633 Broadway, floor 7
New York, NY 10019-6785

Gender: ___ M ___ F

Age: ___ Under 30 ___ 31–40 ___ 41–50 ___ Over 50

Education: ___ High school ___ College ___ Graduate/Professional

What is your occupation?

_____

How did you hear about this guide?
___ Friend or relative
___ Newspaper, magazine, or Internet
___ Radio or TV
___ Recommended at bookstore
___ Recommended by librarian
___ Picked it up on my own
___ Familiar with the *Unofficial Guide*™ travel series

Did you go to the bookstore specifically for a book on alternative medicine? Yes ___ No ___

Have you used any other *Unofficial Guides*™? Yes ___ No ___

If Yes, which ones?

_____
_____
_____

What other book(s) on alternative medicine have you purchased?

_____

_____

Was this book:
___ more helpful than other(s)
___ less helpful than other(s)

Do you think this book was worth its price?
Yes ___   No ___

Did this book cover all topics related to alternative medicine adequately?   Yes ___   No ___

Please explain your answer:

_____

_____

_____

Were there any specific sections in this book that were of particular help to you?   Yes ___   No ___

Please explain your answer:

_____

_____

_____

On a scale of 1 to 10, with 10 being the best rating, how would you rate this guide? ___

What other titles would you like to see published in the _Unofficial Guide_™ series?

_____

_____

Are _Unofficial Guides_™ readily available in your area?   Yes ___   No ___

Other comments:

_____

_____

_____

Get the inside scoop . . . with the
Unofficial Guides™!

The Unofficial Guide to Alternative Medicine
 ISBN: 0-02-862526-9 Price: $15.95

The Unofficial Guide to Buying a Home
 ISBN: 0-02-862461-0 Price: $15.95

The Unofficial Guide to Buying or Leasing a Car
 ISBN: 0-02-862524-2 Price: $15.95

The Unofficial Guide to Childcare
 ISBN: 0-02-862457-2 Price: $15.95

The Unofficial Guide to Cosmetic Surgery
 ISBN: 0-02-862522-6 Price: $15.95

The Unofficial Guide to Dieting Safely
 ISBN: 0-02-862521-8 Price: $15.95

The Unofficial Guide to Divorce
 ISBN: 0-02-862455-6 Price: $15.95

The Unofficial Guide to Eldercare
 ISBN: 0-02-862456-4 Price: $15.95

The Unofficial Guide to Hiring Contractors
 ISBN: 0-02-862460-2 Price: $15.95

The Unofficial Guide to Investing
 ISBN: 0-02-862458-0 Price: $15.95

The Unofficial Guide to Planning Your Wedding
 ISBN: 0-02-862459-9 Price: $15.95

All books in the *Unofficial Guide™* series are available at your local bookseller, or by calling 1-800-428-5331.

About the Authors

Debra Fulghum Bruce and Dr. Harris H. McIlwain can tell you everything you need to know about alternative medicine. Debra is a Florida-based health journalist pursuing a Ph.D. in Health Communications. She has written more than 2,500 articles for women's and health magazines, such as *Woman's Day, Prevention,* and *Success.* She is the co-author of 28 books, and her promotional ventures include ongoing weekly seminars and a new fitness video, *Flexible Fitness: An Arthritis Workout,* starring Linda Lavin. In addition, she has sampled many of the alternative therapies she writes about in this book.

Married and the father of six young adults, Harris H. McIlwain, M.D., a board certified rheumatologist and gerontologist, is a graduate of Emory University Medical School and has been in practice in Florida for more than 20 years. As a founding partner of Tampa Medical Group, PA, McIlwain has three large arthritis and pain clinics in Tampa and Brandon, Florida. He is the coauthor of 13 books on aging, disease prevention, and pain relief. McIlwain has been interviewed more than 1,000 times in the past three years on television and radio talk shows across the nation and also in national and international publications such as *Vogue, US News and World Report, Glamour, GQ, McCall's, Prevention, Men's Health, New Choices, California Senior, Elan, Woman's World Weekly,* and more.

Together, Debra and Dr. McIlwain have written many other health books, including *Super Bone Boosters, The Osteoporosis Cure, Winning with Arthritis, Winning with Back Pain,* and *My Parent My Turn.*